Adaptive Design
Methods in
Clinical Trials
Second Edition

Chapman & Hall/CRC Biostatistics Series

Chapman & Hall/CRC Biostatistics Series

Chapman & Hall/CRC Biostatistics Series

Adaptive Design Methods in Clinical Trials

Second Edition

Shein-Chung Chow

Mark Chang

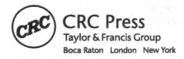

CRC Press
Taylor & Francis Group
Boca Raton London New York

CRC Press is an imprint of the
Taylor & Francis Group, an **informa** business

A CHAPMAN & HALL BOOK

CRC Press
Taylor & Francis Group
6000 Broken Sound Parkway NW, Suite 300
Boca Raton, FL 33487-2742

First issued in paperback 2022

© 2012 by Taylor & Francis Group, LLC
CRC Press is an imprint of Taylor & Francis Group, an Informa business

No claim to original U.S. Government works

Version Date: 20111028

ISBN 13: 978-1-03-247760-2 (pbk)
ISBN 13: 978-1-4398-3987-4 (hbk)

DOI: 10.1201/b11505

Publisher's Note
The publisher has gone to great lengths to ensure the quality of this reprint but points out that some imperfections in the original copies may be apparent.

**Visit the Taylor & Francis Web site at
http://www.taylorandfrancis.com**

**and the CRC Press Web site at
http://www.crcpress.com**

Contents

Preface to the First Edition

In recent years, the use of adaptive design methods in clinical trials has attracted much attention from clinical investigators and biostatisticians. Adaptations (i.e., modifications or changes) made to the trial and/or statistical procedures of on-going clinical trials based on accrued data have been in practice for years in clinical research and development. In the past several decades, we have adopted statistical procedures in the literature and applied them directly to the design of clinical trials originally planned by ignoring the fact that adaptations, modifications, and/or changes have been made to the trials. As pointed out by the U.S. Food and Drug Administration (FDA), these procedures, however, may not be motivated by best clinical trial practice. Consequently, they may not be the best tools to handle certain situations. Adaptive design methods in clinical research and development are attractive to clinical scientists and researchers because of the following reasons. First, it reflects medical practice in the real world. Second, it is ethical with respect to both efficacy and safety (toxicity) of the test treatment under investigation. Third, it is not only flexible but also efficient in clinical development, especially for early phase clinical development. However, there are issues regarding the adjustments of treatment estimations and p-values. In addition, it is also a concern that the use of adaptive design methods in a clinical trial may have led to a totally different trial that is unable to address the scientific/medical questions the trial is intended to answer.

In practice, there exists no universal definition of adaptive design methods in clinical research until recently PhRMA gave a formal definition. Most literature focuses on adaptive randomization with respect to covariate, treatment, and/or clinical response, adaptive group sequential design for interim analysis, and sample size re-assessment. In this book, our definition is broader. Adaptive design methods include any adaptations, modifications, or changes of trial and/or statistical procedures that are made during the conduct of the trials. Although adaptive design methods are flexible and useful in clinical research, little or no regulatory guidances/guidelines are available. The purpose of this book is to provide a comprehensive and unified presentation of the principles and methodologies in adaptive design and analysis with respect to adaptations made to trial and/or statistical procedures based on accrued data of on-going clinical trials. In addition, this book is intended to give a well-balanced summary of current regulatory perspectives and recently developed statistical methods in this area. It is our goal to provide a complete, comprehensive and updated reference and textbook in the area of adaptive design and analysis in clinical research and development.

Chapter 1 provides an introduction to basic concepts regarding the use of adaptive design methods in clinical trials and some statistical considerations of adaptive design methods. Chapter 2 focuses on the impact on target patient population as the result of protocol amendments. Also included in this chapter is the generalization of statistical inference, which is drawn based on data collected from the actual patient population as the result of protocol amendments, to the originally planned target patient population. Several adaptive randomization procedures that are commonly employed in clinical trials are reviewed in Chapter 3. Chapter 4 studies the use of adaptive design methods in the case where hypotheses are modified during the conduct of clinical trials. Chapter 5 provides an overall review of adaptive design methods for dose selection especially in dose finding and dose response relationship studies in early clinical development. Chapter 6 introduces the commonly used adaptive group sequential design methods in clinical trials. Blinded procedures for sample size re-estimation are given in Chapter 7. Statistical tests for seamless phase II/III adaptive designs and statistical inference for switching from one treatment to another adaptively and the corresponding practical issues that one may encounter are studied in Chapter 8 and Chapter 9, respectively. Bayesian approach for the use of adaptive design methods in clinical trials are outlined in Chapter 10. Chapter 11 provides an introduction to the methodology of clinical trial simulation for evaluation of the performance of the adaptive design methods under various adaptive designs that are commonly used in clinical development. Case studies regarding the implementation of adaptive group sequential design, adaptive dose-escalation design, and seamless phase II/III adaptive trial design in clinical trials are discussed in Chapter 12.

From Taylor & Francis, we would like to thank David Grubbs and Dr. Sunil Nair for providing us the opportunity to work on this book. We would like to thank colleagues from the Department of Biostatistics and Bioinformatics and Duke Clinical Research Institute (DCRI) of Duke University School of Medicine and Millennium Pharmaceuticals, Inc. for their support during the preparation of this book. We wish to express our gratitude to the following individuals for their encouragement and support: Roberts Califf, M.D. and John Hamilton, M.D. of Duke Clinical Research Institute and Duke University Medical Center, Nancy Simonian, M.D., Jane Porter, M.S., Andy Boral, M.D. and Jim Gilbert, M.D. of Millennium Pharmaceuticals, Inc., Greg Campbell, Ph.D. of the U.S. Food and Drug Administration, and many friends from the academia, the pharmaceutical industry, and regulatory agencies.

Finally, the views expressed are those of the authors and not necessarily those of Duke University School of Medicine and Millennium Pharmaceuticals, Inc. We are solely responsible for the contents and errors of this edition. Any comments and suggestions will be very much appreciated

Shein-Chung Chow, Ph.D.
Duke University School of Medicine, Durham, NC

Mark Chang, Ph.D.
Millennium Pharmaceuticals, Inc., Cambridge, MA

Preface

Many statistical and/or scientific issues in the area of adaptive clinical trial design have attracted considerable attention from clinical scientists and researchers from academia, the regulatory agencies, and the pharmaceutical industry since the first edition of this book was published in 2006. Most recently, the U.S. Food and Drug Administration (FDA) released a draft guidance for comments, which has generated more issues/concerns when utilizing adaptive design methods in clinical trials. These statistical and/or scientific issues include (i) the feasibility of the use of adaptive design methods in clinical trials, (ii) the validity and integrity of the commonly considered adaptive designs such as adaptive dose finding design and two-stage seamless adaptive designs, and (iii) the search for appropriate statistical methods under complicated adaptive designs (or less well-understood designs). As a result, there was a need for a second edition of this book to provide a comprehensive and unified summary of the vast and continuously growing literature and research activities on regulatory requirements, scientific and practical issues, and statistical methodology.

This revision maintains the same overall objectives and level of presentation as the first edition. Similar to the first edition, the new edition focuses on the concepts rather than technical details. It is written from a practical viewpoint at a basic mathematical and statistical level. Feedback from the first edition was gratifying. We received many positive comments from clinical scientists and researchers from academia, the regulatory agencies, including the FDA, and the pharmaceutical industry. Accordingly, we have kept our intuitive writing style as well as the emphasis on the concepts via numerous examples and illustrations.

We have improved the second edition in the following ways. First, several chapters/sections such as the chapters of protocol amendment and clinical trial simulation are updated to reflect recent developments since the first edition. Both chapters have major revisions. Second, five new chapters are added. These chapters include (i) Two-Stage Adaptive Design (Chapter 9), (ii) Biomarker Adaptive Trials (Chapter 12), (iii) Target Clinical Trials (Chapter 13), (iv) Sample Size and Power Estimation (Chapter 14), and (v) Regulatory Perspectives - A Review of FDA Draft Guidance on Adaptive Clinical Trial Design (Chapter 16).

From Taylor & Francis, we would like to thank Mr. David Grubbs for providing us with the opportunity to work on the revision of this book. We would like to thank colleagues from Duke University School of Medicine, AMAG Pharmaceuticals, and many friends from academia, the pharmaceutical industry, and regulatory agencies for their support during the preparation of the revision of this book. In particular, we wish to express our gratitude to the following individuals for their encouragement and support: Robert Califf, M.D., Robert Hurrington, M.D., Ralph Corey, M.D., John Sundy, M.D., Ph.D., Ken Weinhold, Ph.D., and Liz DeLong, Ph.D. from Duke University Medical Center.

Finally, the views expressed are those of the authors and not necessarily those of Duke University School of Medicine or AMAG Pharmaceuticals, Inc. We are solely responsible for the contents and errors of this book. Any comments and suggestions that will lead to improvement of future revisions are very much appreciated.

Shein-Chung Chow, Ph.D.
Duke University School of Medicine, Durham, NC

Mark Chang, Ph.D.
AMAG Pharmaceuticals, Lexington, MA

Chapter 1

Introduction

In clinical research, the ultimate goal of a clinical trial is to evaluate the effect (e.g., efficacy and safety) of a test treatment as compared to a control (e.g., a placebo control, a standard therapy, or an active control agent). To ensure the success of a clinical trial, a well-designed study protocol is essential. A protocol is a plan that details how a clinical trial is to be carried out and how the data are to be collected and analyzed. It is an extremely critical and the most important document in clinical trials, since it ensures the quality and integrity of the clinical investigation in terms of its planning, execution, conduct, and the analysis of the data of clinical trials. During the conduct of a clinical trial, adherence to the protocol is crucial. Any protocol deviations and/or violations may introduce bias and variation to the data collected from the trial. Consequently, the conclusion drawn based on the analysis results of the data may not be reliable and hence may be biased or misleading. For marketing approval of a new drug product, the United States Food and Drug Administration (FDA) requires that at least two adequate and well-controlled clinical trials be conducted to provide substantial evidence regarding the effectiveness of the drug product under investigation (FDA, 1988). However, under certain circumstances, the FDA Modernization Act (FDAMA) of 1997 includes a provision (Section 115 of FDAMA) to allow data from a single adequate and well-controlled clinical trial to establish effectiveness for risk/benefit assessment of drug and biological candidates for approval. The FDA indicates that substantial evidence regarding the effectiveness and safety of the drug product under investigation can only be provided through the conduct of adequate and well-controlled clinical studies. According to the FDA 1988 guideline for *Format and Content of the Clinical and Statistical Sections of New Drug Applications*, an adequate and well-controlled study is defined as a study that meets the characteristics of the following: (i) objectives, (ii) methods of analysis, (iii) design, (iv) selection of subjects, (v) assignment of subjects, (vi) participants of studies, (vii) assessment of responses (viii) assessment of effect. In the study protocol, it is essential to clearly state the study objectives of the study. Specific hypotheses that reflect the study objectives should be provided in the study protocol. The study design must be valid in order to provide a fair and unbiased assessment of the treatment effect as compared to a control. Target patient population should be defined through the inclusion/exclusion criteria to assure the disease conditions under study. Randomization procedures must be employed to minimize potential bias and to ensure the comparability between treatment groups. Criteria for assessment of the response should be pre-defined and reliable. Appropriate statistical methods should be employed for assessment of the effect. Procedures such as blinding for minimization of bias should be employed to maintain the validity and integrity of the trial.

In clinical trials, it is not uncommon to adjust trial procedures and/or statistical methods at the planning stage and during the conduct of clinical trials. For example, at the planning stage of a clinical trial, as an alternative to the standard randomization procedure, an *adaptive* randomization procedure based on treatment response may be considered for treatment allocation. During the conduct of a clinical trial, some adaptations (i.e., modifications or changes) to trial and/or statistical procedures may be made based on accrued data. Typical examples for adaptations of trial and/or statistical procedures of on-going clinical trials include, but are not limited to, the modification of inclusion/exclusion criteria, the adjustment of study dose or regimen, the extension of treatment duration, changes in study endpoints, and modification in study design such as group sequential design and/or multiple-stage flexible designs. Adaptations to trial and/or statistical procedures of on going clinical trials will certainly have an immediate impact on the target population and consequently, statistical inference on treatment effect of the target patient population. In practice, adaptations or modifications to trial and/or statistical procedures of on-going clinical trails are necessary, which not only reflect real medical practice on the actual patient population with the disease under study, but also increase the probability of success for identifying clinical benefit of the treatment under investigation.

The remainder of this chapter is organized as follows. In the next section, a definition regarding so-called adaptive design is given. Section 1.2 provides regulatory perspectives regarding the use of adaptive design methods in clinical research and development. Sections 1.3 and 1.4 describe the impact of an adaptive design on the target patient population and statistical inference following adaptations of trial and/or statistical procedures, respectively. Practical issues that are commonly encountered when applying adaptive design methods in clinical research and development are briefly outlined in Section 1.5. Section 1.6 presents aims and scope of the book.

1.1   What Is Adaptive Design

On March 16, 2006, the FDA released a Critical Path Opportunities List that outlined 76 initial projects to bridge the gap between the quick pace of new biomedical discoveries and the slower pace at which those discoveries are currently developed into therapies. See, e.g., http://www.fda.gov/oc/initiatives/ criticalpath. The Critical Path Opportunities List consists of six broad topic areas of (i) development of biomarkers, (ii) clinical trial designs, (iii) bioinformatics, (iv) manufacturing, (v) public health needs, and (iv) pediatrics. As indicated in the Critical Path Opportunities Report, biomarker development and streamlining clinical trials are the two most important areas for improving medical product development. The streamlining of clinical trials calls for advancing innovative trial designs such as adaptive designs to improve innovation in clinical development.

In clinical investigation of treatment regimens, it is not uncommon considering adaptations in early phase clinical trials before initiation of large-scale confirmatory phase III trials. An adaptation in clinical trials is referred to as a change or modification made to a clinical trial before and during the conduct of the study. Some commonly seen adaptations include, but are not limited to, (i) relaxation of inclusion/exclusion criteria, (ii) change study endpoints, and (iii) modification of dose and/or treatment duration. In this book, we will refer to the application of adaptations to clinical trials as adaptive design methods in clinical trials. The adaptive design methods are usually developed based on observed treatment effects. To allow wider flexibility, adaptations in clinical investigation of treatment regimen may include changes of sample size, inclusion/exclusion criteria, study dose, study endpoints, and methods for analysis (Liu, Proschan, and Pledger, 2002). Chow, Chang and Pong (2005) define an adaptive design of a clinical trial as a design that allows adaptations or modifications to some aspects (e.g., trial procedures and/or statistical methods) of the trial after its initiation without undermining the validity and integrity of the trial. Trial procedures are referred to as the eligibility criteria, study dose, treatment duration, study endpoints, laboratory testing procedures, diagnostic procedures, criteria for evaluability, and assessment of clinical responses. Statistical methods include randomization scheme, study design selection, study objectives/hypotheses, sample size calculation, data monitoring and interim analysis, statistical analysis plan, and/or methods for data analysis. On the other hand, the PhRMA Working Group refers to an *adaptive design* as a clinical study design that uses accumulating data to decide on how to modify aspects of the study as it continues, without undermining the validity and integrity of the trial (Gallo et al., 2006). As indicated by the PhRMA Working Group, the adaptation is a design feature aimed to enhance the trial, not a remedy for inadequate planning. In other words, changes should be made *by design* and not on an *ad hoc* basis. *By design* changes, however, do not reflect real clinical practice. In addition, it does not allow flexibility.

In its recent draft guidance on *Adaptive Design Clinical Trials for Drugs and Biologics* (February, 2010), the FDA defines an adaptive design clinical study as a study that includes a prospectively planned opportunity for modification of one or more specified aspects of the study design and hypotheses based on analysis of data (usually interim data) from subjects in the study. The FDA emphasizes that one of the major characteristics of an adaptive design is the prospectively planned opportunity. Changes should be made based on analysis of data (usually interim data). In the draft guidance, the FDA classifies adaptive designs as either *well-understood designs* or *less well understood designs* depending upon the nature of adaptations either blinded or unblinded (FDA, 2010a). The FDA's definition excludes changes made through protocol amendments. Thus, it does not reflect real practice in clinical trials. Note that in many cases, an adaptive design is also known as a *flexible* design (EMEA, 2002, 2006).

Adaptive design methods are very attractive to clinical researchers and/or sponsors due to their flexibility especially when there are priority changes for budget/resources and timeline constraints, scientific/statistical justifications for study validity and integrity, medical considerations for safety, regulatory concerns for review/approval, and/or business strategies for go/no-go decisions. However, there is little or no information available in regulatory requirements as to what level of flexibility in modifications of trial procedures and/or statistical procedures of on-going clinical trials would be acceptable. It is a concern that the application of adaptive design methods may result in a totally different clinical trial that is unable to address the scientific/medical questions/hypotheses the clinical trial is intended to answer. In addition, an adaptive design suffers from the following disadvantages. First, it may result in a major difference between the actual patient population as the result of adaptations made to the trial and/or statistical procedures and the (originally) target patient population. The actual patient population under study could be a moving target depending upon the frequency and extent of modifications (flexibility) made to study parameters. Second, statistical inference such as confidence interval and/or p-values on the treatment effect of the test treatment under study may not be reliable. Consequently, the observed clinical results may not be reproducible. In recent years, the use of adaptive design methods in clinical trials has attracted much attention from clinical scientists and biostatisticians.

In practice, adaptation or modification made to the trial and/or statistical procedures during the conduct of a clinical trial based on accrued data is usually recommended by the investigator, the sponsor, or an independent data monitoring committee. Although the adaptation or modification is flexible and attractive, it may introduce bias and consequently has an impact on statistical inference on the assessment of treatment effect for the target patient population under study. The complexity could be substantial depending upon the adaptation employed. Basically, adaptation employed can be classified into three categories: namely prospective (by design) adaptation, concurrent (or on-going ad hoc) adaptation (by protocol amendment), and retrospective adaptation (after end of the conduct of the trial before database lock and/or unblinding) (see also Table 1.1.1). As can be seen, the on-going ad hoc adaptation has higher flexibility, while prospective adaptation is less flexible. Both types of adaptation require a careful planning. It should be noted that statistical methods for certain kinds of adaptation may not be available in the literature. As a result, some studies with complicated adaptation may be more successful than others.

Table 1.1.1: Types of Adaptation in Clinical Trials

Adaptation	Examples
Prospective (by design)	Interim analysis
	Stop trial early due to safety, futility/efficacy
	Sample size re-estimation
	etc.
On-going (ad hoc)	Inclusion/exclusion criteria
	Dose or dose regimen
	Treatment duration
	etc.
Retrospective*	Study endpoint
	Switch from superiority to non-inferiority
	etc.

* Adaptation at the end of the study prior to database lock or unblinding.

Depending upon the types of adaptation or modification made, commonly employed adaptive design methods in clinical trials include, but are not limited to: (i) a group sequential design, (ii) a sample size re-estimation (or an N-adjustable) design, (iii) an seamless (e.g., phase I/II or phase II/III) adaptive design, (iv) a drop-the-loser (or pick-the-winner) design, (v) an adaptive randomization design, (vi) an adaptive dose finding (escalation) design, (vii) a biomarker-adaptive design, (viii) an adaptive treatment-switching design, (ix) an adaptive-hypotheses design, and (x) any combinations of the above (see also, Chow and Chang, 2008; Pong and Chow, 2010).

A group sequential design is an adaptive design that allows for prematurely terminating a trial due to safety, efficacy or futility based on interim analysis results, while a sample size re-estimation (N-adjustable) design is referred to as an adaptive design that allows for sample size adjustment or re-estimation based on the observed data at interim. An seamless (say phase II/III) adaptive trial design is referred to a program that addresses within a single trial objectives that are normally achieved through separate trials in phases IIb and III (Inoue, Thall, and Berry, 2002; Gallo et al., 2006). An seamless phase II/III adaptive design would combine two separate trials (i.e., a phase IIb trial and a phase III trial) into one trial and would use data from patients enrolled before and after the adaptation in the final analysis (Maca et al., 2006). A drop-the-loser (pick-the-winner) design is a multiple-stage adaptive design that allows dropping the inferior treatment groups (or selecting the most promising treatment group). Adaptive randomization design refers to a design that allows modification of randomization schedules. Adaptive dose finding (escalation) design is often used in early phase clinical development to identify the maximum tolerable dose, which is usually considered the optimal dose for later phase clinical trials. Biomarker-adaptive design is a design that allows for adaptations based on the response of biomarkers such as genomic markers. Thus, biomarker-adaptive design is sometimes known as an enrichment design for target clinical trials or biomarker-guide (genomic-guide) clinical trial design. Adaptive treatment-switching design is a design that allows the investigator to switch a patient's treatment from an initial assignment to an alternative treatment if there is evidence of lack of efficacy or safety of the initial treatment. Adaptive-hypotheses design refers to a design that allows change in hypotheses based on interim analysis results. Any combinations of the above adaptive designs are usually referred to as multiple adaptive designs.

Table 1.1.2: Summary of Flexibility/Benefits of Various Less Well-Understood Adaptive Designs

Adaptive Randomization Design	Unequal probability of treatment assignment Assign subjects to more promising treatment arm	Randomization schedule not available prior to the conduct of the trial Not feasible for large trials or trials with long treatment duration Statistical inference is often difficult if not impossible, to obtain
Adaptive Dose Finding Design*	Drop inferior dose group early Modify/add additional dose groups Increase the probability of correctly identifying the MTD with limited number of subjects	Selection of initial dose Selection of dose range under study Selection criteria and decision rule Risk of dropping promising dose groups
Two-stage Seamless Adaptive Design (either phase I/II or II/III)	Combine two studies into a single study Fully utilize data collected from both stages Reduce lead time between studies Shorten the development time Additional adaptations such as drop-the-loser, adaptive randomization, and adaptive hypotheses may be applied at the end of the 1st stage	The control of the overall type I error rate? Sample size calculation/ allocation How to perform a combined analysis based on data collected from both stages Is the O'Brian-Fleming type of boundaries feasible?

* Adaptive dose escalation designs for cancer trials

While enjoying the flexibility and possible benefits of adaptive design methods in clinical trials, it should be noted that more flexibilities could lead to a less well-understood design as described in the FDA draft guidance. A less well-understood adaptive design is often more flexible and yet more complicated. Under a complicated and less well-understood adaptive design, statistical inference is often difficult, if not impossible, to obtain although valid statistical inferences for some less well-understood designs are available in the literature. As an example, Table 1.1.2 provides a summary of flexibilities and possible benefits of some less well-understood adaptive designs such as an adaptive randomization design, an adaptive dose finding design, and a two-stage phase I/II (or phase II/III) seamless adaptive design that are commonly considered in pharmaceutical/clinical research and development.

In recent years, the use of these adaptive designs has received much attention. Many journals have published special issues on adaptive design. These journals included, but are not limited to, Biometrics (Vol. 62, No. 3), Statistics in Medicine (Vol. 25, No. 19), Biometrical Journal (Vol. 48, No. 4), Pharmaceutical Statistics (Vol. 5, No. 2), and Journal of Biopharmaceutical Statistics (Vol. 15, No. 4, Vol. 17, No. 6, and Vol. 20, No. 6). These special issues and theme topics cover many statistical issues related to the use of adaptive design methods, adaptive dose finding, and review of the recent FDA draft guidance on adaptive clinical trial designs (see e.g., Hung et al., 2005; Proschan, 2005; Krams et al., 2007; Hung et al., 2007; Wang, 2010; Benda et al., 2010; Gallo et al., 2010; Cheng and Chow, 2010). This book is intended to address concerns and/or practical issues that one may encounter when applying adaptive design methods in clinical trials.

1.2   Regulatory Perspectives

As pointed out by the FDA, modification of the design of an experiment based on accrued data has been in practice for hundreds, if not thousands, of years in medical research. In the past, we had a tendency to adopt statistical procedures in the literature and applied them directly to the design of clinical trials (Lan, 2002). However, since these procedures were not motivated by clinical trial practice, they may not be the best tools to handle certain situations. The impact of any adaptations made to trial and/or statistical methods before, during, and after the conduct of trial could be substantial.

The flexibility in design and analysis of clinical trials in early phases of the drug development is very attractive to clinical researchers/scientists and the sponsors. However, its use in late phase II or phase III clinical investigation has led to regulatory concern regarding its limitation of interpretation and extrapolation from trial results. As there is an increasing need for the flexibility in design and analysis of clinical trials, the European Agency for the Evaluation of Medicinal Products (EMEA) published a concept paper on points to consider on methodological issues in confirmatory clinical trials with flexible design and analysis plan (EMEA, 2002, 2006). The EMEA's points to consider intend to discuss pre-requisites and conditions under which the methods could be acceptable in confirmatory phase III trials for regulatory decision making.

Principal pre-requisite for all considerations is that methods under investigation can provide correct p-values, unbiased estimates, and confidence intervals for the treatment comparison(s) in an actual clinical trial. As a result, the use of an adaptive design not only raises importance of well-known problems of studies with interim analyses (e.g., lack of a sufficient safety database after early termination and over-running), but also bears new challenges to clinical researchers.

From a regulatory point of view, blinded review of the database at interim analyses is a key issue in adaptive design. During these blinded reviews, often the statistical analysis plan is largely modified. At the same time, more study protocols are submitted, where little or no information on statistical methods is provided and relevant decisions are deferred to a statistical analysis or even the blinded review, which has led to a serious regulatory concern regarding the validity and integrity of the trial. In addition, what the resultant actual patient population of the study is after the adaptations of the trial procedures especially when the inclusion/exclusion criteria are made is a challenge to the regulatory review and approval process. A commonly asked question is whether the adaptive design methods have resulted in a totally different trial with a totally different target patient population. In this case, is the usual regulatory review and approval process still applicable? However, there is little or no information in regulatory guidances or guidelines regarding regulatory requirement or perception as to the degree of flexibility that would be accepted by the regulatory agencies. In practice, it is suggested that regulatory acceptance should be justified based on the validity of statistical inference of the target patient population.

It should be noted that although adaptations of trial and/or statistical procedures are often documented through protocol amendments, standard statistical methods may not be appropriate and may lead to invalid inference/conclusion regarding the target patient population. As a result, it is recommended that appropriate adaptive statistical methods be employed. Although several adaptive design methods for obtaining valid statistical inference on treatment effect available in the literature (see, e.g., Hommel, 2001; Liu, Proschan and Pledger, 2002) are useful, they should be performed in a completely objective manner. In practice, however, it can be very difficult to reach this objectivity in clinical trials due to external inferences and different interests from the investigators and sponsors.

As a result, it is strongly recommended that a guidance/guideline for adaptive design methods must be developed by the regulatory authorities to avoid every intentional or unintentional manipulation of the adaptive design methods in clinical trials. The guidance/guideline should describe in details not only the standards for use of adaptive design methods in clinical trials, but also the level of modifications in an adaptive design that is acceptable to the regulatory agencies. In addition, any changes in the process of regulatory review/approval should also be clearly indicated in such a guidance/guideline. It should be noted that the adaptive design methods have been used in the review/approval process of regulatory submissions for years though it may not be recognized until recently.

1.3 Target Patient Population

In clinical trials, patient population with certain diseases under study is usually described by the inclusion/exclusion criteria. Patients who meet all inclusion criteria and none of the exclusion criteria are qualified for the study. We will refer to this patient population as the *target* patient population. For a given study endpoint such as clinical response, time to disease progression, or survival in the therapeutic area of oncology, we may denote the target patient population by (μ,σ), where μ is the population mean of the study endpoint and σ denotes the population standard deviation of the study endpoint. For a comparative clinical trial comparing a test treatment and a control, the effect size of the test treatment adjusted for standard deviation is defined as

$$\frac{\mu_T - \mu_C}{\sigma},$$

where μ_T and μ_C are the population means for the test treatment and the control, respectively. Based on the collected data, statistical inference such as confidence interval and p-value on the effect size of the test treatment can then be made for the target patient population.

In practice, as indicated earlier, it is not uncommon to modify trial procedures due to some medical and/or practical considerations during the conduct of the trial. Trial procedures of a clinical trial are referred to as operating procedures, testing procedures, and/or diagnostic procedures that are to be employed in the clinical trial. As a result, trial procedures of a clinical trial include, but are not limited to, the inclusion/exclusion criteria, the selection of study dose or regimen, treatment duration, laboratory testing, diagnostic procedures, and criteria for evaluability. In clinical trials, we refer to statistical procedures of a clinical trial as statistical procedures and/or statistical models/methods that are employed at planning, execution, and conduct of the trial as well as the analysis of the data. Thus, statistical procedures of a clinical trial include power analysis for sample size calculation at planning stage, randomization procedure for treatment allocation prior to treatment, modifications of hypotheses, change in study endpoint, and sample size re-estimation at interim during the conduct of the trial. As indicated in the FDA 1988 guideline and the International Conference on Harmonization (ICH) Good Clinical Practices (GCP) guideline (FDA, 1988; ICH, 1996), a well-designed protocol should detail how the clinical trial is to be carried out. Any deviations from the protocol and/or violations of the protocol will not only distort the original patient population under study, but also introduce bias and variation to the data collected from the trial. Consequently, conclusions drawn based on statistical inference obtained or derived from the analysis results of the data may not be applied to the original target patient population.

In clinical trials, the inclusion/exclusion criteria and study dose or regimen and/or treatment duration are often modified due to slow enrollment and/or safety concern during the conduct of the trial. For example, at screening, we may disqualify too many patients with stringent inclusion/exclusion criteria. Consequently, the enrollments may be too slow to meet the timeline of the study. In this case, a typical approach is to relax the inclusion/exclusion criteria to increase the enrollment. On the other hand, the investigators may wish to have the flexibility to adjust the study dose or regimen to achieve optimal clinical benefit of the test treatment during the trial. The study dose may be reduced when there are significant toxicities and/or adverse experiences. In addition, the investigators may wish to extend the treatment duration to (i) reach best therapeutic effect or (ii) achieve the anticipated event rate based on accrued data during the conduct of trial. These modifications of trial procedures are commonly encountered in clinical trials. Modifications of trial procedures are usually accomplished through protocol amendments, which detail rationales for changes and the impact of the modifications.

Any adaptations made to the trial and/or statistical procedures may introduce bias and/or variation to the data collected from the trial. Consequently, it may result in a similar but slightly different target patient population. We will refer to such a patient population as the *actual* patient population under study. As mentioned earlier, in practice, it is a concern whether adaptations made to the trial and/or statistical procedures could lead to a totally different trial with a totally different target patient population. In addition, it is of interest to determine whether statistical inference obtained based on clinical data collected from the actual patient population could be applied to the originally planned target patient population. These issues will be studied in the next chapter.

1.4   Statistical Inference

As discussed in the previous section, modifications of trial procedures will certainly introduce bias/variation to the data collected from the trial. The sources of these biases and variations can be classified into one of the following four categories: (i) expected and controllable, (ii) expected but not controllable, (iii) unexpected but controllable, and (iv) unexpected and not controllable. For example, additional bias/variation is expected but not controllable when there is a change in study dose or regimen and/or treatment duration. For changes in laboratory testing procedures and/or diagnostic procedures, bias/variation is expected but controllable by (i) having experienced technicians to perform the tests or (ii) conducting appropriate training for inexperienced technicians. Bias/variation due to patient non-compliance to trial procedures is usually unexpected but is controllable by improving the procedure for patient compliance. Additional bias/variation due to unexpected and uncontrollable sources is usually referred to as the random error of the trial.

In practice, appropriate statistical procedures should be employed to identify and eliminate/control these sources of bias/variation whenever possible.

In addition, after the adaptations of the trial procedures especially the inclusion/exclusion criteria, the target patient population has been changed to the actual patient population under study. In this case, how to generalize the conclusion drawn based on statistical inference of the treatment effect derived from clinical data observed from the actual patient population to the original target patient population is a challenge to a clinical scientist. It, however, should be noted that although all modifications of trial procedures and/or statistical procedures are documented through protocol amendments, it does not imply that the collected data are free of bias/variation. Protocol amendments should not only provide rationales for changes but also detail how the data are to be collected and analyzed following the adaptations of trial and/or statistical procedures. In practice, it is not uncommon to observe the following inconsistencies following major adaptations of trial and/or statistical procedures of a clinical trial: (i) a right test for wrong hypotheses, (ii) a wrong test for the right hypotheses, (iii) a wrong test for wrong hypotheses, and (iv) the right test for the right hypotheses but insufficient power. Each of these inconsistencies will result in invalid statistical inference and conclusion regarding the treatment effect under investigation.

Flexibility in statistical procedures of a clinical trial is very attractive to the investigator and/or sponsors. However, it suffers the disadvantage of invalid statistical inference and/or misleading conclusion if the impact is not carefully managed. Liu, Proschan and Pledger (2002) provided a solid theoretical foundation for adaptive design methods in clinical development under which not only a general method for point estimation, confidence interval, hypotheses testing and overall p-value can be obtained, but also the validity can be rigorously established. However, they do not take into consideration the fact that the target patient population has become a moving target patient population as the result of adaptations made to the trial and/or statistical procedures through protocol amendments. This issue will be further discussed in the next chapter.

The ICH GCP guideline suggests that a thoughtful statistical analysis plan (SAP), which details statistical procedures (including models/methods) should be employed for data collection and analysis. Any deviations from the SAP and violations of the SAP could decrease the reliability of the analysis results and consequently the conclusion drawn from these analysis results may not be valid.

In summary, the use of adaptive design methods in clinical trials may have an impact on the statistical inference on the target patient population under study. Statistical inference obtained based on data collected from the actual patient population as the result of modifications made to the trial procedures and/or statistical procedures should be adjusted before it can be applied to the original target patient population.

1.5   Practical Issues

As indicated earlier, the use of adaptive design methods in clinical trials has received much attention because it allows adaptations of trial and/or statistical procedures of on-going clinical trials. The flexibility for adaptations to study parameters is very attractive to clinical scientists and sponsors. However, from regulatory point of view, several questions have been raised. First, what level of adaptations to the trial and/or statistical procedures would be acceptable to the regulatory authorities? Second, what are the regulatory requirements and standards for review and approval process of clinical data obtained from adaptive clinical trials with different levels of adaptations to trial and/or statistical procedures of on-going clinical trials? Third, has the clinical trial become a totally different clinical trial after the adaptations to the trial and/or statistical procedures for addressing the study objectives of the originally planned clinical trial? These concerns are necessarily addressed by the regulatory authorities before the adaptive design methods can be widely accepted in clinical research and development.

In addition, from a scientific/statistical point of view, there are also some concerns regarding (i) whether the modifications to the trial procedures have resulted in a similar but different target patient population? (ii) whether the modifications of hypotheses have distorted the study objectives of the trial? (iii) whether the flexibility in statistical procedures has led to biased assessment of clinical benefit of the treatment under investigation? In this section, practical issues associated with the above questions that are commonly encountered in clinical trials when applying adaptive design methods of on-going clinical trials are briefly described. These issues include a moving target patient population as the result of protocol amendments, adaptive randomization, adaptive hypotheses, adaptive dose-escalation trials, adaptive group sequential designs, adaptive sample size adjustment, seamless phase II/III adaptive trial design, dropping the losers adaptively, adaptive treatment switching, Bayesian and hybrid approaches, clinical trial simulation, and case studies.

Moving Target Patient Population

In clinical trials, it is important to define the patient population with the disease under study. This patient population is usually described based on eligibility criteria, i.e., the inclusion and exclusion criteria. This patient population is referred to as the *target* patient population. As indicated in Chow and Liu (2003), a target patient population is usually roughly defined by the inclusion criteria and then fine tuned by the exclusion criteria to minimize heterogeneity of the patient population. When adaptations are made to the trial and/or statistical procedures, especially the inclusion/exclusion criteria during the conduct of the trial, the mean response of the primary study endpoint of the target patient population may be shifted with heterogeneity in variability. As a result, adaptations made to trial and/or statistical procedures could lead to a similar but different patient population. We will refer to this resultant patient population as the *actual* patient population. In practice, it is a concern that major (or significant) adaptation could result in a totally different patient population. During the conduct of a clinical trial, if adaptations are made frequently, the target patient population is in fact a *moving* target patient population (Chow, Chang, and Pong, 2005; Feng et al., 2007; Yang et al., 2011). As a result, it is difficult to draw an accurate and reliable statistical inference on the moving target patient population. Thus, in practice, it is of interest to determine the impact of adaptive design methods on the target patient population and consequently the corresponding statistical inference and power analysis for sample size calculation. More details are given in the next chapter.

Adaptive Randomization

In clinical trials, randomization models such as the population model, the invoked population model, and the randomization model with the method of complete randomization and permuted-block randomization are commonly used to ensure a balanced allocation of patients to treatment within either a fixed total sample size or a pre-specified block size (Chow and Liu, 2003). The population model is referred to as the concept that clinicians can draw conclusions for the target patient population based on the selection of a representative sample drawn from the target patient population by some random procedure (Lehmann, 1975; Lachin, 1988). The invoked population model is referred to as the process of selecting investigators first and then selecting patients at each selected investigator's site. As it can be seen, neither the selection of investigators nor the recruitment of patients at the selected investigator's site is random. However, treatment assignment is random. Thus, the invoked randomization model allows the analysis of the clinical data as if they were obtained under the assumption that the sample is randomly selected from a homogeneous patient population. Randomization model is referred to as the concept of randomization or permutation tests based on the fact that the study site selection and patient selection are not random but the assignment of treatments to patients is random. Randomization model/method is a critical component in clinical trials because statistical inference based on the data collected from the trial relies on the probability distribution of the sample, which in turn depends upon the randomization procedure employed.

In practice, however, it is also of interest to adjust the probability of assignment of patients to treatments during the study to increase the probability of success of the clinical study. This type of randomization is called adaptive randomization because the probability of the treatment to which a current patient being assigned is adjusted based on the assignment of previous patients. Thus, an adaptive randomization design is referred to a design that allows modification of randomization schedules. It should be noted that the randomization codes based on the method of adaptive randomization cannot be prepared before the study begins. This is because the randomization process is performed at the time a patient is enrolled in the study, whereas adaptive randomization requires information on previously randomized patients. In practice, the method of adaptive randomization is often applied with respect to treatment, covariate, or clinical response. Therefore, the adaptive randomization is known as treatment-adaptive randomization, covariate-adaptive randomization, or response-adaptive randomization.

In practice, adaptive randomization may not be feasible for a large trial or a trial with a relatively long treatment duration. In addition, adaptive randomization procedures could have an impact on sample size required for achieving a desired statistical power and consequently statistical inference on the treatment effect, which is often difficult if not impossible to obtain, under investigation. More details regarding the adaptive randomization procedures described above and their impact on sample size calculation and statistical inference is given in Chapter 3 of this book.

Adaptive Hypotheses

An adaptive hypotheses design is a design that allows change in hypotheses based on interim analysis results, which is often considered before database lock and/or prior to data unblinding. As indicated by Hommel (2001), modifications of hypotheses during the conduct of a clinical trial commonly occur due to the following reasons that (i) an investigational method has not yet been validated at the planning stage of the study, (ii) information from other studies is necessary for planning the next stage of the study, (iii) there is a need to include new doses, and (iv) recommendations from a pre-established data safety monitoring committee (Hommel, 2001). In clinical research, it is not uncommon to have more than one set of hypotheses for an intended clinical trial. These hypotheses may be classified as primary hypotheses and secondary hypotheses depending upon whether they are the primary study objectives or secondary study objectives. In practice, a pre-specified overall type I error rate is usually controlled by testing the primary hypotheses. However, if the investigator is interested in controlling the overall type I error rate for testing secondary hypotheses, then techniques for multiple testing are commonly employed.

Following the ideas of Bauer (1999), Kieser, Bauer, and Lehmacher (1999), and Bauer and Kieser (1999) for general multiple testing problem, Hommel (2001) applied the same techniques to obtain more flexible strategies for adaptive modifications of hypotheses based on accrued data at interim by changing weights of hypotheses, changing an a prior order, or even including new hypotheses. The method proposed by Hommel (2001) enjoys the following advantages. First, it is a very general method in the sense that any type of multiple testing problems can be applied. Second, it is mathematically correct. Third, it is extremely flexible which allows not only changes to design, but also changes to the choice of hypotheses or weights for them during the course of the study. In addition, it also allows the addition of new hypotheses.

In clinical trials, commonly seen adaptive hypotheses include (i) switch from a superiority hypothesis to a non-inferiority hypothesis and (ii) change in study endpoints, e.g., switch primary and secondary endpoints (Chang and Chow, 2007). Modifications of hypotheses can certainly have an impact on sample size calculation and statistical inference for assessment of treatment effect. More discussions are given in Chapter 4 of this book.

Adaptive Dose Finding (Escalation) Trials

In clinical research, the *response* in a dose response study could be a biological response for safety or efficacy. For example, in a dose-toxicity study, the goal is to determine the maximum tolerable dose (MTD). On the other hand, in a dose-efficacy response study, the primary objective is usually to address one or more of the following questions: (i) Is there any evidence of the drug effect?, (ii) What is the nature of the dose-response?, and (iii) What is the optimal dose? In practice, it is always a concern as to how to evaluate dose-response relationship with limited resources within a relatively tight time-frame? This concern leads to a proposed design that allows fewer patients to be exposed to the toxicity and more patients to be treated at potential efficacious dose levels. Such a design also allows pharmaceutical companies to fully utilize their resources for development of more new drug products.

A typical example is an adaptive dose escalation trial design in early phase of cancer research for identifying the MTD, which is usually considered the optimal dose for later phase clinical trials. Commonly considered adaptive dose escalation trials include (i) adaptations to the traditional "3+3" escalation rule, and (ii) a trial design utilizing the continual re-assessment method (CRM) in conjunction with the Bayesian's approach. An adaptive dose finding design should possess the following good characteristics (i) small size cohort for lower dose levels, (ii) minimize the number of patients at lower dose groups, (iii) majority of patients near the MTD (ideally, the last two dose cohorts under study), (iv) flexibility for dose de-escalation, (v) limited dose jump if CRM is used, (vi) higher probability of reaching the MTD, (vii) lower probability of overdosing (if overdosing is a great safety concern), and (viii) should be able to take moderate adverse reaction into consideration.

In Chapter 5, we provide a brief background of dose escalation trials in oncology trials. We will reviewed the continued reassessment method (CRM) proposed by O'Quigley (O'Quigley, Pepe , and Fisher, 1990) in phase I oncology trials. We will study the hybrid frequentist-Bayesian adaptive approach for both efficacy and toxicity (Chang, Chow, and Pong, 2005) in detail.

Group Sequential Design

A group sequential design is an adaptive design that allows for prematurely stopping a trial due to safety, efficacy/futility, or both based on interim analysis results. Thus, a group sequential trial is also known as a flexible trial. In practice, flexible trials are usually referred to as trials that utilize interim monitoring based on group sequential and adaptive methodology for (i) early stopping for clinical benefit or harm, (ii) early stopping for futility, (iii) sample size re-adjustment, and (iv) re-designing the study in mid-stream. In practice, an adaptive group sequential design is very popular due to the following two reasons. First, clinical endpoint is a moving target. The sponsors and/or investigators may change their mind regarding clinically meaningful effect size after the trial starts. Second, it is a common practice to request a small budget at the design and then seek supplemental funding for increasing the sample size after seeing the interim data.

To protect the overall type I error rate in an adaptive design with respect to adaptations in some design parameters, many authors have proposed procedures using observed treatment effects. This leads to the justification for the commonly used two-stage adaptive design, in which the data from both stages are independent and the first data set is used for adaptation (see, e.g., Proschan and Hunsberger, 1995; Cui, Hung, and Wang, 1999; Liu and Chi, 2001). In recent years, the concept of two-stage adaptive design has led to the development of the adaptive group sequential design. The adaptive group sequential design is referred to as a design that uses observed (or estimated) treatment differences at interim analyses to modify the design and sample size adaptively (e.g., Shen and Fisher, 1999; Cui, Hung and Wang, 1999; Posch and Bauer, 1999; Lehmacher and Wassmer, 1999).

In clinical research, it is desirable to speed up the trial and at the same time reduce the cost of the trial. The ultimate goal is to get the products to the marketplace sooner. As a result, flexible methods for adaptive group sequential design and monitoring are the key factors for achieving this goal. With the availability of new technology such as electronic data capture, adaptive group sequential design in conjunction with the new technology will provide an integrated solution to the logistical and statistical complexities of monitoring trials in flexible ways without biasing the final conclusions.

As indicated earlier, the FDA classifies adaptive designs as either *well-understood designs* or *less well-understood designs* depending upon the nature of adaptations either blinded or unblinded (FDA, 2010). The typical (standard) group sequential trial design is considered a well-understood design. It, however, should be noted that the overall type I error rate may not be preserved when (i) additional adaptations (e.g., changes in hypotheses and/or study endpoints) are applied and (ii) there is a shift in target patient population. Further discussion regarding the application of adaptive group sequential designs in clinical trials can be found in Chapter 6.

Seamless Phase II/III Adaptive Design

A phase II clinical trial is often a dose-response study, where the goal is to find the appropriate dose level for the phase III trials. It is desirable that to combine phase II and III together so that the data can be used more efficiently and duration of the drug development can be reduced. A seamless phase II/III trial design is referred to as a program that addresses within a single trial objective that which is normally achieved through separate trials in phases IIb and III (Gallo et al., 2006). A seamless phase II/III adaptive design is a seamless phase II/III trial design that would use data from patients enrolled before and after the adaptation in the final analysis (Maca et al., 2006). Bauer and Kieser

(1999) provide a two-stage method for this purpose, where the investigators can terminate the trial entirely or drop a subset of regimens for lack of efficacy after the first stage. As pointed out by Sampson and Sill (2005), their procedure is highly flexible and the distributional assumptions are kept to a minimum. This results in a usual design in a number of settings. However, because of the generality of the method, it is difficult to construct confidence intervals, if not impossible. Sampson and Sill (2005) derived a uniformly most powerful conditionally unbiased test for normal endpoint. For other types of endpoints, no results match Sampson and Sill's results. Thus, it is suggested that computer trial simulation be used in such cases.

An seamless phase II/III adaptive design has the following good characteristics: (i) it is able to address study objectives of individual (e.g., phase IIb and phase III) studies, (ii) it utilizes data collected from both phases (e.g., phase IIb and phase III) for final analysis. However, there are some concerns regarding (i) whether it is efficient, (ii) the control of overall type I error rate, (iii) power analysis for sample size calculation/allocation, (iv) statistical validity of the combined analysis if the study objectives/endpoints are different at different phases. Chow and Tu (2008) classified (two-stage) adaptive seamless designs into four categories depending upon the study objectives and study endpoints used at different stages. More information regarding seamless adaptive designs are provided in Chapters 7 and 9.

Adaptive Sample Size Adjustment

As indicated earlier, an adaptive design is very attractive to the sponsors in early clinical development because it allows modifications of the trial to meet specific needs during the trial within limited budget/resources and target timelines. However, an adaptive design suffers from the losing of power for detecting a clinically meaningful difference of the target patient population under the actual patient population due to bias/variation that has been introduced to the trial as the result of changes in study parameters during the conduct of the trial. To account for the expected and/or unexpected bias/variation, statistical procedures for sample size calculation are necessary adjusted for achieving the desired power. For example, if the study dose or regimen and/or treatment duration have been adjusted during the conduct of the trial, not only the actual patient population may be different from the target patient population, but also the baseline for the clinically meaningful difference to be detected may have been changed. In this case, sample size required for achieving the desired power for correctly detecting a clinically meaningful difference based on clinical data collected from the actual patient population definitely needs adjustment.

It should be noted that procedures for sample size calculation based on power analysis of an adaptive design with respect to specific changes in study parameters are very different from the standard methods. The procedures for sample size calculation could be very complicated for a multiple adaptive design (or a combined adaptive design) involving more than one study parameters. In practice, statistical test for a null hypothesis of no treatment difference may not be tractable under a multiple adaptive design. Chapter 8 provides several methods for adaptive sample size adjustment which are useful for multiple adaptive designs.

Adaptive Treatment Switching

For evaluation of the efficacy and safety of a test treatment for progressive disease such as oncology and HIV, a parallel-group active-control randomized clinical trial is often conducted. Under the parallel-group active-control randomized clinical trial, qualified patients are randomly assigned to receive either an active control (a standard therapy or a treatment currently available in the marketplace) or a test treatment under investigation. Patients are allowed to switch from one treatment to another, due to ethical consideration, if there is lack of responses or there is evidence of disease progression. In practice, it is not uncommon that up to 80% of patients may switch from one treatment to another. This certainly has an impact on the evaluation of the efficacy of the test treatment. Despite allowing a switch between two treatments, many clinical studies are to compare the test treatment with the active control agent as if no patients had ever switched. Sommer and Zeger (1991) referred to the treatment effect among patients who complied with treatment as biological efficacy. Branson and Whitehead (2002) widened the concept of biological efficacy to encompass the treatment effect as if all patients adhered to their original randomized treatments in clinical studies allowing treatment switch.

The problem of treatment switching is commonly encountered in cancer trials. In cancer trials, most investigators would allow patients to get off the current treatment and switch to another treatment (either the study treatment or a rescue treatment) when there is progressed disease due to ethical consideration. However, treatment switching during the conduct of the trial has presented a challenge to clinical scientists (especially biostatisticians) regarding the analysis of some primary study endpoints such as median survival time. Under certain assumptions, Shao, Chang, and Chow (2005) proposed a method for estimation of median survival time when treatment switching occurs during the course of the study. Several methods for adaptive treatment switching are reviewed in Chapter 10.

Bayesian and Hybrid Approaches

Drug development is a sequence of drug decision-making processes, where decisions are made based on the constantly updated information. Bayesian approach fits naturally this mechanics. However, in the current regulatory setting, Bayesian approach is not ready as the criteria for approval of a drug. Therefore, it is desirable to use Bayesian approaches to optimize the trial and increase the probability of success under current frequentist criterion for approval. In the near future, it is expected that drug approval criteria will become Bayesian. In addition, full Bayesian is important because it can provide more informative information and optimal criteria for drug approval based on risk-benefit ratio rather than subjectively (arbitrarily) set $\alpha = 0.05$ as frequentist did. More discussion regarding Bayesian approach is provided in Chapter 11.

Biomarker Adaptive Trials

A biomarker-adaptive trial design is a design that allows for adaptation based on the responses of biomarkers such as genomic markers for assessment of treatment effect. A biomarker-adaptive trial design involves (i) qualification and standard (Liu and Chow, 2008), (ii) optimal screening design (Shao and Chow, 2007), (iii) establishment of predictive model, and (iv) validation of the established predictive model. In practice, a biomarker is usually referred to as (i) a classifier marker, (ii) a prognostic marker, or (iii) a predictive marker. It should be noted that a classifier marker usually does not change over the course of study and can be used to identify a patient population who would benefit from the treatment from those do not. A prognostic marker informs the clinical outcomes, independent of treatment, while a predictive marker informs the treatment effect on the clinical endpoint. Predictive marker can be population-specific. That is, a marker can be predictive for population A but not population B.

In practice, classifier marker is commonly used in enrichment process of target clinical trials. The difference between a prognostic marker and a predictive marker can be summarized as (i) that correlation between biomarker and true endpoint make a prognostic marker, and (ii) that correlation between biomarker and true endpoint does not make a predictive biomarker. In clinical trials, it is well recognized that there is a gap between identifying genes that are associated with clinical outcomes and establishing a predictive model between relevant genes and clinical outcomes. More details regarding biomarker-adaptive trials are provided in Chapter 12 of the book.

Target Clinical Trials

After completion of a human genome project, the disease targets at molecular level can be identified. As a result, treatment modality for molecular targets can be developed. In practice, target clinical trials are usually conducted for evaluation of the possibility and feasibility of the individualized treatment of patients. However, the accuracy of diagnostic devices for identification of such molecular targets is usually not perfect. Therefore, some of the patients enrolled in target clinical trials with a positive result by the diagnostic device might not have the specific molecular targets, and hence the treatment effects of the targeted drugs estimated from target clinical trials could be biased for the patient population truly with the molecular targets. Under an enrichment design for target clinical trials, the inference of the treatment effects of the targeted drugs in the patient population truly with molecular targets can be obtained using the EM algorithm and bootstrap technique (Liu et al., 2009). More details can be found in Chapter 13.

Sample Size and Power Estimation

In clinical trials, "How to perform a power analysis for sample size calculation/allocation?" is probably the most commonly asked question when utilizing an adaptive design especially a two-stage adaptive design. As indicated earlier, Chow and Tu (2008) classified two-stage adaptive designs into four categories depending upon the study objectives and the study endpoints used at different stages. A two-stage adaptive design with the same study objectives and study endpoints at different stages is similar to a group sequential design with one planned interim analysis. In this case, sample size calculation/allocation can be performed using the methods based on (i) individual p-values, (ii) sum of p-values, (iii) product of p-values, and (iv) inverse-normal p-values. Sample size and power estimation based on these methods are reviewed in Chapter 14.

For two-stage adaptive designs with different study objectives and/or different study endpoints at different stages, these methods cannot be applied directly. In this case, sample size calculation/allocation should be performed based on appropriate statistical methods as described in Chapter 9 (see also Chow et al., 2007; Lu et al., 2009, 2010). For other complicated adaptive design such as multiple adaptive design which are considered less well-understood designs, sample size calculation should be performed using valid statistical methods.

Clinical Trial Simulation

It should be noted that for a given adaptive design, it is very likely that adaptations will be made to more than one study parameter simultaneously during the conduct of the clinical trial. To assess the impact of changes in specific study parameters, a typical approach is to perform a sensitivity analysis by fixing other study parameters. In practice, the assessment of the overall impact of changes in each study parameter is almost impossible due to possible confounding and/or masking effects among changes in study parameters. As a result, it is suggested that a clinical trial simulation be conducted to examine the individual and/or overall impact of changes in more than one study parameter. In addition, the performance of a given adaptive design can be evaluated through the conduct of a clinical trial simulation in terms of its sensitivity, robustness, and/or empirical probability of reproducibility. It, however, should be noted that a clinical trial simulation should be conducted in such a way that the simulated clinical data should be able to reflect the real situation of the clinical trial after all of the modifications are made to the trial procedures and/or statistical procedures. In practice, it is then suggested that assumptions regarding the sources of bias/variation as the results of modifications of the ongoing trial be identified and be taken into consideration when conducting the clinical trial simulation. More details are provided in Chapter 15 of the book.

Case Studies

As pointed out by Li (2006), the use of adaptive design methods provides a second chance to re-design the trial after seeing data internally or externally at interim. However, it may introduce so-called operational biases such as selection bias, method of evaluations, early withdrawal, or modification of treatments. Consequently, the adaptation employed may inflate type I error rate. Li (2006) suggested a couple of principles when implementing adaptive designs in clinical trials: (i) adaptation should not alter trial conduct, and (ii) type I error should be preserved. Following these principles, some studies with complicated adaptation may be more successful than others. The successful experience for certain adaptive designs in clinical trials is important to investigators in clinical research and development. For illustration purpose, some successful case studies including the implementation of an adaptive group sequential design (Cui, Hung, and Wang, 1999), an adaptive dose-escalation design (Chang and Chow, 2005), and seamless phase II/III adaptive trial design (Maca et al., 2006) are provided in the last chapter of this book.

1.6 Aims and Scope of the Book

This is intended to be the first book entirely devoted to the use of adaptive design methods in clinical trials. It covers all of the statistical issues that may occur at various stages of adaptive design and analysis of clinical trials. It is our goal to provide a useful desk reference and a state-of-the art examination of this area to scientists and researchers engaged in clinical research and development, those in government regulatory agencies who have to make decisions in pharmaceutical review and approval process, and to biostatisticians who provide the statistical support for clinical trials and related clinical investigation. More importantly, we would like to provide graduate students in the areas of clinical development and biostatistics an advanced textbook in the use of adaptive design methods in clinical trials. We hope that this book can serve as a bridge among the pharmaceutical industry, government regulatory agencies, and academia.

The scope of this book covers statistical issues that are commonly encountered when modifications of study procedures and/or statistical procedures are made during the course of the study. In this chapter, the definition, regulatory requirement, target patient population, statistical issues of adaptive design, and analysis for clinical trials have been discussed. In the next chapter, the impact of modifications made to trial procedures and/or statistical procedures on the target patient population, statistical inference, and power analysis for sample size calculation as the result of protocol amendments is discussed. In Chapter 3, various adaptive randomization procedures for treatment allocation will be discussed. Chapter 4 covers adaptive design methods for modifications of hypotheses including the addition of new hypotheses after the review of interim data. Chapter 5 provides an overall review of adaptive design methods for dose selection especially in dose finding and dose-response relationship studies in early clinical development. Chapter 6 introduces the commonly used adaptive group sequential design in clinical trials. Statistical tests for adaptive seamless phase II/III designs are given in Chapter 7. Chapter 8 provides blinded procedures for sample size re-estimation. Chapter 9 explores statistical tests for various types of two-stage adaptive designs, while statistical inference for switching from one treatment to another adaptively and the corresponding practical issues that one may encounter are studied in Chapter 10. Bayesian and hybrid approaches for the use of adaptive design methods in clinical trials are outlined in Chapter 11. Chapter 12 provides an overview of biomarker adaptive trials, while target clinical trials with enrichment processes are discussed in Chapter 13. Chapter 14 summarizes sample size calculation based on individual, sum, and product of p-values in multi-stage adaptive trial designs. Chapter 15 introduces the methodology of clinical trial simulation for evaluation of the performance of the adaptive design methods under various adaptive designs that are commonly used in clinical development . Chapter 16 reviews the recent FDA guidance on adaptive clinical trial design. Some case studies regarding the implementation of adaptive group sequential design, adaptive dose-escalation design and seamless phase II/III adaptive trial design in clinical trials are discussed in the last chapter of this book.

For each chapter, whenever possible, real examples from clinical trials are included to demonstrate the use of adaptive design methods in clinical trials including clinical/statistical concepts, interpretations, and their relationships and interactions. Comparisons regarding the relative merits and disadvantages of the adaptive design methods in clinical research and development are discussed whenever deemed appropriate. In addition, if applicable, topics for future research are provided. All computations in this book are performed using 8.20 of SAS. Other statistical packages such as S-plus and R can also be applied.

Chapter 2

Protocol Amendment

2.1 Introduction

In clinical trials, it is not uncommon to issue protocol amendments during the conduct of a clinical trial due to various reasons such as slow enrollment and/or safety concerns. For slow enrollment, the investigator may modify the entry eligibility criteria (e.g., inclusion and/or exclusion criteria) in order to expedite patient enrollment in a timely fashion. On the other hand, during the conduct of a clinical trial, it is possible that additional safety information becomes available. This additional safety information may come from either similar clinical trials conducted simultaneously (by the same investigator or different investigators) or clinical results newly published at leading medical journals in the therapeutic areas. With this additional safety information, protocol amendment is necessarily issued for patient protection. For Good Clinical Practice (GCP), before protocol amendments can be issued, description, rationales, and clinical/statistical justification regarding the changes to be made should be provided to ensure the validity and integrity of the clinical trial. As the result of the changes or modifications, the originally targeted patient population under study could have been shifted to a similar but different patient population. If changes or modifications are made frequently during the conduct of the trial, the target patient population is in fact a moving target patient population. This raises the controversial issue regarding the validity of the statistical inference drawn based on data collected before and after protocol amendment.

In practice, there is a risk that major (or significant) modifications made to the trial procedures and/or statistical procedures could lead to a totally different trial, which is unable to address the scientific/medical questions that the clinical trial is intended to answer. In clinical trials, most investigators consider protocol amendment a God-sent gift which allows the flexibility to make any changes/modifications to the on-going clinical trials. It, however, should be recognized that protocol amendments have potential risks for introducing additional bias/variation to the on-going clinical trial. Thus, it is important to identify, control, and hopefully minimize/eliminate the sources of bias/variation whenever possible. In practice, it is then of particular interest to measure the impact of changes or modifications that were made to the trial procedures and/or statistical methods on statistical inference of the treatment effect under investigation after the protocol amendment. This raises another controversial issue regarding (1) the impact of changes made, and (2) the degree of changes that is allowed in a protocol amendment.

In current practice, standard statistical methods are applied to the data collected from the actual patient population regardless of the frequency of changes (protocol amendments) that have been made during the conduct of the trial provided that the overall type I error is controlled at the pre-specified level of significance. This, however, has raised a serious regulatory/statistical concern as to whether the resultant statistical inference (e.g., independent estimates, confidence intervals, and p-values) drawn on the originally planned target patient population based on the clinical data from the actual patient population (as the result of the modifications made via protocol amendments) is accurate and reliable. After some modifications are made to the trial procedures and/or statistical methods, not only the target patient population may have become a similar but different patient population, but also the sample size may not achieve the desired power for detection of a clinically important effect size of the test treatment at the end of the study. In practice, we expect to lose power when the modifications have led to a shift in mean response and/or inflation of variability of the response of the primary study endpoint. As a result, the originally planned sample size may have to be adjusted. Thus, it is suggested that the relative efficiency of each protocol amendment be taken into consideration for derivation of an adjusted factor for sample size in order to achieve the desired power.

In the next section, the concept of a moving target patient population as the result of protocol amendments is introduced. Also included in the section is the derivation of a sensitivity index for measuring the degree of population shift. Section 2.3 discusses the method with covariate adjustment proposed by Chow and Shao (2005). Inference based on mixture distribution is described in Section 2.4. In Section 2.5, sample size adjustment after protocol amendment is discussed. A brief concluding remark is given in the last section.

2.2   Moving Target Patient Population

In practice, for a given clinical trial, it is not uncommon to have 3-5 protocol amendments after the initiation of the clinical trial. In some cases, we may have even up to 12 protocol amendments in a single clinical trial. One of the major impacts of frequent protocol amendments is that the target patient population may have been shifted during the process, which may have resulted in a totally different target patient population at the end of the trial. A typical example is the case when significant adaptation (modification) is applied to inclusion/exclusion criteria of the study. Denote by (μ, σ) the *target* patient population. After a given protocol amendment, the resultant (actual) patient population may have been shifted to (μ_1, σ_1), where $\mu_1 = \mu + \varepsilon$ is the population mean of the primary study endpoint and $\sigma_1 = C\sigma$ $(C > 0)$ is the population standard deviation of the primary study endpoint. The shift in target patient population can be characterized by

$$E_1 \left| \frac{\mu_1}{\sigma_1} \right| = \left| \frac{\mu + \epsilon}{C\sigma} \right| = |\Delta| \left| \frac{\mu}{\sigma} \right| = |\Delta| E$$

where $\Delta = (1 + \varepsilon/\mu)/C$, and E and E_1 are the effect size before and after population shift, respectively. Chow, Shao, and Hu (2002) and Chow and Chang (2008) refer to Δ as a sensitivity index measuring the change in effect size between the actual patient population and the original target patient population.

Similarly, denote by (μ_i, σ_i), the actual patient population after the ith modification of trial procedure, where $\mu_i = \mu + \varepsilon_i$ and $\sigma_i = C_i\sigma$, $i = 0, 1, ..., K$. Note that $i = 0$ reduces to the original target patient population (μ, σ). That is, when $i = 0$, $\varepsilon_0 = 0$ and $C_0 = 1$. After K protocol amendments, the resultant actual patient population becomes (μ_K, σ_K), where

$$\mu_K = \mu + \sum_{i=1}^{K} \varepsilon_i \text{ and } \sigma_K = \prod_{i=1}^{K} C_i\sigma.$$

It should be noted that (ε_i, C_i), $i = 1, ..., K$ are in fact random variables. As a result, the resultant actual patient population is a *moving* target patient population rather than a *fixed* target patient population. In addition, sample sizes before and after protocol amendments and the number of protocol amendments issued for a given clinical trial are also random variables. Thus, one of the controversial issues that is commonly encountered in clinical trials with several protocol amendments during the conduct of the trials is *How to assess the treatment effect while the target patient population is a moving target?*

Table 2.1 provides a summary of the impacts of various scenarios of location shift (i.e., change in ε) and scale shift (change in C, either inflation or deflation of variability). As it can be seen from Table 2.2.1, there is a masking effect between location shift and scale shift. In other words, shift in location could be offset by the inflation or deflation of variability. As a result, the sensitivity index remains unchanged while the target patient population has been shifted. One of the controversial issues in this regard is that whether the conclusion drawn (by ignoring the population shift) at the end of the trial is accurate and reliable.

Table 2.2.1: Changes in Sensitivity Index

	Inflation of Variability		Deflation of Variability	
$\varepsilon/\mu(\%)$	$C(\%)$	Δ	$C(\%)$	Δ
−20	120	0.667	80	1.000
−10	120	0.750	80	1.125
−5	120	0.792	80	1.188
0	120	0.833	80	1.250
5	120	0.875	80	1.313
10	120	0.917	80	1.375
20	120	1.000	80	1.500

As indicated in Chow and Chang (2008), the impact of protocol amendments on statistical inference due to shift in target patient population (moving target patient population) can be studied through a model that links the moving population means with some covariates (Chow and Shao, 2005). However, in many cases, such covariates may not exist or exist but are not observable. In this case, it is suggested that inference on Δ be considered to measure the degree of shift in location and scale of patient population based on a mixture distribution by assuming the location or scale parameter is random (Chow, Chang, and Pong, 2005). These methods will be described in the subsequent sections.

2.3   Analysis with Covariate Adjustment

As indicated earlier, statistical methods for analyzing clinical data should be modified when there are protocol amendments during the trial, since any protocol deviations and/or violations may introduce bias to the trial. As a result, conclusions drawn based on the analysis of data ignoring that there are possible shifts in target patient population could be biased and hence misleading. To overcome this problem, Chow and Shao (2005) proposed to model the population deviations due to protocol amendments using some relevant covariates and developed a valid statistical inference which is described below.

2.3.1   Continuous study endpoint

Suppose that there are a total of K possible protocol amendments. Let μ_k be the mean of the study endpoint after the kth protocol amendment, $k = 1, ..., K$. Suppose that, for each k, clinical data are observed from n_k patients so that the sample mean $\bar{y}_k$ is an unbiased estimator of μ_k, $k = 0, 1, ..., K$. Now, let x be a (possibly multivariate) covariate whose values are distinct from different protocol amendments. To derive statistical inference for μ_0 (the population mean for the original target patient population), Chow and Shao (2005) assumed the following

$$\mu_k = \beta_0 + \beta' x_k, \ k = 0, 1, ..., K, \tag{2.1}$$

where β_0 is an unknown parameter, β is an unknown parameter vector whose dimension is the same as x, β' denotes the transpose of β, and x_k is the value of x under the kth amendment (or the original protocol when $k = 0$). If values of x are different within a fixed population (say P_k, patient population after the kth protocol amendment), then x_k is a characteristic of x such as the average of all values of x within P_k.

Under model (2.1), parameters β_0 and β can be unbiasedly estimated by

$$\begin{pmatrix} \hat{\beta}_0 \\ \hat{\beta} \end{pmatrix} = (X'WX)^{-1}X'W\bar{y},\tag{2.2}$$

where $\bar{y} = (\bar{y}_0, \bar{y}_1, ..., \bar{y}_K)'$, X is a matrix whose kth row is $(1, x_k')$, $k = 0, 1, ..., K$, and W is a diagonal matrix whose diagonal elements are $n_0, n_1, ..., n_K$. It is assumed that the dimension of x is less or equal to K so that $(X'WX)^{-1}$ is well defined. To estimate μ_0, we consider the following unbiased estimator $\hat{\mu}_0 = \hat{\beta}_0 + \hat{\beta}'x_0$. Chow and Shao (2005) indicated that $\hat{\mu}_0$ is distributed as $N(\mu_0, \sigma^2 c_0)$ with $c_0 = (1, x_0)(X'WX)^{-1}(1, x_0)'$. Let s_k^2 be the sample variance based on the data from population P_k, $k = 0, 1, ..., K$. Then, $(n_k - 1)s_k^2/\sigma^2$ has the chi-square distribution with $n_k - 1$ degrees of freedom and consequently, $(N - K)s^2/\sigma^2$ has the chi-square distribution with $N - K$ degrees of freedom, where

$$s^2 = \sum_{k=0}^{K} (n_k - 1)s_k^2/(N - K)$$

and $N = \sum_k n_k$. Confidence intervals for μ_0 and testing hypotheses related to μ_0 can be carried out using the t-statistic $t = (\hat{\mu}_0 - \mu_0)/\sqrt{c_0 s^2}$.

Note that when $P_k's$ have different standard deviations and/or data from P_k are not normally distributed, we may consider an approximation by assuming that all $n_k's$ are large. Thus, by the central limit theorem, it can be shown that $\hat{\mu}_0$ is approximately normally distributed with mean μ_0 and variance

$$\tau^2 = (1, x_0)(X'WX)^{-1}X'W\Sigma X(X'WX)^{-1}(1, x_0)',\tag{2.3}$$

Where Σ is the diagonal matrix whose kth diagonal element is the population variance of P_k, $k = 0, 1, ..., K$. Large sample statistical inference can be made by using the z-statistic $z = (\hat{\mu}_0 - \mu_0)/\hat{\tau}$ (which is approximately distributed as the standard normal), where $\hat{\tau}$ is the same as τ with the kth diagonal element of Σ estimated by s_k^2, $k = 0, 1, ..., K$.

Note that the above statistical inference for μ_0 is a conditional inference. In their paper, Chow and Shao (2005) also derived unconditional inference for μ_0 under certain assumptions. In addition, Chow and Pong (2009) considered an alternative approach with random coefficients under model (9.1) using a Bayesian approach may be considered for obtaining inference on μ_0.

2.3.2   Binary response

As indicated, the statistical inference for μ_0 described above is for continuous endpoint. Following a similar idea, Yang, Chi, and Chow (2011) derived statistical inference for μ_0 assuming that the study endpoint is a binary response. Their method is briefly summarized below.

Let Y_{ij} be the binary response from the jth subject after the ith amendment; $Y_{ij} = 1$ if subject j after amendment i exhibits the response of interest, and 0 otherwise, for $i = 0, 1, ..., k$ and $j = 1, ..., n_i$. Note that the subscript 0 for i indicates that the values related to the original patient population. Let p_i denote the response rate of the patient population after the ith amendment,. Ignoring the possible population deviations results in a pooled estimator

$$\bar{p} = \sum_{i=0}^{k} \sum_{j=1}^{n_i} Y_{ij} / \sum_{i=0}^{k} n_i,,$$

which may be biased for the original defined response rate p_0. In many clinical trials, the protocol amendments are made with respect to one or a few relevant covariates. Modifying entry criteria, for example, may involve patient demographics such as age or body weight and patient characteristics such as disease status or medical history. This section develops statistical inference procedure for the original response rate p_0 based on a covariate-adjusted model.

Estimation of the single response rate. Let X_{ij} be the corresponding covariate for the jth subject after the ith amendment (or the original protocol when $i = 0$). Throughout this article we assume that the response rates for different patient populations can be related by the following model

$$p_i = \frac{\exp(\beta_0 + \beta_1 v_i)}{1 + \exp(\beta_0 + \beta_1 v_i)}, \ i = 0, 1, ..., k,$$

Where β_0 and β_1 are unknown parameters, and v_i is the true mean of the random covariate under the ith amendment. Under the above model, the maximum likelihood estimates for the parameters β_0 and β_1, however cannot be obtained directly because the v_i's are unknown. One approach to estimate β_0 and β_1 is to replace v_i by $\bar{X}_i$, the sample mean under the ith amendment (see Chow and Shao, 2005). Consequently, we specify a logistic model for estimating $\beta = (\beta_0, \beta_1)^T$ as

$$P(Y_{ij} = 1 | \bar{X}_i = \bar{x}_i) = \frac{\exp(\beta_0 + \beta_1 \bar{x}_i)}{1 + \exp(\beta_0 + \beta_1 \bar{x}_i)}. \tag{2.4}$$

Suppose that X_{ij}, $j = 1, 2, ..., n_i$, $i = 0, 1, ..., k$, are independent random variables with means v_i. Thus the sample means $\bar{X}_i$, $i = 0, 1, ..., k$, are independent random variables with means v_i. Let $f_{\bar{X}_i}(\bar{x}_i)$ denote the probability density function of $\bar{X}_i$. In the development that follows, the $f_{\bar{X}_i}(\bar{x}_i)$ are assumed independent of β_0 or β_1.

Since the conditional distribution of Y_{ij} given $\bar{x}_i$ is Bernoulli distribution with parameter defined in (13.4) and $f_{\bar{X}_i}(\bar{x}_i)$ is the probability density function of $\bar{X}_i$, the likelihood function of observing y_{ij} ($j = 1, 2, ..., n_i$) and $\bar{x}_i$ under the ith amendment is given by

$$\ell_i = \prod_{j=1}^{n_i} \left[\left(\frac{\exp(\beta_0 + \beta_1 \bar{x}_i)}{1 + \exp(\beta_0 + \beta_1 \bar{x}_i)} \right)^{y_{ij}} \left(\frac{1}{1 + \exp(\beta_0 + \beta_1 \bar{x}_i)} \right)^{1-y_{ij}} \right] \times f_{\bar{X}_i}(\bar{x}_i)$$

Therefore, the joint likelihood function is $\ell = \coprod_{i=0}^{k} \ell_i$ and the log likelihood function is given by

$$l(\beta) = l_1(\beta) + \sum_{i=0}^{k} \ln f_{\bar{X}_i}(\bar{x}_i), \qquad (2.5)$$

where

$$l_1(\beta) = \sum_{i=0}^{k} \sum_{j=1}^{n_i}$$
$$\times \left[y_{ij} \ln \left(\frac{\exp(\beta_0 + \beta_1 \bar{x}_i)}{1 + \exp(\beta_0 + \beta_1 \bar{x}_i)} \right) + (1 - y_{ij}) \ln \left(\frac{1}{1 + \exp(\beta_0 + \beta_1 \bar{x}_i)} \right) \right]$$

Because $f_{\bar{X}_i}(\bar{x}_i)$ does not depend on β_0 or β_1, the maximum likelihood estimate $\beta = (\beta_0, \beta_1)^T$, which maximize $l_1(\beta)$ also maximize $l(\beta)$. Thus, the data can be analyzed using a fixed-covariate model. By considering the covariate as a random variable, a simple closed-form estimate of the asymptotic covariance matrix of maximum likelihood estimate of the parameters can be obtained to calculate the sample size required to test hypotheses about the parameters (see Demidenko, 2007). On the basis of the estimate $\hat{\beta}$, we propose to estimate p_0 by

$$\hat{p}_0 = \exp(\hat{\beta}_0 + \hat{\beta}_1 \bar{X}_0)/(1 + \exp(\hat{\beta}_0 + \hat{\beta}_1 \bar{X}_0))$$

For inference on p_0, we need to derive the asymptotic distribution of $\hat{p}_0$. In this case, the limiting results regarding the maximum likelihood estimators are obtained as the number of protocol amendments is finite and the numbers of observations from the distinct amendments become large. Assuming that $n_i/N \to r_i$ as $n_i \to \infty$, where $N = \sum_{i=0}^{k} n_i$, and k is a finite constant, it can be shown that

$$\sqrt{N}(\hat{\beta} - \beta) \xrightarrow{d} N(0, I^{-1}), \qquad (2.6)$$

where

$$I = \begin{bmatrix} \sum_{i=0}^{k} r_i \dfrac{\exp(\beta_0 + \beta_1 v_i)}{(1 + \exp(\beta_0 + \beta_1 v_i))^2} & \sum_{i=0}^{k} r_i \dfrac{v_i \exp(\beta_0 + \beta_1 v_i)}{(1 + \exp(\beta_0 + \beta_1 v_i))^2} \\ \sum_{i=0}^{k} r_i \dfrac{v_i \exp(\beta_0 + \beta_1 v_i)}{(1 + \exp(\beta_0 + \beta_1 v_i))^2} & \sum_{i=0}^{k} r_i \dfrac{v_i^2 \exp(\beta_0 + \beta_1 v_i)}{(1 + \exp(\beta_0 + \beta_1 v_i))^2} \end{bmatrix}.$$

The proof of (2.6) is given in the Appendix. Moreover, by the delta method and Slutsky's theorem, it follows that $\sqrt{N}(\hat{p}_0 - p_0)$ is asymptotically normal distributed with mean 0 and variance

$$V = [\exp(\beta_0 + \beta_1 v_0)/(1 + \exp(\beta_0 + \beta_1 v_0))]^2 (1, v_0)_{\mathbf{I}^{-1}} (1, v_0)^T$$

Let $\hat{V}$ be the ML estimator of V with β_0, β_1, v_i, and r_i replaced by $\beta_0, \beta_1, \bar{X}_i$, and n_i/N, respectively. It is known that $\bar{X}_i \xrightarrow{p} v_i$ and $\hat{\beta} \xrightarrow{p} \beta$ by the Weak Law of Large Number and the consistency of a maximum likelihood estimator. Thus, we have $\hat{V} \xrightarrow{p} V$. Then, it can be shown that $\sqrt{N}(\hat{p}_0 - p_0)/\sqrt{\hat{V}}$ is asymptotically distributed as a standard normal distribution by Slutsky's theorem. Based on this result, an approximate $100(1 - \alpha)\%$ confidence interval of p_0 is given by $(\hat{p}_0 - z_{\alpha/2}\sqrt{\hat{V}/N}, \hat{p}_0 + z_{\alpha/2}\sqrt{\hat{V}/N})$, where $z_{\alpha/2}$ is the $100(1 - \alpha/2)$ percentile of a standard normal distribution.

Comparison for two treatments. In clinical trials, it is often of interest to compare two treatments, i.e., a test treatment vs. an active control or placebo. Let Y_{tij} and X_{tij} be the response and the corresponding relevant covariate for the jth subject after the ith amendment under the tth treatment ($t = 1, 2, i = 0, 1, ..., k, j = 1, 2, ..., n_{ti}$). For each amendment, patients selected by the same criteria are randomly allocated to either the test treatment $D_1 = 1$ or control treatment $D_2 = 0$ groups. In this particular case, the true mean values of the covariate for the two treatment groups are the same under each amendment. Therefore, the relationships between the binary response and the covariate for both treatment groups can be described by a single model,

$$p_{ti} = \frac{\exp(\beta_1 + \beta_2 D_t + \beta_3 \nu_i + \beta_4 D_t \nu_i)}{1 + \exp(\beta_1 + \beta_2 D_t + \beta_3 \nu_i + \beta_4 D_t \nu_i)}, t = 1, 2, i = 0, 1, ..., k.$$

Hence, the response rates for the test treatment and the control treatment are

$$p_{1i} = \frac{\exp(\beta_1 + \beta_2 + (\beta_3 + \beta_4)\nu_i)}{1 + \exp(\beta_1 + \beta_2 + (\beta_3 + \beta_4)\nu_i)} \quad \text{and} \quad p_{2i} = \frac{\exp(\beta_1 + \beta_3 \nu_i)}{1 + \exp(\beta_1 + \beta_3 \nu_i)},$$

respectively.

Similar to the single treatment study described previously, the joint likelihood function of $\boldsymbol{\beta} = (\beta_1, \cdots, \beta_4)^T$ is given by

$$\prod_{t=1}^{2} \prod_{i=0}^{k} \prod_{j=1}^{n_{ti}} \left[\left(\frac{\exp(\beta^T z^{(ti)})}{1 + \exp(\beta^T z^{(ti)})} \right)^{y_{tij}} \left(\frac{1}{1 + \exp(\beta^T z^{(ti)})} \right)^{1 - y_{tij}} \times f_{\bar{X}_{\cdot i}}(\bar{x}_{\cdot i}) \right],$$

where $f_{\bar{X}_{\cdot i}}(\bar{x}_{\cdot i})$ is the probability density function of $\bar{X}_{\cdot i} = \sum_{t=1}^{2} \sum_{j=1}^{n_{ti}} X_{tij}$ and $z^{(ti)} = (1, D_t, \bar{x}_{\cdot i}, D_t \bar{x}_{\cdot i})^T$. The log likelihood function is then given by

$$l(\beta) = \sum_{t=1}^{2} \sum_{i=0}^{k} \sum_{j=1}^{n_{ti}} \left[y_{tij} \ln \left(\frac{\exp(\beta^T z^{(ti)})}{1 + \exp(\beta^T z^{(ti)})} \right) \right.$$

$$\left. + (1 - y_{tij}) \ln \left(\frac{1}{1 + \exp(\beta^T z^{(ti)})} \right) + \ln f_{\bar{X}_{\cdot i}}(\bar{x}_{\cdot i}) \right]. \qquad (2.7)$$

Given the resulting the maximum likelihood estimate $\hat{\beta} = (\hat{\beta}_1, \cdots, \hat{\beta}_4)^T$, we obtain the estimate of p_{10} and p_{20} as follows

$$\hat{p}_{10} = \frac{\exp(\hat{\beta}_1 + \hat{\beta}_2 + (\hat{\beta}_3 + \hat{\beta}_4)\bar{X}_{\cdot 0})}{1 + \exp(\hat{\beta}_1 + \hat{\beta}_2 + (\hat{\beta}_3 + \hat{\beta}_4)\bar{X}_{\cdot 0})}, \quad \hat{p}_{20} = \frac{\exp(\hat{\beta}_1 + \hat{\beta}_3\bar{X}_{\cdot 0})}{1 + \exp(\hat{\beta}_1 + \hat{\beta}_3\bar{X}_{\cdot 0})}.$$

Let $n_{t\cdot} = \sum_{i=0}^{k} n_{ti}$ be the sample size for the tth treatment group, and let $N = n_1 + n_2$ be the total sample size. When $n_{ti}/n_{t\cdot} \to r_{ti}$ and $n_{i\cdot}/N \to c$ as all n_{ti} tend to infinity, it is shown by the similar derivation for single response rate shown above that

$$\frac{\sqrt{N}((\hat{p}_{10} - \hat{p}_{20}) - (p_{10} - p_{20}))}{\sqrt{\hat{V}_d}} \xrightarrow{d} N(0,1),$$

where $\hat{V}_d = \varphi^T \left(\sum_{t=1}^{2} \sum_{i=0}^{k} n_{ti} \hat{I}^{(ti)}/N \right)^{-1} \varphi$,

$$\phi^T \begin{pmatrix} \hat{p}_{10}(1 - \hat{p}_{10}) - \hat{p}_{20}(1 - \hat{p}_{20}) \\ \hat{p}_{10}(1 - \hat{p}_{10}) \\ \bar{X}_0(\hat{p}_{10}(1 - \hat{p}_{10}) - \hat{p}_{20}(1 - \hat{p}_{20})) \\ \bar{X}_0(\hat{p}_{10}(1 - \hat{p}_{10})) \end{pmatrix},$$

and

$$\hat{I}^{(ti)} = \hat{p}_{ti}(1 - \hat{p}_{ti}) \begin{bmatrix} 1 & D_t & \bar{X}_{\cdot i} & D_t\bar{X}_{\cdot i} \\ D_t & D_t^2 & D_t\bar{X}_{\cdot i} & D_t^2\bar{X}_{\cdot i} \\ \bar{X}_{\cdot i} & D_t\bar{X}_{\cdot i} & \bar{X}_{\cdot i}^2 & D_t\bar{X}_{\cdot i}^2 \\ D_t\bar{X}_{\cdot i} & D_t^2\bar{X}_{\cdot i} & D_t\bar{X}_{\cdot i}^2 & D_t^2\bar{X}_{\cdot i}^2 \end{bmatrix}.$$

As indicated by Chow et al. (2007), the problem of testing superiority and non-inferiority can be unified by the following hypotheses:

$$H_0 : p_{10} - p_{20} \leq \delta \quad \text{vs.} \quad H_a : p_{10} - p_{20} > \delta \tag{2.8}$$

where δ is the superiority or non-inferiority margin. When $\delta > 0$, the rejection of the null hypothesis indicates the superiority of the test treatment over the control. When $\delta < 0$, the rejection of the null hypothesis indicates the non-inferiority of the test treatment against the control. Under the null hypothesis, the test statistic

$$T = \frac{\sqrt{N}(\hat{p}_{10} - \hat{p}_{20} - \delta)}{\sqrt{\hat{V}_d}} \tag{2.9}$$

approximately follows a standard normal distribution when all n_{ti} are sufficiently large. Thus, we reject the null hypothesis at the α level of significance if $T > z_\alpha$ For testing equivalence, the following hypotheses are considered:

$$H_0 : |p_{10} - p_{20}| \geq \delta \quad \text{vs.} \quad H_a : |p_{10} - p_{20}| < \delta. \tag{2.10}$$

where δ is the equivalence limit. Thus the null hypothesis is rejected at a significance level α and the test treatment is concluded to be equivalent to the control if

$$\frac{\sqrt{N}(\hat{p}_{10} - \hat{p}_{20} - \delta)}{\sqrt{\hat{V}_d}} < -z_\alpha \quad \text{and} \quad \frac{\sqrt{N}(\hat{p}_{10} - \hat{p}_{20} + \delta)}{\sqrt{\hat{V}_d}} > z_\alpha.$$

2.4   Assessment of Sensitivity Index

The primary assumption of the above approaches is that there is a relationship between $\mu'_{ik}s$ and a covariate vector x. As indicated earlier, such covariates may not exist or may not be observable in practice. In this case, Chow, Chang, and Pong (2005) suggested assessing the sensitivity index and consequently deriving a unconditional inference for the original target patient population assuming that the shift parameter (i.e., ε) and/or the scale parameter (i.e., C) is random. Thus, the shift and scale parameters (i.e., ε and C) of the target population after a protocol amendment is made can be estimated by

$$\hat{\varepsilon} = \hat{\mu}_{Actual} - \hat{\mu} \ \text{ and } \ \hat{C} = \hat{\sigma}_{Actual}/\hat{\sigma},$$

Respectively, where $(\hat{\mu}, \hat{\sigma})$ and $(\hat{\mu}_{Actual}, \hat{\sigma}_{Actual})$ are some estimates of (μ, σ) and $(\mu_{Actual}, \sigma_{Actual})$, respectively. As a result, the sensitivity index can be estimated by

$$\hat{\Delta} = \frac{1 + \hat{\varepsilon}/\hat{\mu}}{\hat{C}}.$$

2.4.1   The case where ε is random and C is fixed

Estimates for μ and σ can be obtained based on data collected prior to any protocol amendments is issued. Assume that the response variable x is distributed as $N(\mu, \sigma^2)$. Let $x_{ji}, \quad i = 1, ..., n_j; \ j = 0, ..., m$ be the response of the ith patient after the jth protocol amendment. As a result, the total number of patients is given by $n = \sum_{j=0}^{m} n_j$. Note that n_0 is the number of patients in the study prior to any protocol amendments. Based on $x_{0i}, \ i = 1, ..., n_0$, the maximum likelihood estimates of μ and σ^2 can be obtained as follows

$$\hat{\mu} = \frac{1}{n_0} \sum_{i=1}^{n_0} x_{0i}, \ \text{ and } \ \hat{\sigma}^2 = \frac{1}{n_0} \sum_{i=1}^{n_0} (x_{0i} - \hat{\mu})^2.$$

To obtain estimates for μ_{Actual} and σ_{Actual}, Chow, Chang, and Pong (2005) considered the case where μ_{Actual} is random and σ_{Actual} is fixed. For convenience's sake, we set $\mu_{Actual} = \mu$ and $\sigma_{Actual} = \sigma$ for the derivation of ε and C. Assume that x conditional on μ, i.e., $x|_{\mu=\mu_{Actual}}$ follows a normal distribution $N(\mu, \sigma^2)$. That is,

$$x|_{\mu=\mu_{Actual}} \ \sim \ N(\mu, \sigma^2),$$

where μ is distributed as $N(\mu_\mu, \sigma_\mu^2)$ and σ, μ_μ, and σ_μ are some unknown constants. Thus, the unconditional distribution of x is a mixed normal distribution given below

$$\int N(x; \mu, \sigma^2) N(\mu; \mu_\mu, \sigma_\mu^2) d\mu = \frac{1}{\sqrt{2\pi\sigma^2}} \frac{1}{\sqrt{2\pi\sigma_\mu^2}} \int_{-\infty}^{\infty} e^{-\frac{(x-\mu)^2}{2\sigma^2} - \frac{(\mu-\mu_\mu)^2}{2\sigma_\mu^2}} d\mu,$$

where $x \in (-\infty, \infty)$. It can be verified that the above mixed normal distribution is a normal distribution with mean μ_μ and variance $\sigma^2 + \sigma_\mu^2$. In other words, x is distributed as $N(\mu_\mu, \sigma^2 + \sigma_\mu^2)$. See Theorem 2.1 below.

Theorem 2.1 Suppose that $X|_\mu \sim N(\mu, \sigma^2)$ and $\mu \sim N(\mu_\mu, \sigma_\mu^2)$, then we have

$$X \sim N(\mu_\mu, \sigma^2 + \sigma_\mu^2). \tag{2.11}$$

Proof. Consider the following characteristic function of a normal distribution $N(t; \mu, \sigma^2)$

$$\phi_0(w) = \frac{1}{\sqrt{2\pi\sigma^2}} \int_{-\infty}^{\infty} e^{iwt - \frac{1}{2\sigma^2}(t-\mu)^2} \, dt = e^{iw\mu - \frac{1}{2}\sigma^2 w^2}.$$

For distribution $X|_\mu \sim N(\mu, \sigma^2)$ and $\mu \sim N(\mu_\mu, \sigma_\mu^2)$, the characteristic function after exchanging the order of the two integrations is given by

$$\phi(w) = \int_{-\infty}^{\infty} e^{iw\mu - \frac{1}{2}\sigma^2 w^2} N(\mu; \mu_\mu, \sigma_\mu^2) d\mu$$

$$= \int_{-\infty}^{\infty} e^{iw\mu - \frac{\mu - \mu_\mu}{2\sigma_\mu^2} - \frac{1}{2}\sigma^2 w^2} \, d\mu.$$

Note that

$$\int_{-\infty}^{\infty} e^{iw\mu - \frac{\mu - \mu_\mu}{2\sigma_\mu^2}} \, d\mu = e^{iw\mu - \frac{1}{2}\sigma^2 w^2}$$

is the characteristic function of the normal distribution. It follows that

$$\phi(w) = e^{iw\mu - \frac{1}{2}\sigma^2 w^2},$$

which is the characteristic function of $N(\mu_\mu, \sigma^2 + \sigma_\mu^2)$. This completes the proof.

Based on the above theorem, the maximum likelihood estimates of σ^2, μ_μ, and σ_μ^2 can be obtained as follows:

$$\tilde{\mu}_\mu = \frac{1}{m+1} \sum_{j=0}^{m} \tilde{\mu}_j, \quad \tilde{\sigma}_\mu^2 = \frac{1}{m+1} \sum_{j=0}^{m} (\tilde{\mu}_j - \tilde{\mu}_\mu)^2, \tag{2.12}$$

and

$$\tilde{\sigma}^2 = \frac{1}{n} \sum_{j=0}^{m} \sum_{i=1}^{n_j} (x_{ji} - \tilde{\mu}_j)^2,$$

where

$$\tilde{\mu}_j = \frac{1}{n_j} \sum_{i=1}^{n_j} x_{ji}.$$

Based on these MLE's, estimates of the shift parameter (i.e., ε) and the scale parameter (i.e., C) can be obtained as follows: $\tilde{\varepsilon} = \tilde{\mu} - \hat{\mu}$ and $\tilde{C} = \tilde{\sigma}/\hat{\sigma}$, respectively. Consequently, the sensitivity index can be estimated by simply replacing ε, μ, and C with their corresponding estimates $\tilde{\varepsilon}$, $\tilde{\mu}$, and $\tilde{C}$.

2.4.2   The case where ε is fixed and C is random

Similarly, set $\mu_{actual} = \mu$ and $\sigma_{actual} = \sigma$ and assume that $x|_{\sigma=\sigma_{actual}}$ follows a normal distribution $N(\mu, \sigma^2)$, that is

$$x|_{\sigma=\sigma_{actual}} \sim N(\mu, \sigma^2),$$

where σ^2 is distributed as $IG(\alpha, \lambda)$, so μ, α and λ are unknown parameters we are interested in.

Theorem 2.2 Suppose that $x|_{\sigma=\sigma_{actual}} \sim N(\mu, \sigma^2)$ and $\sigma^2 \sim IG(\alpha, \lambda)$, then

$$x \sim f(x) = \frac{\Gamma(\alpha+1/2)}{\Gamma(\alpha)} \frac{1}{\sqrt{2\pi\lambda}} [1 + \frac{(x-\mu)^2}{2\lambda}]^{-(\alpha+\frac{1}{2})}. \tag{2.13}$$

That is, x is a non-central $t-distribution$, where $\mu \in R$ is location parameter, λ/α is scale parameter and 2α is freedom degree.

Proof: $f(x, \sigma^2) = f(x|\sigma^2)f(\sigma^2)$

$$= \frac{1}{\sqrt{2\pi}\sigma} \frac{\lambda^\alpha}{\Gamma(a)} (\frac{1}{\sigma^2})^{\alpha+1} \exp\{-\frac{(x-\mu)^2 + 2\lambda}{2\sigma^2}\}$$

$$f(x) = \int_0^{+\infty} f(x, \sigma^2)d\sigma^2$$

$$= \frac{1}{\sqrt{2\pi}} \frac{\lambda^\alpha}{\Gamma(a)} \int_0^{+\infty} (\frac{1}{\sigma^2})^{\alpha+\frac{3}{2}} \exp\{-\frac{(x-\mu)^2 + 2\lambda}{2\sigma^2}\}d\sigma^2$$

$$= \frac{1}{\sqrt{2\pi}} \frac{\lambda^\alpha}{\Gamma(a)} \int_0^{+\infty} t^{\alpha-\frac{1}{2}} \exp\{-\frac{(x-\mu)^2 + 2\lambda}{2}t\}dt$$

$$= \frac{\Gamma(\alpha+1/2)}{\Gamma(\alpha)} \frac{1}{\sqrt{2\pi\lambda}} [1 + \frac{(x-\mu)^2}{2\lambda}]^{-(\alpha+\frac{1}{2})}.$$

Thus, X follows a non-central t-distribution. Hence, we have $E(x) = \mu$ and $var(x) = \lambda/(\alpha - 1)$. This completes the proof.

Based the above theorem, the maximum likelihood estimation of the parameters μ, α and λ can be obtained as follows. Suppose that the observations satisfy the following conditions.

(1) $(x_{ji}|\mu, \sigma_i^2) \sim N(\mu, \sigma_i^2), i = 0, \cdots, m, j = 1, \cdots n_i$, and given σ_i^2, $x_{1i}, \cdots, x_{n_i i}$ are i.i.d.

(2) $\{x_{ji}, j = 1, \cdots, n_i\}, i = 0, \cdots, m$ are independent.

(3) $\sigma_i^2 \sim IG(\alpha, \lambda),$.

the likelihood function is given by

$$f(x_{01}, \cdots, x_{mn_m}) = \prod_{i=0}^{m} \int_0^{\infty} \prod_{j=1}^{n_i} f(x_{ij}|\sigma_i^2) f(\sigma_i^2) d\sigma_i^2$$

$$= \prod_{i=0}^{m} \prod_{j=1}^{n_i} \frac{\Gamma(\alpha + \frac{1}{2})}{\Gamma(\alpha)} \frac{1}{\sqrt{2\pi\lambda}} [1 + \frac{(x_{ij} - \mu)^2}{2\lambda}]^{-(\alpha + \frac{1}{2})}$$

$$= \prod_{i=0}^{m} \int_0^{\infty} \prod_{j=1}^{n_i} \frac{1}{\sqrt{2\pi}\sigma_i} \exp\{-\frac{(x_{ij} - \mu)^2}{2\sigma_i^2}\} \frac{\lambda^{\alpha}}{\Gamma(\alpha)} \exp\{-\frac{\lambda}{\sigma_i^2}\} d\sigma_i^2.$$

(2.14)

Thus, the log-likelihood function is:

$$L = \ln f(x_{01}, \cdots, x_{mn_m})$$
$$= n \ln \Gamma(\alpha + \frac{1}{2}) - n \ln \Gamma(\alpha) - \frac{n}{2} \ln 2\pi\lambda - (\alpha + \frac{1}{2}) \sum_{i=0}^{m} \sum_{j=1}^{n_i} \ln[1 + \frac{(x_{ij} - \mu)^2}{2\lambda}].$$

(2.15)

Based on (2.15), we can obtain the derivatives of the unknown parameters μ, α and λ, as follow:

$$\frac{\partial L}{\partial \mu} = \sum_{i=0}^{m} \sum_{j=1}^{n_i} \frac{(x_{ij} - \mu)}{1 + (x_{ij} - \mu)^2/2\lambda} = 0$$

$$\frac{\partial L}{\partial \alpha} = n\Psi(\alpha + \frac{1}{2}) - n\Psi(\alpha) - \sum_{i=0}^{m} \sum_{j=1}^{n_i} \ln[1 + \frac{(x_{ij} - \mu)^2}{2\lambda}] = 0$$

$$\frac{\partial L}{\partial \lambda} = -n + \frac{(\alpha + 1/2)}{\lambda} \sum_{i=0}^{m} \sum_{j=1}^{n_i} \frac{(x_{ij} - \mu)^2}{1 + (x_{ij} - \mu)^2/2\lambda}$$

where the $\Psi(\alpha) = \Gamma'(\alpha)/\Gamma(\alpha)$ is digamma function.

Define

$$w_{ij} = [1 + (x_{ij} - \mu)^2/2\lambda]^{-1}.$$ (2.16)

Then the maximum likelihood estimation of the parameters μ, α and λ be decided by

$$\overset{\wedge}{\mu} = \sum_{i=0}^{m} \sum_{j=1}^{n_i} w_{ij} x_{ij} \bigg/ \sum_{i=0}^{m} \sum_{j=1}^{n_i} w_{ij}.$$ (2.17)

$$\overset{\wedge}{\lambda} = (\overset{\wedge}{\alpha} + \frac{1}{2}) \frac{1}{n} \sum_{i=0}^{m} \sum_{j=1}^{n_i} w_{ij} (x_{ij} - \overset{\wedge}{\mu})^2.$$ (2.18)

Digamma function may be approximated as in Johnson and Kotz (1972) $\psi(\alpha) \doteq \ln(\alpha - 0.5)$, employing a Taylor expansion we find

$$\overset{\wedge}{\alpha} = 0.5 + n \bigg/ 2 \sum_{i=0}^{m} \sum_{j=1}^{n_i} \ln w_{ij}^{-1}$$ (2.19)

The maximum likelihood estimates of μ, α and λ can be obtained by (2.14)-(2.16). In fact it is difficult to solve the equation from (2.14)-(2.16) directly, but there are some published giving the maximum likelihood estimation of the location parameter and freedom degree in central t distribution, according to the (2.14)-(2.16), the estimation of the scale parameter in non-central t distribution could be obtained.

Lu, Chow, and Zhang (2010) used the moment estimation to obtain the estimation of the parameters μ, α and λ. The observations

$$(x_{ij}|\mu, \sigma_i^2) \sim N(\mu, \sigma_i^2), i = 0, \cdots, m, j = 1, \cdots n_i,$$

and x_{ij} independent, according to the Theorem 1, x is a non-central $t-$ $distribution$, mean $= E(x) = \mu$ and variance $= var(x) = \lambda/(\alpha - 1)$, if $\alpha > 1$; even central moment

$$\mu_k(x) = \mu_{k-2}(x) \cdot [2\lambda(k-1)/(2\alpha - k)] \text{ if } \alpha > k/2$$

since the fourth moment does not exist for $\alpha \leq 2$, moreover the variance of the estimator of α is infinite if $\alpha \leq 4$. Under the background of the medical research, we assume $\alpha > 4$ is held, the obvious choices are sample mean, variance and the fourth moment employed, the moment estimation of the parameters could be obtained

$$\hat{\mu} = \frac{1}{n} \sum_{i=1}^{n} x_i,$$

$$\hat{\alpha} = [3(S_n^2)^2 - 2S_n^4]/[3(S_n^2)^2 - S_n^4],$$

$$\hat{\lambda} = -S_n^2 S_n^4/[3(S_n^2)^2 - S_n^4].$$

We now examine the large-sample behavior of maximum likelihood estimates, further differentiability assumption is required, under the condition of Normal distribution and IG-distribution, requirement can be satisfied. Cox and Snell (1968) have derived a general formula for the second order bias of the maximum likelihood estimator of the vector:

$$b(\hat{\beta}_s) = \sum_{r,t,u} k^{s,r} k^{t,u} \{\frac{1}{2}k_{rtu} + k_{rt,u}) \tag{2.20}$$

where set parameter vector $\theta = (\beta_r, \beta_s, \beta_t) = (\mu, \alpha, \lambda)^T$ and r, s, t, u index the parameter space (μ, α, λ) and we use the standard notation for the moments of the derivatives of the log-likelihood function: $k_{rs} = E[U_{rs}]$, $k_{rst} = E[U_{rst}]$, $k_{rs,t} = E[U_{rs}U_t]$, where $U_r = \partial l/\partial \beta_r, U_{rs} = \partial^2 l/\partial \beta_r \partial \beta_s, U_{rst} = \partial^3 l/\partial \beta_r \beta_s \beta_t$. Also, $k^{r,s}$ denotes the general (r, s) element of the inverse of the information matrix, the information matrix itself having its general (r, s) element given by

$k_{rs} = -E[U^]_{rs}$. The fisher information matrix would be:

$$I(\theta) = n \begin{pmatrix} \dfrac{\alpha(2\alpha+1)}{\lambda(2\alpha+3)} & 0 & 0 \\[2ex] 0 & \Psi'(\alpha) - \Psi'(\alpha+\frac{1}{2}) & \dfrac{\alpha(\lambda-1)-1}{\lambda(\alpha+1)} \\[2ex] 0 & \dfrac{\alpha(\lambda-1)-1}{\lambda(\alpha+1)} & \dfrac{\alpha}{\lambda^2(2\alpha+3)} \end{pmatrix} \tag{2.21}$$

that $k_{\lambda\lambda\alpha} = k_{\lambda\alpha\lambda} = k_{\alpha\lambda\lambda} = -(4\alpha+3)/(2\alpha+1)(2\alpha+3)\lambda^2, k_{\alpha\alpha\alpha} = \Psi"(\alpha+\frac{1}{2}) - \Psi"(\alpha)$

$k_{\mu\mu\lambda} = k_{\mu\lambda\mu} = k_{\lambda\mu\mu} = 4\alpha(\alpha+1)^2/\lambda^2(2\alpha+3)(2\alpha+5)k_{\mu\mu\alpha} = k_{\mu\alpha\mu} = k_{\alpha\mu\mu} = -2\alpha/\lambda(2\alpha+3)$ when r, s, t take others value in parameter space except the enumerated above $k_{rst} = 0$ and $k_{rs,t} = 0$, where r, s, t index the parameter space. The bias of the maximum likelihood estimate of the parameter α is :

$$b(\hat{\alpha}) = A_1\{B_1 C_1 - D_1 + E_1 F_1\}/nM^2 \tag{2.22}$$

where $M = \{[\psi'(\alpha) - \psi'(\alpha+\frac{1}{2})][\frac{\alpha}{\lambda^2(2\alpha+3)} - \frac{1}{\lambda^2(2\alpha+1)^2}]\}\frac{\alpha}{\lambda}\frac{2\alpha+1}{2\alpha+3}$ is determinant of the inverse information matrix $I^{-1}(\theta)$, $A_1 = \frac{\alpha^2}{2\lambda^6(2\alpha+3)^3}$, $B_1 = \frac{\alpha(2\alpha+1)(12\alpha+21)}{2\alpha+5}$,

$$C_1 = (\psi'(\alpha) - \psi'(\alpha+\frac{1}{2})), \quad D_1 = \frac{2(4\alpha+3)}{2\alpha+1}, \quad E_1 = \frac{\alpha^2(2\alpha+1)^2}{(2\alpha+3)},$$

$$F_1 = \psi"(\alpha+\frac{1}{2}) - \psi"(\alpha)$$

at the same time we have:

$$b(\hat{\lambda}) = (A_2 C_1^2 + B_2 F_1 - E_2 C_1)/nM^2 \tag{2.23}$$

where $A_2 = \frac{2\alpha^3(2\alpha+1)^2(5\alpha+8)}{\lambda^5(2\alpha+3)^3(2\alpha+5)}$ $B_2 = \frac{\alpha^3(2\alpha+1)}{\lambda^5(2\alpha+3)^3}$, $C_2 = \frac{\alpha^2(14\alpha+9)}{\lambda^5(2\alpha+3)^3}$, the maximum likelihood estimator of α has n^{-1} order bias, it's same to the estimator of λ, and we also obtain the bias of parameter μ is $b(\hat{\mu}) = 0$, obviously it is the unbiased estimate of the parameter μ.

Under the case of μ_{actual} is fixed and σ_{actual} is random we'll focus on statistical inference on ε, C and Δ to illustrate the impact on statistical inference of the actual patient population after m protocol amendment.

2.5 Sample Size Adjustment

In clinical trials, for a given target patient population, sample size calculation is usually performed based on a test statistic (which is derived under the null hypothesis) evaluated under an alternative hypothesis. After protocol amendments, the target patient population may have been shifted to an *actual* patient population. In this case, the original sample size may have to be adjusted in

order to achieve the desired power for assessment of the treatment effect for the
original patient population. For clinical evaluation of efficacy and safety, statistical inference such as hypotheses testing is usually considered. In practice,
the commonly considered hypotheses testing includes (i) testing for equality,
(ii) testing for non-inferiority, (iii) testing for superiority, and (iv) testing for
equivalence. The hypotheses are summarized below

$$
\begin{aligned}
&\text{Equality: } H_0 : \mu_1 = \mu_2 \text{ vs. } H_a : \mu_1 - \mu_2 = \delta \neq 0, \\
&\text{Non - inferiority: } H_0 : \mu_1 - \mu_2 \leq \delta \text{ vs. } H_a : \mu_1 - \mu_2 > \delta, \\
&\text{Superiority: } H_0 : \mu_1 - \mu_2 \leq \delta \text{ vs. } H_a : \mu_1 - \mu_2 > \delta, \\
&\text{Equivalence: } H_0 : |\mu_1 - \mu_2| > \delta \text{ vs. } H_a : |\mu_1 - \mu_2| \leq \delta,
\end{aligned}
\tag{2.24}
$$

where δ is a clinically meaningful difference (for testing equality), a non-
inferiority margin (for testing non-inferiority), a superiority margin (for testing
superiority), and a equivalence limit (for testing equivalence), respectively.

Let $n_{Classic}$ and n_{Actual} be the sample size based on the original patient population and the actual patient population as the result of protocol amendments.
Also, let $n_{Actual} = Rn_{Classic}$, where R is the adjustment factor. Following the
procedures described in Chow, Shao, and Wang (2008), sample sizes for both
$n_{Classic}$ and n_{Actual} can be obtained. For example, Table 2.5.1 provides formulas for sample size adjustment based on covariate-adjusted model for binary
response endpoint, while Tables 2.5.2 and 2.5.3 give sample size adjustments
based on random location shift and random scale shift, respectively.

2.6   Concluding Remarks

As indicated, the investigator has the flexibility to modify or change the study
protocol during the conduct of the clinical trial by issuing protocol amendments. This flexibility gives the investigator (i) the opportunity to correct (mi-
nor changes) the assumptions early, and (ii) the chance to re-design (major
changes) the study. It is well recognized that the abuse of this flexibility may
result in a moving target patient population, which makes the intended trial
almost impossible to address the medical or scientific questions that the study
intends to answer. Thus far, regulatory agencies do not have regulations regarding the issue of protocol amendments after the initiation of a clinical trial. It
is suggested that regulatory guideline/guidance regarding (i) levels of changes,
and (ii) number of protocol amendments that are allowed be developed in order
to maintain the validity and integrity of the intended study. In addition, it is
also suggested that a sensitivity analysis should be conducted for evaluating
the possible impact due to protocol amendments.

As pointed out by Chow and Chang (2008), the impact on statistical inference due to protocol amendments could be substantial especially when there
are major modifications, which have resulted in a significant shift in mean response and/or inflation of the variability of response of the study parameters.

Table 2.5.1: Sample Size Adjustment Based on Covariate-adjusted Model

Test	Hypothesis	Non-adjustment	Adjustment
Superiority	$H_0: p_{10} - p_{20} \leq \delta$ $H_a: p_{10} - p_{20} > \delta$	$N_{Classic} = \frac{(z_\alpha + z_\gamma)^2}{(p_{10} - p_{20} - \delta)^2} \cdot \left[\frac{p_{10}(1 - p_{10})}{w} + \frac{p_{20}(1 - p_{20})}{1 - w}\right]$	$N_{Actual} = \frac{(z_\alpha + z_\gamma)^2 \tilde{V}_d}{(p_{10} - p_{20} - \delta)^2}$
Non-inferiority	$H_0: p_{10} - p_{20} \leq -\delta$ $H_a: p_{10} - p_{20} > -\delta$	$N_{Classic} = \frac{(z_\alpha + z_\gamma)^2}{(p_{10} - p_{20} + \delta)^2} \cdot \left[\frac{p_{10}(1 - p_{10})}{w} + \frac{p_{20}(1 - p_{20})}{1 - w}\right]$	$N_{Actual} = \frac{(z_\alpha + z_\gamma)^2 \tilde{V}_d}{(p_{10} - p_{20} + \delta)^2}$
Equivalence	$H_0: |p_{10} - p_{20}| \geq \delta$ $H_a: |p_{10} - p_{20}| < \delta$	$N_{Classic} = \frac{(z_\alpha + z_\gamma)^2}{(\delta - |p_{10} - p_{20}|)^2} \cdot \left[\frac{p_{10}(1 - p_{10})}{w} + \frac{p_{20}(1 - p_{20})}{1 - w}\right]$	$N_{Actual} = \frac{(z_\alpha + z_{\gamma/2})^2 \tilde{V}_d}{(\delta - |p_{10} - p_{20}|)^2}$

w is the proportion of patients for the first treatment.

$\tilde{V}_d = [g'(\beta)]^T \left(w \sum_{i=0}^{k} \rho_{1i} I^{(1i)} + (1 - w) \sum_{i=0}^{k} \rho_{2i} I^{(2i)}\right)^{-1} g'(\beta)$ where $w = n_{1.}/N$, $\rho_{ti} = n_{ti}/n_{t.}$ and

$$g'(\beta) = \begin{pmatrix} p_{10}(1 - p_{10}) - p_{20}(1 - p_{20}) \\ p_{10}(1 - p_{10}) \\ \nu_0(p_{10}(1 - p_{10}) - p_{20}(1 - p_{20})) \\ \nu_0(p_{10}(1 - p_{10})) \end{pmatrix}.$$

Table 2.5.2: Sample Size Adjustment Based on Random Location Shift

Test	Hypothesis	Non-adjustment	Adjustment
Equality	$H_0: \mu_1 - \mu_2 = 0$ $H_a: \mu_1 - \mu_2 \neq 0$	$N_{Classic} = \dfrac{2(z_{\alpha/2}+z_\beta)^2 \tilde\sigma^2}{(\mu_1-\mu_2)^2}$	$N_{Actual} = \dfrac{2(m+1)(z_{\alpha/2}+z_\beta)^2 \tilde\sigma^2}{(m+1)(\mu_1-\mu_2)^2 - 2(z_{\alpha/2}+z_\beta)^2 \tilde\sigma_\mu^2}$
Non-inferiority /Superiority	$H_0: \mu_1 - \mu_2 \leq \delta$ $H_a: \mu_1 - \mu_2 > \delta$	$N_{Classic} = \dfrac{2(z_\alpha+z_\beta)^2 \tilde\sigma^2}{(\mu_1-\mu_2-\delta)^2}$	$N_{Actual} = \dfrac{2(m+1)(z_\alpha+z_\beta)^2 \tilde\sigma^2}{(m+1)(\mu_1-\mu_2-\delta)^2 - (z_\alpha+z_\beta)^2 \tilde\sigma_\mu^2}$
Equivalence	$H_0: |\mu_1 - \mu_2| \geq \delta$ $H_a: |\mu_1 - \mu_2| < \delta$	$N_{Classic} = \dfrac{2(z_\alpha+z_{\beta/2})^2 \tilde\sigma^2}{(|\mu_1-\mu_2|-\delta)^2}$	$N_{Actual} = \dfrac{2(m+1)(z_{\alpha/2}+z_\beta)^2 \tilde\sigma^2}{(m+1)(|\mu_1-\mu_2|-\delta)^2 - (z_{\alpha/2}+z_\beta)^2 \tilde\sigma_\mu^2}$

Table 2.5.3: Sample Size Adjustment Based on Random Scale Shift

Test	Hypothesis	Non-adjustment	Adjustment
Equality	$H_0: \mu_1 - \mu_2 = 0$ $H_a: \mu_1 - \mu_2 \neq 0$	$N_{Classic} = \dfrac{2(z_{\alpha/2}+z_\beta)^2 \bar{\bar\sigma}^2}{(\mu_1-\mu_2)^2}$	$N_{Actual} = \dfrac{2(z_{1-\alpha/2}+z_{1-\beta})^2(m+1)\bar{\bar v}\bar{\bar\sigma}^2 \sum_{j=0}^m (V_{1j}^{(t)})^2}{(\mu_1-\mu_2)^2(\bar v-2)\left(\sum_{j=0}^m V_{1j}^{(t)}\right)^2}$
Non-inferiority /Superiority	$H_0: \mu_1 - \mu_2 \leq \delta$ $H_a: \mu_1 - \mu_2 > \delta$	$N_{Classic} = \dfrac{2(z_\alpha+z_\beta)^2 \bar{\bar\sigma}^2}{(\mu_1-\mu_2-\delta)^2}$	$N_{Actual} = \dfrac{2(z_\alpha+z_\beta)^2(m+1)\bar{\bar v}\bar{\bar\sigma}^2 \sum_{j=0}^m (V_{1j}^{(t)})^2}{(\mu_1-\mu_2-\delta)^2(\bar v-2)\left(\sum_{j=0}^m V_{1j}^{(t)}\right)^2}$
Equivalence	$H_0: |\mu_1 - \mu_2| \geq \delta$ $H_a: |\mu_1 - \mu_2| < \delta$	$N_{Classic} = \dfrac{2(z_\alpha+z_{\beta/2})^2 \bar{\bar\sigma}^2}{(|\mu_1-\mu_2|-\delta)^2}$	$N_{Actual} = \dfrac{2(z_\alpha+z_{\beta/2})^2(m+1)\bar{\bar v}\bar{\bar\sigma}^2 \sum_{j=0}^m (V_{1j}^{(t)})^2}{(|\mu_1-\mu_2|-\delta)^2(\bar v-2)\left(\sum_{j=0}^m V_{1j}^{(t)}\right)^2}$

$V_{1j}^{(t)} = \dfrac{\nu^{(t)}(\sigma^{(t)})^2 + n_j(\sigma^{(t)})^2}{\nu^{(t)}(\sigma^{(t)})^2 + \sum_{i=1}^{n_j}(x_{ji}-\mu^{(t)})^2}$ where $\{\mu^{(t)}, \sigma^{(t)}, \nu^{(t)}\}$ is the tth step estimate in the EM algorithm.

It is suggested that a sensitivity analysis with respect to changes in study parameters be performed to provide a better understanding on the impact of changes (protocol amendments) in study parameters on statistical inference. Thus, regulatory's guidance on what range of changes in study parameters are considered acceptable is necessarily developed. As indicated earlier, adaptive design methods are very attractive to the clinical researchers and/or sponsors due to their flexibility especially in clinical trials of early clinical development. It, however, should be noted that there is a high risk that a clinical trial using adaptive design methods may fail in terms of its scientific validity and/or its limitation of providing useful information with a desired power especially when the sizes of the trials are relatively small and there are a number of protocol amendments.

As indicated in the previous sections, analysis with covariate adjustment and the assessment of sensitivity index are the two commonly considered approaches when there is population shift due to protocol amendment. For the method of analysis with covariate adjustment, an alternative approach by considering random coefficients in model (2.1) and/or Bayesian approach may be useful for obtaining accurate and reliable estimates of the treatment effect of the compound under study. For the assessment of sensitivity index, in addition to the cases where (i) ε is random and C is fixed, and (ii) ε is fixed and C is random, there are other cases such as (iii) both ε and C are random, (ii) sample sizes before and after protocol amendments are random variables, and (iii) the number of protocol amendments is also a random variable that remain unchanged.

In addition, statistically it is a challenge to clinical researchers when there are missing values. The causes of missing values could be due to the causes that are related to or unrelated to the changes or modifications made in the protocol amendments. In this case, missing values must be handled carefully to provide an unbiased assessment and interpretation of the treatment effect. When there is a population shift either in location parameter or scale parameter, the standard methods for assessment of treatment effect are necessarily modified. For example, the standard methods such as the O'Brien-Fleming method in typical group sequential design for controlling the overall type I error rate are not appropriate when there is a population shift due to protocol amendments.

Chapter 3

Adaptive Randomization

Randomization plays an important role in clinical research. For a given clinical trial, appropriate use of randomization procedure not only ensures that the subjects selected for the clinical trial are a truly representative sample of the target patient population under study, but also provides an unbiased and fair assessment regarding the efficacy and safety of the test treatment under investigation. As pointed out in Chow and Liu (2003), statistical inference of the efficacy and safety of a test treatment under study relies on the probability distribution of the primary study endpoints of the trial, which in turn depends on the randomization model/method employed for the trial. Inadequate randomization model/method may violate the primary distribution assumption and consequently distort statistical inference. As a result, the conclusion drawn based on the clinical data collected from the trial may be biased and/or misleading.

Based on the allocation probability (i.e., the probability of assigning a patient to a treatment), the randomization procedures that are commonly employed in clinical trials can be classified into four categories: conventional randomization, treatment-adaptive randomization, covariate-adaptive randomization, and response-adaptive randomization. The conventional randomization refers to any randomization procedures with a constant treatment allocation probability. Commonly used conventional randomization procedures include simple (or complete) randomization, stratified randomization, and cluster randomization. Unlike the conventional randomization procedures, treatment allocation probabilities for adaptive randomization procedures usually vary over time depending upon the cumulative information on the previously assigned patients. Similar to the conventional randomization procedures, treatment-adaptive randomization procedures can also be prepared in advance. For covariate-adaptive randomization and response-adaptive randomization procedures, the randomization codes are usually generated in a dynamically real time fashion. This is because the randomization procedure is based on the patient information on covariates or response observed up to the time when the randomization is performed. Treatment-adaptive randomization and covariate-adaptive randomization are usually considered to reduce treatment imbalance or deviation from the target sample size ratio between treatment groups. On the other hand, a response-adaptive randomization procedure emphasizes ethical consideration, i.e., it is desirable to provide patients with better/best treatment based on the knowledge about the treatment effect at that moment.

In practice, conventional randomization procedures could result in severe treatment imbalance at some time point during the trial or at the end of the trial, especially when there is a time-dependent heterogeneous covariance that related to treatment responses. Treatment imbalance could decrease statistical power for demonstration of treatment effect of the intended trial and consequently the validity of the trial. In this chapter, we attempt to provide a comprehensive review of various randomization procedures from each category.

In the next section, the conventional randomization procedures are briefly reviewed. In Section 3.2 we introduce some commonly used treatment-adaptive randomization procedures in clinical trials. Several covariate-adaptive randomization procedures and response-adaptive randomization methods are discussed in Section 3.3 and Section 3.4, respectively. In Section 3.5, some practical issues in adaptive randomization are examined. A brief summary is given in the last section of this chapter.

3.1   Conventional Randomization

As mentioned earlier, the treatment allocation probability of conventional randomization procedures is a fixed constant. As a result, it allows the experimenters to prepare the randomization codes in advance. The conventional randomization procedures are commonly employed in clinical trials, particularly in double-blind randomized clinical trials. In what follows, we introduce some commonly employed conventional randomization procedures, namely, simple randomization, stratified randomization and cluster randomization.

Simple Randomization

Simple (or complete) randomization is probably one of the most commonly employed conventional randomization procedures in clinical trials. Consider a clinical trial for comparing the efficacy and safety of k treatments in treating patients with certain diseases. For a simple randomization, each patient is randomly assigned to each of the k treatment groups with a fixed allocation probability p_i $(i = 1, ..., k)$, where $\sum_{i=1}^{k} p_i = 1$. The allocation probabilities are often expressed as the ratio between the sample size (n_i) of the ith treatment group and the overall sample size ($n = \sum_{i=1}^{k} n_i$), i.e., $p_i = \frac{n_i}{n}$, which is usually referred to as the *sample size ratio* of the ith treatment group. In the interest of treatment balance, an equal allocation probability for each treatment group (i.e., $p_i = p$ for all i) is usually considered which has the following advantages. First, it has the most (optimal) statistical power for correct detection of a clinically meaningful difference under the condition of equal variances. Second, it is ethical in the sense of equal toxic (Lachin, 1988). In practice, however, it is may be of interest to have an unequal allocation between treatment groups. For example, it may be desirable to assign more patients to the treatment group than a placebo group. It, however, should be noted that a balanced design may not achieve the optimal power when there is heterogeneity in variance between treatment groups. The optimal power can only be achieved when the sample size ratio is proportional to the standard deviation of the group.

The simple (complete) randomization for a two-arm parallel group clinical trial can be easily performed assuming that the treatment assignments are independent Bernoulli random variables with a success probability of 0.5. In practice, treatment imbalance inevitably occurs even by chance alone. Since this treatment imbalance could result in a decrease in power for detecting a clinically meaningful difference, it is of interest to examine the probability of imbalance. Denote the two treatments under study by treatment A and treatment B, respectively. Let $D_n = N_A(n) - N_B(n)$ be the measure of the imbalance in treatment assignment at stage n, where $N_A(n)$ and $N_B(n)$ are the sample size of treatment A and treatment B at stage n, respectively. Then, the *imbalance* D_n is asymptotically normally distributed with mean 0 and variance n. Therefore, the probability of imbalance, for a real value $r > 0$, is given by (see, e.g., Rosenberger et al., 2001; Rosenberger and Lachin, 2002)

$$P(|D_n| > r) = 2 \left[1 - \Phi \left(\frac{r}{\sqrt{n}} \right) \right]. \qquad (3.1)$$

The sample size for a unbalanced design with homogeneous variance is given by

$$n = \frac{1}{R} \frac{2(z_{1-\alpha/2} + z_{1-\beta})^2 \sigma^2}{\delta^2},$$

where the relative efficiency R is a function of sample size ratio $k = \frac{n_2}{n_1}$ between the two groups, i.e.,

$$R = \frac{4}{2 + k + 1/k}.$$

Let

$$r = n_2 - n_1 = \frac{k-1}{1+k} n.$$

Then

$$P(|D_n| > r) = 2 \left[1 - \Phi \left(\frac{k-1}{1+k} \sqrt{n} \right) \right].$$

Table 3.1.1: Relative Efficiencies

Sample size ratio, k	Relative efficiency, R	Pr(efficiency< R)
1	1	1
1.5	0.96	0.11
2	0.89	0.01
2.5	0.82	0.001

Note: n=64.

As it can be seen from Table 3.1.1 that $\Pr(R < 0.96)=11\%$ and $\Pr(R < 0.89) = 1\%$. Thus, $\Pr(0.89 < R < 0.96) = 10\%$.

Stratified Randomization

As discussed above, simple (complete) randomization does not assure the balance between treatment groups. The impact of treatment imbalance could be substantial. In practice, treatment imbalance could become very critical especially when there are important covariates. In this case, stratified randomization is usually recommended to reduce treatment imbalance. For a stratified randomization, the target patient population is divided into several homogenous strata, which are usually determined by some combinations of covariates (e.g., patient demographics or patient characteristics). In each stratum, a simple (complete) randomization is then employed. Similarly, treatment imbalance of stratified randomization for a clinical trail comparing two treatment groups can be characterized by the following probability of imbalance asymptotically (see, e.g., Hallstron and Davis, 1988)

$$P(|D| > r) = 2 \left[1 - \Phi \left(\frac{r}{\sqrt{Var(D)}} \right) \right], \tag{3.2}$$

where

$$Var(D) = \frac{\sum_{i=1}^{s} b_i + s}{6},$$

s is the number of strata, b_i is the size of the ith block, and

$$D = \sum_{i=1}^{s} |N_i - 2A_i|,$$

in which N_i and A_i are the number of patients and the number of patients in treatment A within the ith stratum, respectively.

When the number of strata is large, it is difficult to achieve treatment balance across all stages. This imbalance will decrease the power of statistical analysis such as the analysis of covariance (ANCOVA).

Cluster Randomization

In certain trials, the appropriate unit of randomization may be some aggregate of individuals. This form of randomization is known as cluster randomization or group randomization. Cluster randomization is employed by necessity in trials in which the intervention is by nature designed to be applied at the cluster level such as community-based interventions. In the simple cluster randomization, the degree of imbalance can be derived based on simple randomization, i.e.,

$$P(|D_{n_{cluster}}| > r) = 2\left[1 - \Phi\left(\frac{r}{\sqrt{n_{cluster}}}\right)\right],$$

where

$$D_{n_{cluster}} = N_{cluster\ A}(n_{cluster}) - N_{cluster\ B}(n_{cluster}).$$

The number of clusters $N_{cluster} = N/k$ where k is the number of subjects within each cluster. Then

$$D_{n_{cluster}} = D_{n/k} = \frac{N_A(n/k)}{k} - \frac{N_B(n/k)}{k}.$$

Thus we have

$$P(|D_n|/k > r) = 2\left[1 - \Phi\left(\frac{r}{\sqrt{n}}\right)\right].$$

It can be written as

$$P(|D_n| > r) = 2\left[1 - \Phi\left(\frac{r}{k\sqrt{n}}\right)\right].$$

It should be noted that the analysis for a cluster randomized trial is very different from that of individual subject based randomization trial. A cluster-randomization trial requires both adequate number of individual subjects and clusters.

Remarks For a given sample size, the statistically most powerful design is defined as a design with allocation probabilities proportional to the standard deviation of the group. For binary responses, Neyman's treatment allocation with the following allocation ratio leads to a most powerful design

$$r = n_a/n_b = \left(\frac{p_a}{p_b}\frac{1-p_a}{1-p_b}\right)^{\frac{1}{2}}, \tag{3.3}$$

where p_a and p_b are the proportions for treatment A and treatment B, respectively. Note that for the most powerful design, the target imbalance is $r_0 \neq 0$ and the power of a design can be measured by the quantity

$$P(|D| > r - r_0).$$

3.2   Treatment-Adaptive Randomization

Treatment-adaptive randomization is also known as variance-adaptive randomization. The purpose of a treatment-adaptive randomization is to achieve a
more balanced design or to reduce the deviation from the target treatment
allocation ratio by utilizing a varied allocation probability. Commonly used
treatment-adaptive randomization models in clinical research and development
include *block randomization, a biased-coin model*, and various *urn models*. To
introduce these randomization procedures, consider a two-arm parallel group
randomized clinical trial comparing a test treatment (A) with a control (B).

Block Randomization

In block-randomization the allocation probability is a fixed constant before any
of the two treatment groups reach its target number. However, after the target
number is reached in one of the two treatment groups, all the future patients
in the trial will be assigned to the other treatment group. As a result, block
randomization is a deterministic randomization procedure. It should be noted
that although the block size of the block randomization can vary, a small block
size will reduce the randomness. The minimum block size commonly chosen in
clinical trials is two, which leads to an alternative assignment of the two treatments. In variance-adaptive randomization, the imbalance can be reduced or
eliminated when the target number of patients is exactly randomized. Note that
when there are two treatment groups, the block-randomization is sometimes referred to as a *truncated binomial randomization*. The allocation probability is
defined as

$$P = \begin{cases} 0 & \text{if } N_A(j-1) = n/2, \\ 1 & \text{if } N_B(j-1) = n/2, \\ 0.5 & \text{otherwise}, \end{cases} \quad .$$

where $N_A(j-1)$ and $N_B(j-2)$ are the sample size of treatment A and treatment
B at stage $j-1$, respectively and $n/2$ is the target number for each group.

Efron's Biased-Coin Model

Efron (1971) proposed a biased-coin design to balance treatment assignment.
The allocation rule to treatment A is defined as follows:

$$P(\delta_j | \Delta_{j-1}) = \begin{cases} 0.5 & \text{if } N_A(j) = N_B(j), \\ p & \text{if } N_A(j) < N_B(j), \\ 1-p & \text{if } N_A(j) > N_B(j), \end{cases}$$

where δ_j is a binary indicator for treatment assignment of the jth subject, i.e.,
$\delta_j = 1$ if treatment A is assigned and $\delta_j = 0$ if treatment B is assigned and

$\Delta_{j-1} = \{\delta_1, ..., \delta_{j-1}\}$ is the set of treatment assignment up to subject $j - 1$. The imbalance is measured by

$$|D_n| = |N_A(n) - n|.$$

The limiting balance property can be obtained by random walk method as follows

$$\lim_{m \to \infty} \Pr(|D_{2m}| = 0) = 1 - \frac{1-p}{p},$$

$$\lim_{m \to \infty} \Pr(|D_{2m}| = 1) = 1 - \frac{(1-p)^2}{p^2}.$$

Note that for odd number of patients, the minimum imbalance is 1. It can be seen that as $p \to 1$, we achieve perfect balance. But such a procedure is deterministic.

Lachin Urn Model

Lachin's urn model is another typical example of variance-adaptive randomization. The model is described as follows. Suppose that there are N_A white balls and N_B red balls in an urn initially. A ball is randomly drawn from the urn *without* replacement. If it is a white ball, the patient is assigned to receive treatment A; otherwise, the patient is assigned to receive treatment B. Therefore, if N_A and N_B are the target sample sizes for treatment groups A and B, respectively, the target sample size ratio (or balance) is always reached if the total planned number of patients is reached. The treatment allocation probability for treatment group A in a trial comparing two treatment groups is

$$P(A) = \frac{\frac{n}{2} - N_A(j-1)}{N_A + N_B - (j-1)}.$$

Although Lachin's urn model can result in a *perfect* balance design after all patients are randomized, the maximum imbalance occurs when the half of the treatment allocations are completed, which is given by

$$P_{\max}(|D_n| > r) = 2 \left[1 - \Phi \left(\frac{2r}{n} \sqrt{(n-1)} \right) \right].$$

Friedman-Wei's Urn Model

The Friedman-Wei's urn model is a popular model that can reduce possible treatment imbalance (see, e.g., Friedman, 1949; Wei, 1977; Rosenberger and Lachin, 2002). Friedman-Wei's urn model is described below. Suppose that there is an urn containing a white balls and a red balls. For treatment assignment, a ball is drawn at random and then replaced. If the ball is white, then treatment A is assigned. On the other hand, if a red ball is drawn, then treatment B is assigned. Furthermore, b additional balls of the opposite color of the ball chosen are added to the urn. Note that a and b could be any reasonable nonnegative numbers. This drawing procedure is replaced for each treatment assignment.

Denote a urn design by $UD(a, b)$. The allocation rule for $UD(a, b)$ can then be defined mathematically as follows:

$$P(\delta_j = 1 | \Delta_{j-1}) = \frac{a + bN_B(j-1)}{2a + b(j-1)}. \tag{3.4}$$

Note that $UD(a, 0)$ is nothing but a simple or complete randomization.

Let D_n be the absolute difference in number of subjects between the two treatment groups after the nth treatment assignment. Then D_n forms a stochastic process with possible values $d \in \{0, 1, 2, ..., n\}$. At initial, $D_0 = 0$. The $(n+1)th$ stage transition probabilities are then given by (see also Wei, 1977)

$$Pr(D_{n+1} = d - 1 | D_n = d) = 1/2 + bd[2(2a + bn)], \tag{3.5}$$
$$Pr(D_{n+1} = d + 1 | D_n = d) = 1/2 - bd[2(2a + bn)],$$
$$Pr(D_{n+1} = 1 | D_n = 0) = 1,$$

where $n \geq d \geq 1$. Note that $P(d, n)$ is a monotonically increasing function with respect to d and a monotonically decreasing function with respect to n. $P(d, n)$ tends to $1/2$ as n increases for a fixed $d > 0$. Therefore, the (a, b) forces the trial to be more balanced when severe imbalance occurs. In addition, $UD(a, b)$ can also ensure the balance of a relatively small size trial. It should be noted that $UD(a, b)$ behaves like the complete randomization design as n increases.

The transition probabilities in (3.1) can be used recursively to calculate the probability of an imbalance of degree d at any stage of the trial as

$$Pr(D_{n+1} = d) = Pr(D_{n+1} = d | D_n = d - 1) Pr(D_{n+1} = d - 1) + Pr(D_{n+1} = d | D_n = d + 1) Pr(D_{n+1} = d + 1). \tag{3.7}$$

For a moderate or large n, the probability of imbalance is approximatly Normal distribution, $D_n \sim N\left(0, \frac{n(a+b)}{3b-a}\right)$. As a result, the probability of imbalance for large sample size n can be expressed as

$$P(|D_n| > r) = 2\left\{1 - \Phi\left(r\sqrt{\frac{3b-a}{n(a+b)}}\right)\right\}, \tag{3.8}$$

Remarks

The urn procedure is relative easy to implement. It forces a small scale trial to be balanced but approaches complete randomization as the sample size increases. It has less vulnerability to selection bias than does the permuted-block design, biased-coin design, or random allocation rule. As n increases, the potential selection bias approaches to the complete randomization for which the expected selection bias is zero. The urn design can also be extended to the prospective stratification trial when the number of strata is either small or large.

The urn design can easily be generalized to the case of multiple-group comparisons (Wei, 1978; Wei, Smythe, and Smith 1986). We can even further generalize it using different a and b for difference groups in the urn model.

3.3   Covariate-Adaptive Randomization

The *covariate-adaptive randomization* is usually considered to reduce the covariate imbalance between treatment groups. Thus, the covariate-adaptive randomization is also known as *adaptive stratification*. Allocation probability for the covariate-adaptive randomization is modified over time during the trial based on the cumulative information about baseline covariates and treatment assignments. Covariate-adaptive randomization includes Zelen's model, Pocock-Simon's model, Wei's marginal urn design, minimization, and the Atkinson optimal model, which will be briefly described below.

Zelen's Model

Zelen's model (Zelen, 1974) requires a simple randomization sequence. When the imbalance reaches a certain threshold, the next subject will be forced to be assigned to the group with fewer subjects. Let $N_{ik}(n)$ be the number of patients in stratum $i = 1, 2, ..., s$ of the kth treatment $k = 1, 2$. When patient $n + 1$ in stratum i is ready to be randomized, one computes $D_i(n) = N_{i1}(n) - N_{i2}(n)$. For an integer c, if $|D_i(n)| < c$, then the patient is randomized according to schedule, otherwise, the patient will be assigned to the group with fewer subjects, where the constant can be $c = 2, 3$, or 4 as Zelen suggested.

Pocock-Simon's Model

Similar to the Zelen's model, Pocock and Simon (1975) proposed an alternative covariate-adaptive randomization procedure. We follow Rosenberger and Lachin's descriptions of the method (Rosenberger and Lachin, 2002). Let $N_{ijk}(n)$, $i = 1, ..., I$, $j = 0, 2, ..., n_i$, and $k = 1, 2$ (1 = treatment A, 2= treatment B) be the number of patients in stratum j of covariate i on treatment

k after n patients have been randomized. Note that $\prod_{i=1}^{I} n_i = s$ is the total number of strata in the trial. Suppose the $(n+1)$th patient to be randomized is a member of strata $r_1, ..., r_I$ of covariates $1, ..., I$. Let $D_i(n) = N_{ir_i1} - N_{ir_i2}$. Define the following weighted difference measure $D(n) = \sum_{i=1}^{I} w_i D_i(n)$, where w_i are weights chosen depending on which covariates are deemed of greater importance. If $D(n)$ is less than $1/2$, then the weighted difference measure indicates that B has been favored thus far for that set, $r_1, ..., r_I$, of strata and the patient $n+1$ should be assigned with higher probability to treatment A, and vice versa. If $D(n)$ is greater than $1/2$, Pocock and Simon (1975) suggested biasing a coin with

$$p = \frac{c^* + 1}{3}$$

and implementing the following rule: if $D(n) < 1/2$, then assign the next patient to treatment A with probability p; if $D(n) > 1/2$, then assign the next patient to treatment B with probability p; and if $D(n) = 1/2$, then assign the next patient to treatment A with probability $1/2$. where $c^* \in [1/2,\ 1]$.

Note that if $c^* = 1$, we have a rule very similar to Efron's biased-coin design as described in the previous section. If $c^* = 2$, we have the deterministic minimization method proposed by Taves (1974) (see also Simon, 1979). Note that many other rules could also be derived following the Zelen's rule and Taves's minimization method with a biased-coin twist to give added randomization. Efron (1980) described one of such rules and applied it to a clinical trial in ovarian cancer research.

Pocock and Simon (1975) also generalized their covariate-adaptive randomization procedure to more than two treatments. They suggested the following allocation rule be applied:

$$p_k = c^* - \frac{2(K c^* - 1)k}{K(K+1)}, \quad k = 1, .., K,$$

where K is the number of treatments.

Wei's Marginal Urn Design

In practice, when the number of covariates results in a large number of strata with small stratum sizes, the use of a separate urn in each stratum could result in treatment imbalance within strata. Wei (1978) proposed *marginal urn design* for solving the problem. The idea is that instead of using N urns, one for each unique stratum, he suggested to use the urn with maximum imbalance to do the randomization each time. For a given new subject with covariate values $r(1), ..., r(I)$, treatment imbalance within each of the corresponding urn is calculated. The one with the greatest imbalance is used to generate the treatment assignment for the next subject. A ball from that urn is chosen with replacement. Meanwhile, b balls representing the opposite treatment are added to the urns corresponding to that patient's covariate values. Wei (1978) called this approach a *marginal urn design* because it tends to balance treatment assignments within each category of each covariate marginally, and thus also jointly (Rosenberger and Lachin, 2002).

Imbalance Minimization Model

Imbalance minimization allocation has been advocated as an alternative to the stratified randomization when there are large numbers of prognostic variables under the imbalance minimization model (Birkett, 1985). The allocation of a patient is determined as follows. A new patient is first classified according to the prognostic variables of interest. He/she is then tentatively assigned to each treatment group in turn and a summary measure of the resulting treatment imbalance is calculated. The measure of imbalance is obtained by summing the absolute value of excess number of patients receiving one treatment rather than other treatment within every level of each prognostic variable. The two measures are compared and final allocation is made to that group that minimizes that imbalance measurement. As indicated by Birkett (1985), the imbalance minimization would help gain the power.

Although minimization has been widely used in clinical trials, it is a concern that the potential risk of enabling the investigator to break the code due to the deterministic nature of the allocation which may bias the enrollment of patients (Ravaris et al., 1976; Gillis and Ratkowsky, 1978; Weinthrau et al., 1977).

Atkinson Optimal Model

Atkinson (1982) considered a linear regression model to minimize the variance of treatment contrast in the presence of important covariates. The allocation rule is given by

$$p_k = \frac{d_A(k, \xi_n)}{\sum_{k=1}^{K} d_A(k, \xi_n)}, \tag{3.9}$$

where

$$\xi_n = \arg\max_{\xi} \left\{ |A' M^{-1}(\xi) A|^{-1} \right\}, \tag{3.10}$$

in which $M = X'X$ is the $p \times p$ dispersion matrix from n observations, and A is an $s \times p$ matrix of contrasts, $s < p$. More details regarding Atkinson's optimal model can be found in Atkinson and Donev (1992).

3.4   Response-Adaptive Randomization

Response-adaptive randomization is a randomization technique in which the allocation of patients to treatment groups is based on the response (outcome) of the previous patients. The purpose is to provide the patients better/best treatment based on the knowledge about the treatment effect at that moment. As a result, response-adaptive randomization takes the ethical concern into consideration. The well-known response-adaptive models include play-the-winner (PW) model, randomized play-the-winner (RPW) model, Rosenberger's optimization model, Bandit model, and optimal model with finite population. In what follows, these response-adaptive randomization models will be briefly described.

Play-the-Winner Model

Play-the-winner (PW) model can be easily applied to clinical trials comparing two treatments (e.g., treatment A and treatment B) with binary outcomes (i.e., *success* or *failure*). For PW model, it is assumed that the previous subject's outcome will be available before the next patient is randomized. The treatment assignment is based on treatment response of the previous patient. If a patient responds to treatment A, then the next patient will be assigned to treatment A. Similarly, if a patient responds to treatment B, then the next patient will be assigned treatment B. If the assessment of previous patient is not available, the treatment assignment can be based on the last available patient with response assessment or randomly assigned to treatment A or B. It is obvious that this model lacks randomness.

Randomized Play-the-Winner Model

The randomized play-the-winner (RPW) model is a simple probabilistic model to sequentially randomize subjects in a clinical trial (see, e.g., Rosenberger, 1999; Coad and Rosenberger, 1999). RPW model is useful especially for clinical trials comparing two treatments with binary outcomes. For RPW, it is assumed that the previous subject's outcome will be available before the next patient is randomized. At the start of the clinical trial, an urn contains α_A balls for treatment A and α_B balls for treatment B, where α_A and α_B are positive integers. For convenience's sake, we will denote these balls by either type A or type B balls. When a subject is recruited, a ball is drawn and replaced. If it is a type A ball, the subject receives treatment A; if it is type B, the subject receives treatment B. When a subject's outcome is available, the urn is updated. A success on treatment A or a failure on treatment B will generate an additional b type-B balls in the urn, where b is a positive integer. In this way, the urn builds up more balls representing the more successful (or less successful) treatment.

There are some interesting asymptotic properties with RPW. Let N_a/N be the proportion of subjects assigned to treatment A out of N subjects. Also, let $q_a = 1 - p_a$ and $q_b = 1 - p_b$ be the failure probabilities. Further, let F be the total number of failures. Then, we have (Wei and Durham, 1978)

$$\lim_{N \to \infty} \frac{N_a}{N_b} = \frac{q_b}{q_a}, \tag{3.11}$$

$$\lim_{N \to \infty} \frac{N_a}{N} = \frac{q_b}{q_a + q_b},$$

$$\lim_{N \to \infty} \frac{F}{N} = \frac{2 q_a q_b}{q_a + q_b}.$$

Note that for balanced randomization, $E(F/N) = (q_a + q_b)/2$.

Since treatment assignment is based on response of previous patients in RPW model, it is not optimized with respect to any clinical endpoint. It is reasonable to randomize treatment assignment based on some optimal criteria such as minimizing the expected numbers treatment failures. This leads to the so-called optimal designs.

Optimal RPW Model

Adaptive designs have long been proposed for ethical reasons. The basic idea is to skew allocation probabilities to reflect the response history of patients, hopefully giving a greater than 50% chance of a patient's receiving the treatment performing better thus far in the trial. The optimal randomized play-winner-model (ORPW) is to minimize the number of failures in the trial.

There are three commonly used efficacy endpoints in clinic trials, namely, simple proportion difference $(p_a - p_b)$, the relative risk (p_a/p_b), and the odds ratio $(p_a q_b/p_b q_a)$, where $q_a = 1 - p_a$ and $q_b = 1 - p_b$ are failure rates. These can be estimated consistently by replacing p_a by $\hat{p}_a$ and p_b by $\hat{p}_b$, where $\hat{p}_a$ and $\hat{p}_b$ are the proportions of observed successes in treatment groups A and B, respectively. Suppose that we wish to find the optimal allocation $r = n_a/n_b$ such that it minimizes the expected number of treatment failures $n_a q_a + n_b q_b$ which is mathematically given by

$$r^* = \arg \min_r \{n_a q_a + n_b q_b\} \tag{3.12}$$

$$= \arg \min_r \{\frac{r}{1+r} n \, q_a + \frac{1}{1+r} n \, q_b\}.$$

For simple proportion difference, the asymptotic variance is given by

$$\frac{p_a q_a}{n_a} + \frac{p_b q_b}{n_b} = \frac{(1+r)(p_a \, q_a + r \, p_b \, q_b)}{n \, r} = K, \tag{3.13}$$

where K is some constant. Solving (3.13) for n yields

$$n = \frac{(1+r)(p_a\,q_a + r\,p_b\,q_b)}{rK}.$$ (3.14)

Substituting (3.14) into (3.13), we obtain

$$r^* = \arg\min_r \left\{ \frac{(r\,p_a + q_b)(p_a q_a + r\,p_b q_b)}{r\,K} \right\}.$$ (3.15)

Taking the derivative of (3.14) with respect to r and equating to zero, we have

$$r^* = \left(\frac{p_a}{p_b}\right)^{\frac{1}{2}}.$$

Note that r^* does not depend on K.

Table 3.4.1: Asymptotic Variance with RPW

Measure	r^*	Asymptotic variance
Proportion difference	$\left(\frac{p_a}{p_b}\right)^{\frac{1}{2}}$	$\frac{p_a\,q_a}{n_a} + \frac{p_b\,q_b}{n_b}$
Relative risk	$\left(\frac{p_a}{p_b}\right)^{\frac{1}{2}}\left(\frac{q_b}{q_a}\right)$	$\frac{p_a\,q_b^2}{n_a q_a^3} + \frac{p_b\,q_b}{n_b q_a^2}$
Odds ratio	$\left(\frac{p_b}{p_a}\right)^{\frac{1}{2}}\left(\frac{q_b}{q_a}\right)$	$\frac{p_a\,q_b^2}{n_a q_a^3 p_b^2} + \frac{p_b q_b}{n_b q_a^2 p_b^2}$

Source: Rosenberger and Lachin (2002), p.176.

Note that the limiting allocation for the RPW rule $\left(\frac{q_b}{q_a}\right)$ is not optimal for any of the three measures. It is also interesting to note that none of the optimal allocation rule yields Neyman allocation given by (Melfi and Page, 1998)

$$r^* = \left(\frac{p_a\,q_a}{p_b\,q_b}\right)^{\frac{1}{2}},$$

which minimizes the variance of the difference in sample proportions. Note that Neyman allocation would be unethical when $p_a > p_b$ (i.e., more patients receive the inferior treatment).

Because the optimal allocation depends on the unknown binomial parameters, we must develop a sequential design that can approximate the optimal design. The rule for the proportion difference is to simply replace the unknown success probabilities in the optimal allocation rule by the current estimate of the proportion of successes (i.e., $\hat{p}_{a,n}$ and $\hat{p}_{b,n}$) observed in each treatment group thus far. This leads to the so-called sequential maximum likelihood procedure. Alternatively, we can use Bayesian approach such as Bandit allocation rule, where different optimal criteria can be optionally utilized.

Bandit Model

A bandit allocation rule is a Bayesian's approach that utilizes prior information on unknown parameters in conjunction with incoming data to determine optimal treatment assignment at each stage of the trial (Hardwick and Stout, 1991, 1993, 2002). The weighting of returns is known as discounting, which consists of multiplying the payoff of each outcome by the corresponding element of a discount sequence. The properties of any given bandit allocation rule depends upon the associated discount sequence and prior distribution.

Consider a two-arm bandit (TAB) design for the two proportion difference. The procedure can be described as follows.

(i) Binary outcomes X_{ia} and X_{ib} for the two treatment groups are Bernoulli random variables:

$$X_{ia} \sim B(1, p_a), \tag{3.16}$$

and

$$X_{ib} \sim B(1, p_b), \; i = 1, 2, ..., n.$$

(ii) Prior distribution is assumed to be a beta distribution:

$$p_a \sim Beta(a_0, b_0), \tag{3.17}$$

and

$$p_b \sim Beta(c_0, d_0).$$

(iii) At stage $m \leq n$, the posteriors of p_a and p_b are given by:

$$(p_a | k, i, j) \sim Beta(a, b), \tag{3.18}$$

and

$$(p_b | k, i, j) \sim Beta(c, d),$$

where

$$k = \sum_{i=1}^{m} \delta_{ia}, \; i = \sum_{i=1}^{k} X_{ia}, \text{ and } \; j = \sum_{i=1}^{m-k} X_{ia},$$

and

$$\begin{cases} a = i + a_0, \\ b = k - i - b, \\ c = j + c_0, \\ d = m - k - j + d_0. \end{cases} \tag{3.19}$$

Thus, the posterior means of p_a and p_b at m stage are given by

$$E_m[p_a] = a/(a + b),$$

and

$$E_m[p_b] = c/(c + d),$$

where $E_m[.]$ denotes expectation under the model.

(iv) Two commonly used discount sequences $\{1, \beta_1, \beta_2, ..., \beta_n\}$ are the n-horizon uniform sequence with all $\beta_i = 1$, and the geometric sequence with all $\beta_i = \beta$ $(0 < \beta < 1)$.

(v) Allocation rule, δ, is defined to be a sequence $(\delta_1, \delta_2, ..., \delta_n)$ where $\delta_i = 1$ if the ith subject receives treatment A and $\delta_i = 0$ if the ith subject receives treatment B. It is required that the decision, δ_i at stage i dependent only upon the information available at that time (not the future). The two commonly used allocation rules are: Uniform Bandit and Truncated Gittins Lower Bound.

The *truncation* here refers to a rule that if a state is reached such that the final decision can not be influenced by any further outcomes, then the treatment with the best success rate will be used for all further subjects.

Uniform Bandit   The n-horizon uniform TAB uses prior and accumulated information to minimize the number of failures *during* the trial. Let $F_m(i, j, k, l)$ denote the minimal possible expected number of failures remaining in the trial, if m patients have already been treated and there were i successes and j failures on treatment A, and k successes and l failures on treatment B. (Note that one parameter can be eliminated since $m = i + j + k + l$.) The algorithmic approach is based on the observation that if A were used on next patient, then the expected number of failures for patient $m + 1$ and through n would be

$$F_m^A(i, j, k, l) = E_m[p_a]F_{m+1}(i, j, k, l) + E_m[1 - p_a](1 + F_{m+1}(i, j, k, l)), \quad (3.20)$$

If B were used, we would have

$$F_m^B(i, j, k, l) = E_m[p_b]F_{m+1}(i, j, k, l) + E_m[1 - p_b](1 + F_{m+1}(i, j, k, l)). \quad (3.21)$$

Therefore, F satisfies the recurrence

$$F_m(i, j, k, l) = \min\left\{F_m^A(i, j, k, l), F_m^B(i, j, k, l)\right\}, \quad (3.22)$$

which can be solved by dynamic programming, starting with patient n and proceeding toward the first patient. The computation is at order of $O(n^4)$.

Gittins Lower Bound   According to a theorem of Gittins and John (Berry and Fristedt, 1985), for bandit problems with geometric discount and independent arms, for each arm there exists an index with the property that, at given stage, it is optimal to select, at the next stage, the arm with the higher index. The index for an arm, the Gittins Index, is a function only of the posterior distribution and discount factor β. The existence of Gittins index removes many computation difficulties associated with other Bandit problems.

Remarks For a small sample, the allocation rule can be implemented by means of dynamic programming (Hardwick and Stout, 1991). Sequential treatment allocation can also be done based on other optimal criteria. For example, Hardwick and Stout (2002) developed allocation rule based on maximizing the likelihood of making the correct decision by utilizing a curtailed equal allocation rule with a minimal expected sample size. The optimization is given for any fixed $|p_a - p_b| = \Delta$ among the curtailed (pruned) equal allocation rule. The pruning refers to a rule whereby, if a state is reached such that the sign of the final observed difference in success rate for the two groups will not be influenced by any further outcomes, then the trial will be stopped. The pruning could result in an insufficient sample size or power for clinical trials.

Rosenberger et al.(2001) using computer simulations compared the ORPW, Neyman allocation, the RPW rule, and equal allocation. They found out that RPW rule tends to highly variable for larger value p_a and p_b. The adaptive structure of sequential designs includes dependencies that could result in extra-binomial variability. This increased variability will decrease power to some extent. ORPW reduces the expected number of failures from equal allocation and reduces the expected failures by around 3 or 4 when p_a and p_b are small to moderate. When p_a and p_b are large, there are more moderate reductions and it is questionable whether adaptive designs would improve much over equal allocation when a test is based on proportion difference. For the RPW design, for example, if $p_a = 0.7$ and $p_b = 0.9$ with a sample size of 192, the RPW design has power 0.88 for z_1 with t expected 31.5 failures, while equal allocation design for 162 patients has power 0.90 with 32.4 failures.

The RPW rule does not require instantaneous outcomes, or even that they are available before randomization of the next subject. Investigators can update the urn when a subject's outcome is ascertained. The effect of this will "slow" the adaptation, and hence there will be less benefit to subjects, particularly those recruited early. If delay of the response is so significant, it could be practically impossible to implement RPW rule.

Bandit Model for Finite Population

Bandit allocation rule discussed in the previous section is optimal in the sense that it minimizes the number of failures in the trial. In what follows, we will discuss an optimal criterion in the scope of the entire patient population with the disease and compare five different randomization procedures (Berry and Eick, 1995) with this criterion.

Suppose that the 'patient horizon' is N. Each of N patients is to be treated with one of two treatments, A or B. Treatment allocation is sequential for the first n patients, and the responses are dichotomous and immediate. Let Z_j, $j = 1, ..., N$, denote the response of patient j; $Z_j = 1$ if success and $Z_j = 0$ if failure. The probability of a success with treatment A is p_a and with B is p_b. We have that

$$E[Z_j | p_a, p_b] = \begin{cases} P[Z_j = 1 | p_a, p_b] = p_a, & \text{If patient } j \text{ receives treatment A} \\ P[Z_j = 1 | p_a, p_b] = p_b, & \text{If patient } j \text{ receives treatment B.} \end{cases}$$

Since treatment allocation for patients 1 to n is sequential, treatment assignment can depend upon the responses of all previously treated patients. However, treatment assignment for patients $n + 1$ to N can depend only on the responses of patients 1 to n. In all the procedures we consider, these latter patients receive the treatment with the larger fraction of successes among the first n. (If the two observed success proportions are equal then the treatment with the greater number of observations is given to patients $n + 1$ to N.) Let D be the class of all treatment allocation procedures satisfying these restrictions.

The conditional worth (W) of procedure $\tau \in D$ (given p_a and p_b) is

$$W_\delta(p_a, p_b) = E_\delta \left[\sum_{j=1}^{N} Z_j | p_a, p_b \right], \tag{3.23}$$

where the distribution of the $Z_j s$ is determined by τ. This can be no greater than $N \max\{p_a, p_b\}$. The conditional expected successes lost (ESL) using τ is:

$$L_\tau(p_a, p_b) = N \max\{p_a, p_b\} - W_\tau(p_a, p_b). \tag{3.24}$$

This function is obviously non-negative for all τ.

Allocation Procedures Berry and Eick (1995) considered four adaptive procedures and compare them with a balanced randomized design or equal randomization (ER). All of these procedures are members of D. We describe the procedures on the basis of the way they allocate treatments to the first n patients. We assume for convenience that n is an even integer.

Procedure ER: Half of the first n patients are randomly assigned to treatment A and the other half to B. For comparison purposes, it does not matter whether patients are randomized in pairs, or in blocks of larger size.

Procedure JB (J. Bather): Treatments A and B are randomly assigned to patients 1 and 2 so that one patient receives each. Suppose that during the trial m patients have been treated, $2 \leq m < n$, and assume that s_a, f_a, s_b, f_b successes and failures have been observed on A and B, respectively ($s_a + f_a + s_b + f_b = m$). Define

$$\lambda(k) = (4 + \sqrt{k})/(15k). \tag{3.25}$$

Let $\lambda_a = \lambda(s_a + f_a)$ and $\lambda_b = \lambda(s_b + f_b)$. Procedure JB randomizes between the respective treatments except that the randomization probabilities depend upon the previously observed response. Let

$$q = \frac{s_a}{s_a + f_a} - \frac{s_b}{s_b + f_b} + 2(\lambda_a - \lambda_b),$$ (3.26)

then under procedure JB, the next patient (patient $m + 1$) receives treatment A with probability

$$\frac{\lambda_a}{\lambda_a + \lambda_b} \exp(q/\lambda_a) \text{ for } q \leq 0$$

and

$$1 - \frac{\lambda_b}{\lambda_a + \lambda_b} \exp(q/\lambda_b) \text{ when } q > 0.$$

Procedure TAB is the two-armed bandit procedure where randomization of the first n patients are randomized based on the current probability distribution of (p_a, p_b) assuming a uniform prior density on (p_a, p_b):

$$\pi(p_a, p_b) = 1 \text{ on } (0,1) \text{x}(0,1)$$ (3.27)

The next patient receives treatment A with probability equal to the current probability that $p_a > p_b$. This probability is

$$\int_0^1 \int_0^1 u^{s_a}(1-u)^{f_a} v^{s_b}(1-v)^{f_b} \, du dv \, \{B(s_a + 1, \ f_a + 1)B(s_b + 1, \ f_b + 1)\}^{-1}$$

(3.28)

where $B(.,.)$ is the complete beta function:

$$B(a,b) = \int_0^1 u^{a-1}(1-u)^{b-1} du.$$ (3.29)

Procedure PW (Play-the-winner/Switch-from-loser): The first patient receives treatment A and B with a equal probability 0.5. For patients 2 to n, the treatment given to the previous patient is used again if it was successful; otherwise the other treatment is used.

Procedure RB (Robust Bayes): This strategy is optimal in the following two-arm bandit problem. Suppose that the uniform prior density of (p_a, p_b) is given, the discount sequence of $\beta = \{1, \beta_1, \beta_2, ..., \beta_n\}$ is defined by

$$\beta_i = \begin{cases} 1 & \text{for } 1 \leq i \leq n, \\ N - n & \text{for } i = n + 1, \\ 0 & \text{for } i > n + 1. \end{cases}$$ (3.30)

That means that all N patients have equal weights. The first n patients each have a weight of $N - n$. Procedure RB maximizes

$$\int_0^1 \int_0^1 W_\tau(p_a, p_b; \boldsymbol{\beta}) \, dp_a dp_b \tag{3.31}$$

over all $\delta \in D$, where

$$W_\delta(p_a, p_b; \boldsymbol{\beta}) = E_\delta[\sum_{j=1}^N \beta_j Z_j | p_a, p_b].$$

This maximum can be found using dynamic programming. The starting point is after the n patients in the trial have responded. The subsequent expected number of the successes is $N - n$ times the maximum of the current expected values of p_a and p_b. If both treatments are judged equally effective at any stage, then procedure RB randomizes the next treatment assignment.

Procedure RB comprises a dynamic programming process. The symmetry of the uniform prior distribution implies that the treatments are initially equivalent. For the first patient, one is chosen at random. If the first patient has a success, then the second patient receives the same treatment. If the first patient has a failure, then the second patient receives the other treatment. Thus, procedure RB imitates procedure PW for the first two treatment assignments. The same treatment is used as long as it is successful, again imitating PW. However, after a failure, switching to the other treatment may or may not be optimal. If the data sufficiently strongly favor the treatment that has just failed, then that treatment will be used again.

When following procedure RB, if the current probability of success for treatment A (which is the current expected value of p_a), is greater than that for treatment B, then treatment A may or may not be optimal for the next patient. If the current number of patients on treatment A, $s_a + f_a$ is smaller than the number of patients on B, $s_b + f_b$, then A is indeed optimal. However, if $s_a + f_a$ is greater than $s_b + f_b$, then, for sufficiently large N, treatment B is optimal irrespective of the current expected values of p_a and p_b. Procedure RB tends to assign the currently superior treatment, but less so for large N than for small N. As N increases, gathering information early on by balancing the treatment assignment is important. Thus, assignment to the two treatments tends to be more balanced when N is large than when it is small.

Some comparisons between these procedures are possible without detailed calculations. Procedure ER is designed to obtain information from the first n patients that will help patients outside the trial. Because it gives maximal information about $p_a - p_b$, its performance relative to the other procedures will improve as N increases.

Procedure RB is designed to perform well on the *average* for any n, N, p_a, and p_b. Of the five procedures described, it alone specifically uses the value of N, giving it an advantage over the other procedures.

Procedure PW ignores most of the accumulating data; its treatment assignments are based not on sufficient statistics but only on the result for the previous patient. On the other hand, since PW tends to allocate patients to both of the treatments except when one or both p's are close to 1 – it should perform well when N is large.

Procedures JB and TAB are quite similar. Both randomize allocations so that the currently superior treatment is more likely to be assigned.

As indicated above, RB minimizes (4) over all procedures in D. Thus, procedures PW, JB, and TAB will not perform better than RB when averaged over p_a and p_b. However, they might outperform RB for some N and some moderately large set of (p_a, p_b). The computer simulations showed that they do not.

Remarks Berry and Eick (1995) conducted computer simulations compared the five methods mentioned above with N =100, 1000, 10,000 and 100,000. Their main conclusion is that a balanced randomized design is nearly optimal when the disease is relatively common, e.g., when N is moderately large (such as N $\geq$ 10,000). However, when a substantial portion of patients is involved in the trial (as with a rare form of cancer), then adaptive procedures can perform substantially better than a balanced randomization. There are many relevant questions that need to be answered before these adaptive allocations can take advantage practically. These questions include (i) How relevant is the condition? (ii) How effective are the treatments A and B? (iii) Are other effective treatments available? (iv) How long will it take to discover a new treatment that is clearly superior to both A and B? (v) What effect will the results of the current trial have on practitioners? (There is a sociological aspect of this last question that might favor a randomized procedure when the decision is a close one; namely, it is so widely accepted.) In addition, if Bayesian's approach is used, should p_a and p_b have different priorities because the control is using an approved drug?

Adaptive Models for Ordinal and Continuous Outcomes

Ordinal Outcome Ivanova and Flournoy (2001) developed an urn model, called Ternary urn model, for categorical outcome. In this section, we will introduce an urn model for ordinal outcome. This model can fall into Rosenberger's treatment effect mapping model, whose allocation rule is given by

$$P(\delta_j | \Delta_{j-1}) = g(E_j)$$

where g is a function of treatment effect E_{j-1} at stage j.

We propose here a response-adaptive model with ordinal outcomes for multiple treatments. Suppose there are K treatment groups in the trial and the primary response is ordinal with M categories. Without loss of generality, let $C_j (j = 1, .., M)$ be the integer scales for the ordinal response with a higher score indicating a desired outcome). Our response adaptive urn model is defined as follows. There are K types of balls in a urn, initially a_i balls of type i. The treatment assignment for a patient is determined by the ball type randomly drawn from the urn with replacement. If a ball of type k is drawn from the urn, the patient will be assigned treatment k. Then observe the response for all the patients treated. If a patient with treatment i had response C_j at stage n (n patients have been treated), then $n\, C_j$ balls of type i will be added to the urn. Repeat this procedure for treatment assignment to all patients in the trial.

Normal Outcome   Let Y_i be a continuous variable representing the response of the ith patient, treated with either A or B following the adaptive design. Assume responses to be instantaneous and normally distributed. Suppose μ_a and μ_b are population characteristics representing the treatment effects A and B respectively (Assume a larger value μ indicates a better result). For the ith patient, we define an indicator variable δ_i which takes the value 1 or 0 according as the patient is treated by A or B. Then, the adaptive allocation rule is described as follows:

For the initial two patients, we randomly assign one to each treatment A or B. For patient i +1 ($2 < i \leq n$), we assign him/her to treatment A with a probability of

$$P_a(\delta_{i+1}|\delta_1, .., \delta_i, Y_1, ..., Y_i) = \left[\Phi(\frac{\hat{\mu}_a - \hat{\mu}_b}{\hat{\sigma}_p\sqrt{\frac{1}{i_a} + \frac{1}{i_b}}}) \right]^\alpha , \qquad (3.32)$$

where α is constant that can be determined by optimal criteria later, $\Phi(\bullet)$ is the standard normal cumulative distribution function, i_a and i_b are number of patients in treatment A and B at state i, the pooled variance

$$\hat{\sigma}_p^2 = \frac{(i_a - 1)\hat{\sigma}_a^2 - (i_b - 1)\hat{\sigma}_b^2}{i_a - i_b - 2},$$

and $\hat{\mu}_a = \bar{Y}_a$ and $\hat{\mu}_b = \bar{Y}_b$. Note that Bandyopadhyay and Biswas (1997) suggested using the allocation probability $\Phi(\frac{\hat{\mu}_a - \hat{\mu}_b}{T})$, where T is a constant.

Survival Outcome   Rosenberger and Seshaiyer (1997) proposed a treatment effect mapping g(S)=0.5(1+S), where S is the centered and scaled logrank test. We suggest using the optimal model proposed in the previous section since logrank test statistic is normally distributed.

3.5 Issues with Adaptive Randomization

Rosenberger and Lachin (2002) discussed the issues with adaptive design. They classified the bias into accrual bias and selection bias as summarized below.

Accrual Bias

RPW or other adaptive designs may lead to a unique type of bias, i.e., accrual bias, by which volunteers may wish to be recruited later in the study to take the advantage of benefit from previous outcomes. Earlier subjects mostly have higher probabilities of receiving the inferior treatment.

Accidental Bias

Efron (1971) introduced the term accidental bias to describe the bias in estimation of treatment effect induced by an unobserved covariate. The bias in estimation of treatment, $(E(\hat{\alpha}) - \alpha)^2$, is minimized when treatment assignment is balanced, where α and $\hat{\alpha}$ are the true treatment effect and estimated treatment effect through linear regression, respectively. The bound of the bias due to unbalance treatment assignments is controlled by the eigenvalue of covariance matrix of treatment assignment sequence. The eigenvalues for different randomization models are presented in Table 3.5.1.

Table 3.5.1: Accidental Bias for Various Randomization Models

Model name	Maximum Eigenvalue, λ_{max}
Complete random	1
Lachin's allocation rule	$1+\frac{1}{n-1}$
Stratified Lachin' allocation rule	$1+\frac{1}{m-1}$
Truncated binomial model	$\sqrt{\pi n/3} \leq \lambda_{max} \leq \sqrt{n/2}$
Friedman-Wei's urn model	$1+\frac{2}{3}\frac{\ln n}{n}+O(n^{-1})$

Note: n= sample size, and m = sample size with each stratum.

Accidental bias does not appear to be a serious problem for any of the randomization models discussed so far except for the truncated binomial design. More details regarding the accidental bias can be found in Rosenberger and Lachin (2002).

Selection Bias

Selection bias refers to biases that are introduced into an unmasked study because an investigator may be able to guess the treatment assignment of future patients based on knowing the treatments assigned to the past patients. Patients usually enter a trial sequentially over time. Staggered entry allows the possibility for a study investigator to alter the composition of the groups attempting to guess which treatment will be assigned next. Based on whichev treatment is guessed to be assigned next, the investigator can then choose t next patient scheduled for randomization to be one whom the investigator co siders to be better suited for that treatment. One of the principal concerns an unmasked study is that a study investigator might attempt to "beat t randomization" and recruit patients in a manner such that each patient is a signed to whichever treatment group the investigator feels is best suited to th individual patient.

Blackwell and Hodges (1957) developed a model for selection bias. Usi this model the selection bias can be measured by the so-called *expected b factor*.

$$E(F) = E(G - n/2), \tag{3.}$$

where G is total number of correct guesses (A better to B better), n/2 is t number of patients in each of the two groups.

Blackwell and Hodges (1957) showed that the optimal strategy for the perimeter upon randomizing the jth patient is to guess treatment A wh $N_A(j-1) < N_B(j-1)$ and B when $N_A(j-1) > N_B(j-1)$. When there tie, the experimenter guesses with equal probability. This is called *converge strategy*.   The expected bias factor under convergence strategy for vari randomization models are presented in Table 3.5.2.

Table 3.5.2: Expected Selection Bias Factor Under Convergence Strategy

Model	Maximum Eigenvalue, $\lambda_{\max}$
Complete random	0
Lachin's allocation rule	$\dfrac{2^{n-1}}{\binom{n}{n/2}} - \dfrac{1}{2}$
Stratified Lachin's allocation rule	$M\left(\dfrac{2^{m-1}}{\binom{m}{m/2}} - \dfrac{1}{2}\right)$
Truncated binomial model	$\dfrac{n}{2^{n+1}}\binom{n}{n/2}$
Friedman-Wei's urn model	$\sum_{i=1}^{n}\left[\dfrac{1}{2} + \dfrac{\beta E(|D_{i-1}|)}{2(2\alpha+\beta(i-1))}\right] - \dfrac{n}{2}$

Note: n = sample size, m = # of patients/block, and M = number of block

Inferential Analysis

Analyses based on a randomization model are completely different from t ditional analyses using hypotheses tests of population parameters under

Neyman-Pearson paradigm. The most commonly used basis for the development of a statistical test is the concept of a population model, where it assumed that the sample of patients is representative of a reference population and that the patient responses to treatment are independent and identically distributed from a distribution dependent on unknown population parameters. A null hypothesis under a population model is typically based on the equality of parameters from known distributions. Permutation tests or randomization tests are nonparametric tests. The null hypothesis of a permutation test is that the assignment of treatment A vs. B have no effect on the responses of the n patients randomized in the study. The essential feature of a permutation test is that randomization null hypothesis, the set of observed responses is assumed to be a set of deterministic values that are unaffected by treatment. The observed difference between the treatment groups depends only upon the way in which the n patients were randomized. Permutation tests are assumption-free, but depend explicitly upon the particular randomization procedure used.

A number of questions arise to the permutation test. (1) What measure of extremeness, or test statistic, should be used? The most general family of permutation tests is the family of linear rank tests. Linear rank tests are used often in clinical trials, and the family includes such tests as the traditional Wilcoxon rank-sum test and the logrank test. (2) Which set of permutations of the randomization sequence should be used for comparison? (3) If the analysis of a clinical trial is based on a randomization model that does not in any way involve the notion of a population, how can results of the trial be generalized to determine the best care for future patients? However, this weakness exists in the population model too.

Power and Sample Size

For the urn $UD(\alpha, \beta)$ design, if the total sample size n $=$ 2m is specified, a perfectly balanced design with $n_a = n_b = m$ will minimize the quantity

$$\eta = [1/n_a + 1/n_b]$$

which is $\eta = 2/m$. If n is not know beforehand, it is interesting to know how many extra observations are needed for $UD(0, \beta)$ to reduce η to be less than or equal to $2/m$. That is, we continue taking observations until n_a and n_b satisfy

$$\frac{1}{n_a} + \frac{1}{n_b} \leq \frac{2}{m} \tag{3.41}$$

If we write $n_a + n_b = 2m + \nu$, then ν is the number of additional observations required by the $UD(0, \beta)$ to satisfy this condition. It follows (Wei, 1978) that for any given ν and large m,

$$\Pr(\nu \leq z) \approx \Phi[(3z)^{1/2}] - \Phi[-(3z)^{1/2}] \tag{3.42}$$

For large m, $\Pr[\nu \leq 4]$ is approximately 0.9995, and thus the $UD(0, \beta)$ needs at most 4 extra observations to satisfy the above inequality, i.e., to yield the same efficiency as the perfectly balanced randomization allocation rule.

3.6 Summary

In this chapter, we have discussed several types of adaptive randomization. Theoretically, outcomes (efficacy or safety) with a response-dependent randomization are not independent. Therefore, the population-based inferential analysis method distinguishes the two types of adaptive designs. However, the randomization based analysis (permutation test) can be used under both adaptive randomizations. When a test statistic for the non-adaptive randomized trial is going to be used for an adaptive randomization trial, the corresponding power/sample size calculation for the non-adaptive randomization trial can also be used. For small sample size, permutation can be used for the inferential analysis, confidence interval estimation, and power/sample size estimation. An adaptive randomization can be either optimal or intuitive one. The outcome can be binary, ordinal, or continuous. The adaptive approach can be Bayesian's or non-Bayesian's. Our discussions have been focused on the cases with two treatment groups, but it can be easily expanded to multiple arms.

Chapter 4

Adaptive Hypotheses

Modifications of hypotheses of on-going clinical trials based on accrued data can certainly have an impact on statistical power for testing the treatment effect with the pre-selected sample size. Modifications of hypotheses of on-going trials commonly occur during the conduct of a clinical trial due to the following reasons that (i) an investigational method has not yet been validated at the planning stage of the study, (ii) information from other studies is necessary for planning the next stage of the study, (iii) there is a need to include new doses, and (iv) recommendations from a pre-established data monitoring committee (DMC). In addition, to increase the probability of success, the sponsors may switch a superiority hypothesis (originally planned) to a non-inferiority hypothesis. In this chapter, we will refer to adaptive hypotheses as modifications of hypotheses of on-going trials based on accrued data. Depending upon the clinically meaningful difference (e.g., effect size, non-inferiority margin or equivalence limit) to be detected, sample size is necessarily adjusted for achieving the desired power when adaptive hypotheses are applied during the conduct of a clinical trial.

In this chapter, we will examine the impact of a modification to hypotheses on the type I error rate, the statistical power of the test, and sample size for achieving the desired power. For a given clinical trial, the situations where hypotheses are modified as deemed appropriate by the investigator or as recommended by an independent DMC or data safety monitoring board (DSMB) after the review of interim data during the conduct of the clinical trial are described in the next section. In Section 4.2, the choice of non-inferiority margin, change in statistical inference, and impact on sample size calculation when switching from a superiority hypothesis to a non-inferiority hypothesis are discussed. Multiple hypotheses such as independent vs. dependent and/or primary vs. secondary hypotheses are discussed in Section 4.3. Also included in this section is a proposed decision theory approach for testing multiple hypotheses. A brief concluding remark is given in the last section.

4.1   Modifications of Hypotheses

In clinical trials with planned data monitoring for safety and interim analyses for efficacy, a recommendation for modifying or changing the hypotheses is commonly made after the review of interim data. The purpose for such a recommendation is to ensure the success of the clinical trials for identifying possible best clinical benefits to the patients who enter the clinical trials. In practice, the following situations are commonly encountered.

The first commonly seen situation for modifying hypotheses during the conduct of an active controlled clinical trial is switching a superiority hypothesis to a non-inferiority hypothesis. For a promising compound, the sponsor would prefer an aggressive approach for planning a superiority study. The study is usually powered to compare the promising compound with an active control agent. However, the interim analysis results may not support superiority at interim analysis. In this case, instead of declaring the failure of the superiority trial, the independent data monitoring committee may recommend to switch from testing the superiority hypothesis to testing a non-inferiority hypothesis. The switch from a superiority hypothesis to a non-inferiority hypothesis will certainly increase the probability of success of the trial because the study objective has been modified to establishing non-inferiority rather than showing superiority as compared to the active control. Note that the concept of switching a superiority hypothesis to a non-inferiority hypothesis is acceptable to the regulatory agency such as the U.S. FDA provided that the impact of the switch on statistical issues (e.g., the determination of non-inferiority margin) and inference (e.g., appropriate statistical methods) on the assessment of treatment effect is well justified. More details regarding the switch from a superiority hypothesis to a non-inferiority hypothesis are given in the next section.

Another commonly seen situation where the hypotheses are modified during the conduct of a clinical trial is the switch from a single hypothesis to a composite hypothesis or multiple hypotheses. A composite hypothesis is defined as a hypothesis that involves more than one study endpoint. These study endpoint may or may not be independent. In many clinical trials, in addition to the primary study endpoint, some clinical benefits may be observed based on the analysis/review of the interim data from secondary endpoints for efficacy and/or safety. It is then of particular interest to the sponsor to change testing a single hypothesis for the primary study endpoint to testing a composite hypothesis for the primary endpoint in conjunction with several secondary endpoints for clinical benefits or multiple hypotheses for the primary endpoint and the secondary endpoints. More details regarding testing multiple hypotheses are given in Section 4.3.

Other situations where the hypotheses are modified during the conduct of a clinical trial include (i) change in hypotheses due to the switch in study endpoints, (ii) dropping ineffective treatment arms, and (iii) interchange between the null hypothesis and the alternative hypothesis. These situations are briefly described below.

In cancer trials, there is no universal agreement regarding which study endpoint should be used as the primary study endpoint for evaluation of the test treatment under investigation. Study endpoints such as response rate, time to disease progression, and survival are commonly used study endpoints for cancer clinical trials (see Williams, Pazdur, and Temple, 2004). A typical approach is to choose one study endpoint as the primary endpoint for efficacy. Power analysis for sample size calculation is then performed based on the primary endpoint and other study endpoints are considered as secondary endpoints for clinical benefits. After the review of the interim data, the investigator may consider to switch the primary endpoint to a secondary endpoint if no evidence of substantial efficacy in terms of the originally selected primary endpoint (e.g., response rate) is observed but a significant improvement in efficacy is detected in one of the secondary endpoints (e.g., time to disease progression or median survival time).

For clinical trials comparing several treatments or several doses of the same treatment with a placebo or an active control agent, a parallel-group design is usually considered. After the review of the interim data, it is desirable to drop the treatment groups or the dose groups, which either show no efficacy or exhibit serious safety problems based on ethical consideration. It is also desirable to modify the dose and/or dose regimen for patients who are still on the study for best clinical results. As a result, hypotheses and the corresponding statistical methods for testing treatment effect are necessarily modified for a valid and fair assessment of the effect of the test treatment under investigation. More details regarding dropping the losers are discussed in Chapter 7.

In some cases, we may consider to switch the null hypothesis and the alternative hypothesis. For example, a pharmaceutical company may conduct a bioavailability study to study the relative bioavailability of a newly developed formulation as compared to the approved formulation by testing the null hypothesis of bioinequivalence against the alternative hypothesis of bioequivalence. The idea is to reject the null hypothesis and conclude the alternative hypothesis. After the review of the interim data, the sponsor realizes that the relative bioavailabilities between the two formulations are not similar. As a result, instead of establishing bioequivalence, the sponsor may wish to demonstrate superiority in bioavailability for the new formulation.

4.2   Switch from Superiority to Noninferiority

As indicated in the previous section, it is not uncommon to switch from a superiority hypothesis (the originally planned hypothesis) to a noninferiority hypothesis during the conduct of clinical trial in clinical trials. The purpose of this switching is to increase the probability of success. For testing superiority, if we fail to reject the null hypothesis of nonsuperiority, the trial is considered a failure. On the other hand, the rejection of the null hypothesis of inferiority provides the opportunity for testing superiority without paying any statistical penalty due to closed testing procedure.

When comparing a test treatment with a standard therapy or an active control agent, as indicated by Chow, Shao and Wang (2003), the problem of testing non-inferiority and superiority can be unified by the following hypotheses:

$$H_0 : \epsilon \leq \delta \quad vs. \quad H_a : \epsilon > \delta,$$

where $\epsilon = \mu_2 - \mu_1$ is the difference in mean responses between the test treatment (μ_2) and the active control agent (μ_1), δ is the clinical superiority or noninferiority margin. In practice, when $\delta > 0$, the rejection of the null hypothesis indicates *clinical* superiority over the reference drug product. When $\delta < 0$, the rejection of the null hypothesis implies noninferiority against the reference drug product. Note that when $\delta = 0$, the above hypotheses are referred to as hypotheses for testing *statistical* superiority which is usually misused with that of clinical superiority.

Noninferiority Margin

One of the major considerations in a noninferiority test is the selection of the noninferiority margin. A different choice of noninferiority margin may affect the method of analyzing clinical data and consequently may alter the conclusion of the clinical study. As pointed out in the guideline by the International Conference on Harmonization (ICH), the determination of noninferiority margins should be based on both statistical reasoning and clinical judgment. Despite the existence of some studies, there is no established rule or gold standard for determination of noninferiority margins in active control trials.

According to the ICH E10 Guideline, a noninferiority margin may be selected based on past experience in placebo control trials with valid design under conditions similar to those planned for the new trial and the determination of a noninferiority margin should not only reflect uncertainties in the evidence on which the choice is based, but also be suitably conservative. Furthermore, as a basic frequentist statistical principle, the hypothesis of noninferiority should be formulated with population parameters, not estimates from historical trials. Along these lines, Chow and Shao (2006) proposed a method of selecting noninferiority margins with some statistical justification. Our proposed noninferiority margin depends on population parameters including parameters related to the placebo control if it were not replaced by the active control. Unless a fixed (constant) noninferiority margin can be chosen based on clinical judgment, a fixed noninferiority margin not depending on population parameters is rarely suitable. Intuitively, the noninferiority margin should be small when the effect of the active control agent relative to placebo is small or the variation in the population under investigation is large. Chow and Shao's approach ensures that the efficacy of the test therapy is superior to placebo when non-inferiority is concluded. When it is necessary/desired, their approach can produce a non-inferiority margin that ensures that the efficacy of the test therapy relative to placebo can be established with great confidence.

Because the proposed non-inferiority margin depends on population parameters, the non-inferiority test designed for the situation where the non-inferiority margin is fixed has to be modified in order to apply it to the case where the non-inferiority margin is a parameter. In what follows, Chow and Shao's method for determination of non-inferiority margin is described.

Chow and Shao's Approach Let θ_T, θ_A, and θ_P be the unknown population efficacy parameters associated with the test therapy, the active control agent, and the placebo, respectively. Also, let $\delta \geq 0$ be a non-inferiority margin. Without loss of generality, we assume that a large value of population efficacy parameter is desired. The hypotheses for non-inferiority can be formulated as

$$H_0 : \theta_T - \theta_A \leq -\delta \quad \text{vs.} \quad H_a : \theta_T - \theta_A > -\delta. \tag{4.1}$$

If δ is a fixed pre-specified value, then standard statistical methods can be applied to testing hypotheses (4.1. In practice, however, δ is often unknown.

There exists an approach that constructs the value of δ based on a placebo-controlled historical trial. For example, $\delta = $ a fraction of the lower limit of the 95% confidence interval for $\theta_A - \theta_P$ based on some historical trial data (see, e.g., CBER/FDA Memorandum, 1999). Although this approach is intuitively conservative, it is not statistically valid because (i) if the lower confidence limit is treated as a fixed value, then the variability in historical data is ignored, and (ii) if the lower confidence limit is treated as a statistic, then this approach violates the basic frequentist statistical principle, i.e., the hypotheses being tested should not involve any estimates from current or past trials.

From statistical point of view, the ICH E10 Guideline suggests that the non-inferiority margin δ should be chosen to satisfy at least the following two criteria:

Criterion 1. The ability to claim that the test therapy is non-inferior to the active control agent and is superior to the placebo (even though the placebo is not considered in the active control trial).

Criterion 2. The non-inferiority margin should be suitably conservative, i.e., variability should be taken into account.

A fixed δ (i.e., it does not depend on any parameters) is rarely suitable under criterion 1. Let $\Delta > 0$ be a *clinical* superiority margin if a placebo-controlled trial is conducted to establish the *clinical* superiority of the test therapy over a placebo control. Since the active control is an established therapy, we may assume that $\theta_A - \theta_P > \Delta$. However, when $\theta_T - \theta_A > -\delta$ (i.e., the test therapy is non-inferior to the active control) for a fixed δ, we cannot ensure that $\theta_T - \theta_P > \Delta$ (i.e., the test therapy is *clinically* superior to the placebo) unless $\delta = 0$.

Thus, it is reasonable to consider non-inferiority margins depending on unknown parameters. Hung et al. (2003) summarized the approach of using the non-inferiority margin of the form

$$\delta = \gamma(\theta_A - \theta_P), \tag{4.2}$$

where γ is a fixed constant between 0 and 1. This is based on the idea of preserving a certain fraction of the active control effect $\theta_A - \theta_P$. The smaller $\theta_A - \theta_P$ is, the smaller δ. How to select the proportion γ, however, is not discussed.

Following the idea of Chow and Shao (2006), we now derive a non-inferiority margin satisfying criterion 1. Let $\Delta > 0$ be a clinical superiority margin if a placebo control is added to the trial. Suppose that the non-inferiority margin δ is proportional to Δ, i.e., $\delta = r\Delta$, where r is a known value chosen in the beginning of the trial. To be conservative, r should be ≤ 1. If the test therapy is not inferior to the active control agent and is superior over the placebo, then both

$$\theta_T - \theta_A > -\delta \quad \text{vs.} \quad \theta_T - \theta_P > \Delta \tag{4.3}$$

should hold. Under the worst scenario, i.e., $\theta_T - \theta_A$ achieves its lower bound $-\delta$, the largest possible δ satisfying (4.3) is given by

$$\delta = \theta_A - \theta_P - \Delta,$$

which leads to

$$\delta = \frac{r}{1+r}(\theta_A - \theta_P). \tag{4.4}$$

From (4.2) and (4.4), $\gamma = r/(r+1)$. If $0 < r \leq 1$, then $0 < \gamma \leq \frac{1}{2}$.

The above argument in determining δ takes Criterion 1 into account, but is not conservative enough, since it does not consider the variability. Let $\hat{\theta}_T$ and $\hat{\theta}_P$ be sample estimators of θ_T and θ_P, respectively, based on data from a placebo-controlled trial. Assume that $\hat{\theta}_T - \hat{\theta}_P$ is normally distributed with mean $\theta_T - \theta_P$ and standard error SE_{T-P} (which is true under certain conditions or approximately true under the central limit theorem for large sample sizes). When $\theta_T = \theta_A - \delta$,

$$P\left(\hat{\theta}_T - \hat{\theta}_P < \Delta\right) = \Phi\left(\frac{\Delta + \delta - (\theta_A - \theta_P)}{SE_{T-P}}\right) \tag{4.5}$$

where Φ denotes the standard normal distribution function. If δ is chosen according to (4.4) and $\theta_T = \theta_A - \delta$, then the probability that $\hat{\theta}_T - \hat{\theta}_P$ is less than Δ is equal to $\frac{1}{2}$. In view of Criterion 2, a value much smaller than $\frac{1}{2}$ for this probability is desired, because it is the probability that the estimated test therapy effect is not superior over that of the placebo.

Since the probability in (4.5) is an increasing function of δ, the smaller δ (the more conservative choice of the non-inferiority margin) is, the smaller the chance that $\hat{\theta}_T - \hat{\theta}_P$ is less than Δ. Setting the probability on the left hand side of (4.5) to ϵ with $0 < \epsilon \leq \frac{1}{2}$, we obtain that

$$\delta = \theta_A - \theta_P - \Delta - z_{1-\epsilon} SE_{T-P},$$

where $z_a = \Phi^{-1}(a)$. Since $\Delta = \delta/r$, we obtain that

$$\delta = \frac{r}{1+r}(\theta_A - \theta_P - z_{1-\epsilon} SE_{T-P}), \tag{4.6}$$

Comparing (4.2) and (4.6), we obtain that

$$\gamma = \frac{r}{1+r}\left(1 - \frac{z_{1-\epsilon} SE_{T-P}}{\theta_A - \theta_P}\right),$$

i.e., the proportion γ in (4.2) is a decreasing function of a type of noise-to-signal ratio (or coefficient of variation).

As indicated by Chow and Shao (2006), the above non-inferiority margin (4.6) can also be derived from a slightly different point of view. Suppose that we actually conduct a placebo-controlled trial with superiority margin Δ to establish the superiority of the test therapy over the placebo. Then, the power of the large sample t-test for hypotheses $\theta_T - \theta_P \leq \Delta$ vs. $\theta_T - \theta_P > \Delta$ is approximately equal to

$$\Phi\left(\frac{\theta_T - \theta_P - \Delta}{SE_{T-P}} - z_{1-\alpha}\right),$$

where α is the level of significance. Assume the worst scenario $\theta_T = \theta_A - \delta$ and that β is a given desired level of power. Then, setting the power to β leads to

$$\frac{\theta_A - \theta_P - \Delta - \delta}{SE_{T-P}} - z_{1-\alpha} = z_\beta,$$

i.e.,

$$\delta = \frac{r}{1+r}[\theta_A - \theta_P - (z_{1-\alpha} + z_\beta)SE_{T-P}]. \tag{4.7}$$

Comparing (4.6) with (4.7), we have

$$z_{1-\epsilon} = z_{1-\alpha} + z_\beta.$$

For $\alpha = 0.05$, the following table gives some examples of values of β, ϵ, and $z_{1-\epsilon}$.

Table 4.2.1: Examples of Values
of β, ϵ and $z_{1-\epsilon}$

β	ϵ	$z_{1-\epsilon}$
0.36	0.1000	1.282
0.50	0.0500	1.645
0.60	0.0290	1.897
0.70	0.0150	2.170
0.75	0.0101	2.320
0.80	0.0064	2.486

As a result, we arrive the following conclusions with respect to the non-inferiority margin given by (4.6).

1. The non-inferiority margin (4.6) takes variability into consideration, i.e., δ is a decreasing function of the standard error of $\hat{\theta}_T - \hat{\theta}_P$. It is an increasing function of the sample sizes, since SE_{T-P} decreases as sample sizes increase. Choosing a non-inferiority margin depending on the sample sizes does not violate the basic frequentist statistical principle. In fact, it cannot be avoided when variability of sample estimators is considered. Statistical analysis, including sample size calculation in the trial planning stage, can still be performed. In the limiting case ($SE_{T-P} \to 0$), the non-inferiority margin in (4.6) is the same as that in (4.4).

2. The ϵ value in (4.6) represents a degree of conservativeness. An arbitrarily chosen ϵ may lead to highly conservative tests. When sample sizes are large (SE_{T-P} is small), one can afford a small ϵ. A reasonable value of ϵ and sample sizes can be determined in the planning stage of the trial.

3. The non-inferiority margin in (4.6) is nonnegative if and only if $\theta_A - \theta_P \geq z_{1-\epsilon} SE_{T-P}$, i.e., the active control effect is substantial or the sample sizes are large. We might take our non-inferiority margin to be the larger of the quantity in (4.6) and 0 to force the non-inferiority margin to be nonnegative. However, it may be wise not to do so. Note that if θ_A is not substantially larger than θ_P, then non-inferiority testing is not justifiable since, even if $\delta = 0$ in (4.1), concluding H_a in (4.1) does not imply the test therapy is superior over the placebo. Using δ in (4.6), testing hypotheses (4.1) converts to testing the superiority of the test therapy over the active control agent when δ is actually negative. In other words, when $\theta_A - \theta_P$ is smaller than a certain margin, our test automatically becomes a superiority test and the property $P(\hat{\theta}_T - \hat{\theta}_P < \Delta) = \epsilon$ (with $\Delta = |\delta|/r$) still holds.

4. In many applications, there is no historical data. In such cases parameters related to placebo are not estimable and, hence, a non-inferiority margin not depending on these parameters is desired. Since the active control

agent is a well established therapy, let us assume that the power of the
level α test showing that the active control agent is superior to placebo
by the margin Δ is at the level η. This means that approximately,

$$\theta_A - \theta_P \geq \Delta + (z_{1-\alpha} + z_\eta)SE_{A-P}.$$

Replacing $\theta_A - \theta_P - \Delta$ in (4.6) by its lower bound given in the previous
expression we obtain the non-inferiority margin

$$\delta = (z_{1-\alpha} + z_\eta)SE_{A-P} - z_{1-\epsilon}SE_{T-P}.$$

To use this non-inferiority margin, we need some information about the
population variance of the placebo group. As an example, consider the
parallel design with two treatments, the test therapy and the active control agent. Assume that the same two-group parallel design would have
been used if a placebo-controlled trial had been conducted. Then

$$SE_{A-P} = \sqrt{\sigma_A^2/n_A + \sigma_P^2/n_P}$$

and

$$SE_{T-P} = \sqrt{\sigma_T^2/n_T + \sigma_P^2/n_P},$$

where σ_k^2 is the asymptotic variance for $\sqrt{n_k}(\hat{\theta}_k - \theta_k)$ and n_k is the sample
size under treatment k. If we assume $\sigma_P/\sqrt{n_P} = c$, then

$$\delta = (z_{1-\alpha} + z_\eta)\sqrt{\frac{\sigma_A^2}{n_A} + c^2} - z_{1-\epsilon}\sqrt{\frac{\sigma_T^2}{n_T} + c^2}. \tag{4.8}$$

Formula (4.8) can be used in two ways. One way is to replace c in (4.8) by
an estimate. When no information from the placebo control is available,
a suggested estimate of c is the smaller of the estimates of $\sigma_T/\sqrt{n_T}$ and
$\sigma_A/\sqrt{n_A}$. The other way is to carry out a sensitivity analysis by using δ
in (4.8) for a number of c values.

Statistical Inference

When the non-inferiority margin depends on unknown population parameters,
statistical tests designed for the case of constant non-inferiority margin may
not be appropriate. Valid statistical tests for hypotheses (4.1) with δ given by
(4.2) are derived in CBER/FDA Memorandum (1999), Holmgren (1999), and
Hung et al. (2003) assuming that (i) γ is known and (ii) historical data from
a placebo-controlled trial are available and the so-called "constancy condition"
holds, i.e., the active control effects are equal in the current and the historical
patient populations. In this section, we derive valid statistical tests for the
non-inferiority margin given in (4.6) or (4.8). We use the same notations as
described in the previous section.

Tests based on historical data under constancy condition   We first consider tests involving the non-inferiority margin (4.6) in the case where historical data for a placebo-controlled trial assessing the effect of the active control agent are available and the constancy condition holds, i.e., the effect $\theta_{A0} - \theta_{P0}$ in the historical trial is the same as $\theta_A - \theta_P$ in the current active control trial, if a placebo control is added to the current trial. It should be emphasized that the constancy condition is a crucial assumption for the validity of the results.

Assume that the two-group parallel design is adopted in both the historical and current trials and that the sample sizes are respectively n_{A0} and n_{P0} for the active control and placebo in the historical trial and n_T and n_A for the test therapy and active control in the current trial. Without the normality assumption on the data, we adopt the large sample inference approach. Let $k = T, A, A0$ and $P0$ be the indexes, respectively, for the test and active control in the current trial and the active control and placebo in the historical trial. Assume that $n_k = l_k n$ for some fixed l_k and that, under appropriate conditions, estimators $\hat{\theta}_k$ for parameters θ_k satisfy

$$\sqrt{n_k}(\hat{\theta}_k - \theta_k) \to_d N(0, \sigma_k^2) \tag{4.9}$$

as $n \to \infty$, where $\to_d$ denotes convergence in distribution. Also, assume that consistent estimators $\hat{\sigma}_k^2$ for σ_k^2 are obtained. The following result can be established.

Theorem 1   We have

$$\frac{\hat{\theta}_T - \hat{\theta}_A + \frac{r}{1+r}(\hat{\theta}_{A0} - \hat{\theta}_{P0} - z_{1-\epsilon}\widehat{SE}_{T-P}) - (\theta_T - \theta_A + \delta)}{\widehat{SE}_{T-C}} \to_d N(0,1),$$
$$\tag{4.10}$$

where

$$\widehat{SE}_{T-P} = \sqrt{\hat{\sigma}_T^2/n_T + \hat{\sigma}_{P0}^2/n_{P0}}$$

is an estimator of $SE_{T-P} = \sqrt{\sigma_T^2/n_T + \sigma_{P0}^2/n_{P0}}$ and $\widehat{SE}_{T-C}$ is an estimator of SE_{T-C}, the standard deviation of $\hat{\theta}_T - \hat{\theta}_A + \frac{r}{1+r}(\hat{\theta}_{A0} - \hat{\theta}_{P0})$, i.e.,

$$\widehat{SE}_{T-C} = \sqrt{\frac{\hat{\sigma}_T^2}{n_T} + \frac{\hat{\sigma}_A^2}{n_A} + \left(\frac{r}{1+r}\right)^2 \left(\frac{\hat{\sigma}_{A0}^2}{n_{A0}} + \frac{\hat{\sigma}_{P0}^2}{n_{P0}}\right)}.$$

Proof: From result (4.9), the independence of data from different groups, and the constancy condition,

$$\frac{\hat{\theta}_T - \hat{\theta}_A + \frac{r}{1+r}(\hat{\theta}_{A0} - \hat{\theta}_{P0}) - [\theta_T - \theta_A \frac{r}{1+r}(\theta_A - \theta_P)]}{SE_{T-C}} \to_d N(0,1). \tag{4.11}$$

From the consistency of $\hat{\sigma}_k^2$ and the fact that $\sqrt{n}SE_{T-C}$ is a fixed constant,

$$\frac{\widehat{SE}_{T-P} - SE_{T-P}}{SE_{T-C}} = \frac{\sqrt{n}(\widehat{SE}_{T-P} - SE_{T-P})}{\sqrt{n}SE_{T-C}} = o_p(1)$$

and

$$\frac{\widehat{SE}_{T-C}}{SE_{T-C}} - 1 = \frac{\sqrt{n}(\widehat{SE}_{T-C} - SE_{T-C})}{\sqrt{n}SE_{T-C}} = o_p(1),$$

where $o_p(1)$ denotes a quantity converging to 0 in probability. Then

$$\frac{\hat{\theta}_T - \hat{\theta}_A + \frac{r}{1+r}(\hat{\theta}_{A0} - \hat{\theta}_{P0} - z_{1-\epsilon}\widehat{SE}_{T-P}) - (\theta_T - \theta_A + \delta)}{\widehat{SE}_{T-C}}$$

$$= \Big\{ \frac{\hat{\theta}_T - \hat{\theta}_A + \frac{r}{1+r}(\hat{\theta}_{A0} - \hat{\theta}_{P0}) - [\theta_T - \theta_A + \frac{r}{1+r}(\theta_A - \theta_P)]}{SE_{T-C}}$$

$$- \frac{r}{1+r}\frac{\widehat{SE}_{T-P} - SE_{T-P}}{SE_{T-C}} \Big\} \frac{SE_{T-C}}{\widehat{SE}_{T-C}}$$

$$= \Big\{ \frac{\hat{\theta}_T - \hat{\theta}_A + \frac{r}{1+r}(\hat{\theta}_{A0} - \hat{\theta}_{P0}) - [\theta_T - \theta_A + \frac{r}{1+r}(\theta_A - \theta_P)]}{SE_{T-C}}$$

$$- o_p(1) \Big\} [1 + o_p(1)]$$

and result (4.10) follows from result (4.11) and Slutsky's theorem.

Then, when the non-inferiority margin in (4.6) is adopted, the null hypothesis H_0 in (4.1) is rejected at approximately level α if

$$\hat{\theta}_T - \hat{\theta}_A + \frac{r}{1+r}(\hat{\theta}_{A0} - \hat{\theta}_{P0} - z_{1-\epsilon}\widehat{SE}_{T-P}) - z_{1-\alpha}\widehat{SE}_{T-C} > 0.$$

Impact on Sample Size

Using result (4.11), we can approximate the power of this test by

$$\Phi\left(\frac{\theta_T - \theta_A + \delta}{SE_{T-C}} - z_{1-\alpha}\right).$$

Using this formula, we can select the sample sizes n_T and n_A to achieve a desired power level (say β), assuming that n_{A0} and n_{P0} are given (in the historical trial). Assume that $n_T/n_A = \lambda$ is chosen. Then n_T should be selected as a solution of

$$\theta_T - \theta_A + \frac{r}{1+r}\left(\theta_A - \theta_P - z_{1-\epsilon}\sqrt{\frac{\sigma_T^2}{n_T} + \frac{\sigma_{P0}^2}{n_{P0}}}\right)$$

$$= (z_{1-\alpha} + z_\beta) \sqrt{\frac{\sigma_T^2}{n_T} + \frac{\lambda \sigma_A^2}{n_T} + \left(\frac{r}{1+r}\right)^2 \left(\frac{\sigma_{A0}^2}{n_{A0}} + \frac{\sigma_{P0}^2}{n_{P0}}\right)}. \tag{4.12}$$

Although equation (4.12) does not have an explicit solution in terms of n_T, its solution can be numerically obtained once initial values for all parameters are given.

Remarks

The constancy condition   The use of historical data usually increases the power of the test for hypotheses with a non-inferiority margin depending on parameters in the historical trial. On the other hand, using historical data without the constancy condition may lead to invalid conclusions. As indicated in Hung et al. (2003), checking the constancy condition is difficult. In this subsection we discuss a method of checking the constancy condition under an assumption much weaker than the constancy condition.

Note that the key is to check whether the active control effect $\theta_A - \theta_P$ in the current trial is the same as $\theta_{A0} - \theta_{P0}$ in the historical trial. If we assume that the placebo effects θ_P and θ_{P0} are the same (which is much weaker than the constancy condition), then we can check whether $\theta_A = \theta_{A0}$ using the data under the active control in the current and historical trials.

Tests without historical data   We now consider tests when non-inferiority margin (4.10) is chosen. Following the same argument as given in the proof of result (4.11), we can establish that

$$\frac{\hat\theta_T - \hat\theta_A + (z_{1-\alpha} + z_\eta)\widehat{SE}_{A-P} - z_{1-\epsilon}\widehat{SE}_{T-P} - (\theta_T - \theta_A + \Delta)}{\widehat{SE}_{T-A}} \to_d N(0,1), \tag{4.13}$$

where

$$\widehat{SE}_{k-l} = \sqrt{\hat\sigma_k^2/n_k + \hat\sigma_l^2/n_l}.$$

Hence, when the non-inferiority margin in (4.10) is adopted, the null hypothesis H_0 in (4.1) is rejected at approximately level α if

$$\hat\theta_T - \hat\theta_A + (z_{1-\alpha} + z_\eta)\widehat{SE}_{A-P} - z_{1-\epsilon}\widehat{SE}_{T-A} - z_{1-\alpha}\sqrt{\frac{\hat\sigma_T^2}{n_T} + \frac{\hat\sigma_A^2}{n_A}} > 0.$$

The power of this test is approximately

$$\Phi\left(\frac{\theta_T - \theta_A + \delta}{SE_{T-A}} - z_{1-\alpha}\right).$$

If $n_T/n_A = \lambda$, then we can select the sample sizes n_T and n_A to achieve a desired power level (say β) by solving

$$\theta_T - \theta_A + (z_{1-\alpha} + z_\eta)\sqrt{\frac{\lambda\sigma_A^2}{n_T} + \frac{\sigma_P^2}{n_P}} - z_{1-\epsilon}\sqrt{\frac{\sigma_T^2}{n_T} + \frac{\sigma_P^2}{n_P}} = (z_{1-\alpha} + z_\beta)\sqrt{\frac{\lambda\sigma_A^2}{n_T} + \frac{\sigma_T^2}{n_T}}.$$

FDA Draft Guidance

Note that in its recent draft guidance on *Noninferiority Clinical Trials*, the FDA recommends two noninferiority margins, namely, M_1 and M_2, where M_1 is the entire effect of the active control assumed to the present in the noninferiority study and M_2 is the largest clinically acceptable difference of the test drug compared to the active control. As indicated by the FDA, M_2 is a clinical judgment which is never greater than M_1, even if for active control drugs with small effects, a clinical judgment might argue that a larger difference is not clinically important. Ruling out a difference between the active control and the test drug that is larger than M_1 is a critical finding that supports the conclusion of effectiveness.

4.3   Concluding Remarks

For large-scale clinical trails, a data safety monitoring committee (DMC) is usually established to monitor safety and/or perform interim efficacy analysis of the trial based on accrual data at some pre-scheduled time or when the trial has achieved certain number of events. Based on the interim results, the DMC may recommend modification of study objectives and/or hypotheses. As an example, suppose that a clinical trial was designed as a superiority trial to establish the superiority of the test treatment as compared to a standard therapy or an active control agent. However, after the review of the interim results, it is determined that the trial will not be able to achieve the study objective of establishing superiority with the observed treatment effect size at interim. The DMC does not recommend stopping the trial based on futility analysis. Instead, the DMC may suggest modifying the hypotheses for testing noninferiority. This modification raises a critical statistical/clinical issue regarding the determination of non-inferiority margin. Chow and Shao (2006) proposed a statistical justification for determining a non-inferiority margin based on accrued data at interim following ICH guidance.

Chapter 5

Adaptive Dose-Escalation Trials

In clinical research, the *response* in a dose response study could be a biological response for safety or efficacy. For example, in a dose-toxicity study, the goal is to determine the maximum tolerable dose (MTD). On the other hand, in a dose-efficacy response study, the primary objective is usually to address one or more of the following questions: (i) Is there any evidence of the drug effect?, (ii) What is the nature of the dose-response?, and (iii) What is the optimal dose? In practice, it is always a concern as to how to evaluate dose-response relationship with limited resources within a relatively tight time-frame. This concern leads to a proposed design that allows fewer patients to be exposed to the toxicity and more patients to be treated at potential efficacious dose levels. Such a design also allows pharmaceutical companies to fully utilize their resources for development of more new drug products (see, e.g., Arbuck, 1996; Babb, Rogatko, and Zacks, 1998; Babb and Rogatko, 2001; Berry et al., 2002; Bretz and Hothorn, 2002; Ivanova, 2006; Ivanova et al., 2009).

The remaining of this chapter is organized as follows. In the next section, we provide a brief background of dose escalation trials. The concepts of the continued reassessment method (CRM) in phase I oncology trials is reviewed in Section 5.2. In Section 5.3, We propose a hybrid frequentist-Bayesian adaptive approach. In Section 5.4, several simulations were conducted to evaluate the performance of the proposed method. The concluding remarks are presented in Section 5.5.

5.1   Introduction

For dose-toxicity studies, the traditional escalation rules (TER), also known as the "3+3" rules, are commonly used in early phase of oncology studies. The "3+3" rule is to enter three patients at a new dose level and then enter another three patients when dose limiting toxicity (DLT) is observed. The assessment of the six patients is then performed to determine whether the trial should be stopped at the level or to increase the dose. Basically, there are two types of the "3+3" rules, namely the traditional escalation rule (TER) and strict traditional escalation rule (STER). TER does not allow dose de-escalation but STER does when two of three patients have DLTs. The "3+3" rules can be generalized to the "m+n" TER and STER escalation rules. Chang and Chow (2006a) provided detailed description of general "m+n" designs with and without dose de-escalation. The corresponding formulas for sample size calculation can be found in Lin and Shih (2001).

Recently, many new methods such as the assessment of dose response using multiple-stage designs (Crowley, 2001) and the continued reassessment method (CRM) (see, e.g., O'Quigley, Pepe, and Fisher, 1990; O'Quigley and Shen, 1996; Babb and Rogatko, 2004) have been developed. For the method of CRM, the dose-response relationship is continually reassessed based on accumulative data collected from the trial. The next patient who enters the trial is then assigned to the potential MTD level. This approach is more efficient than that of the usual TER with respect to the allocation of the MTD. However, the efficiency of CRM may be at risk due to delayed response and/or a constraint on dose-jump in practice (Babb and Rogatko, 2004). In recent years, the use of adaptive design methods for characterizing dose response curve has become very popular (Bauer and Röhmel, 1995). An adaptive design is a dynamic system that allows the investigator to optimize the trial (including design, monitoring, operating, and analysis) with cumulative information observed from the trial. For Bayesian adaptive design for dose response trials, some researchers suggest the use of loss/utility function in conjunction with dose assignment based on minimization/maximization of loss/utility function (e.g., Gasparini and Eisele, 2000; Whitehead, 1997).

In this chapter, we use an adaptive method that combines CRM and utility-adaptive randomization (UAR) for multiple-endpoint trials (Chang, Chow and Pong, 2005). The proposed UAR is similar to response-adaptive randomization (RAR). It is an extension of RAR to multi-endpoint case. In UAR scheme, the probability of assigning a patient to a particular dose level is determined by its normalized utility value (ranging from 0 to 1). The CRM could be a Bayesian, a frequentist, or a hybrid frequentist-Bayesian based approach. This proposed method has the advantage for achieving the optimal design by means of the adaptation to the accrued data of on-going trial. In addition, CRM could provide a better prediction of dose response relationship by selecting an appropriate model as compared to the method simply based on the observed response. In practice, it is not uncommon that the observed response rate is lower in a higher dose group than that in a lower dose group provided that the high dose group, in fact, has a higher response rate. The use of CRM is able to avoid this problem by using a monotonic function such as a logistic function in the model. The proposed adaptive method deals with multiple endpoint in two ways. The first approach is to model each dose-endpoint relationship with or without constraints among the models. Each model usually a monotonic function family such as logistic or some power function. The second approach is to combine the multiple endpoints into a single utility index. Then model the utility using a more flexible function family such as hyper-logistic function as proposed in this chapter.

5.2   CRM in Phase I Oncology Study

CRM is originally used in Phase I oncology trials (O'Quigley, Pepe, and Fisher 1990). The primary goal of phase I oncology trial is not only to assess the dose-toxicity relationship, but also to determine MTD. Due to potential high toxicity of the study drug, in practice usually only a small number of patients (e.g., 3 to 6) are treated at each ascending dose level. The most common approach is the "3+3" TER with a pre-specified sequence for dose escalation. However, this ad hoc approach is found to be inefficient and often underestimate the MTD, especially when the starting dose is too low. The CRM is developed to overcome these limitations. The estimation or prediction from CRM is weighted by number of data points. Therefore, if the data points are mostly around the estimated value then the estimation is more accurate. CRM assigns more patients near MTD; consequently the estimated MTD is much more precise and reliable. In practice, this is the most desirable operating characteristic of the Bayesian CRM. In what follows, we will briefly review the CRM approach.

Dose Toxicity Modeling

In most phase I dose response trials, it is assumed that there is a monotonic relationship between dose and toxicity. This ideal relationship suggests that the biologically inactive dose is lower than the active dose, which is in turn lower than the toxic dose. To characterize this relationship, the choice of an appropriate dose-toxicity model is important. In practice, the logistic model is often utilized

$$p(x) = [1 + b\exp(-ax)]^{-1}$$

where $p(x)$ is the probability of toxicity associated with dose x, and a and b are positive parameters to be determined. Practically, $p(x)$ is equivalent to toxicity rate or dose limiting toxicity (DLT) rate as defined by the Common Toxicity Criteria (CTC) of the United States National Cancer Institute. Denote θ the probability of DLT (or DLT rate) at MTD. Then, the MTD can be expressed as

$$MTD = \frac{1}{a} \ln(\frac{b\theta}{1 - \theta})$$

If we can estimate a and b or their posterior distributions (For common logistic model, b is predetermined.), we will be able to determine the MTD from (2) or provide predictive probabilities for MTD. The choice of toxicity rate at MTD, θ, depends on the nature of the DLT and the type of the target tumor. For an aggressive tumor and a transient and non-life-threatening DLT, θ could be as high as 0.5. For persistent DLT and less aggressive tumors, it could be as low as 0.1 to 0.25. A commonly used value is somewhere between 0 and $1/3 = 0.33$ (Crowley, 2001).

Dose Level Selection

The initial dose given to the first patients in a phase I study should be low enough to avoid severe toxicity but high enough for observing some activity or potential efficacy in humans. The commonly used starting dose is the dose at which 10% mortality (LD_{10}) occurs in mice. The subsequent dose levels are usually selected based on the following multiplicative set

$$x_i = f_{i-1}x_{i-1} \quad (i = 1, 2, ...k),$$

where f_i is called the dose escalation factor. The highest dose level should be selected such that it covers the biologically active dose, but remains lower than the toxic dose. In general, CRM does not require pre-determined dose intervals. However, the use of pre-determined dose is often of practically convenience.

Reassessment of Model Parameters

The key is to estimate the parameter a in the response model (1). An initial assumption or a prior about the parameter is necessary in order to assign patients to the dose level based the dose-toxicity relationship. This estimation of a is continually updated based cumulative data observed from the trial. The estimation method can be a Bayesian or frequentist approach. For Bayesian approach, it leads to the posterior distribution of a. For frequentist approaches such as maximum likelihood estimate or least square estimate are straight forward. Note that Bayesian approach requires a prior distribution about parameter a. It it provides posterior distribution of a and predictive probabilities of MTD. The frequentist, Bayesian and a hybrid frequentist-Bayesian based approaches in conjunction with the response-adaptive randomization will be further discussed in this article.

Assignment of Next Patient

The updated dose-toxicity model is usually used to choose the dose level for the next patient. In other words, the next patient enrolled in the trial is assigned to the current estimated MTD based on dose-response model. Practically, this assignment is subject to safety constraints such as limited dose jump and delayed response. Assignment of patient to the most updated MTD is intuitive. It leads to majority of the patients assigned to the dose levels near MTD, which allows a more precise estimate of MTD with a minimum number of patients.

5.3   Hybrid Frequentist-Bayesian Adaptive Design

When Bayesian is used for multiple-parameter response models, some numerical irregularities cannot be easily resolved. In addition, Bayesian methods require an extensive computation for a multiple-parameter model. To overcome these limitations, a hybrid frequentist and Bayesian method is useful. The use of a utility-adaptive randomization allows the allocation of more patients to the superior dose levels and less patients to the inferior dose levels. This adaptive method is not only optimal ethically but also has a favor benefit/risk ratio (such as benefit-safety and/or benefit-cost).

The Adaptive Model

In this section, we use the adaptive design as outlined in Figure 5.3.1 for dose response trial or Phase II/III combined trials. Start with several dose levels with or without a placebo group, followed by the prediction of the dose-response relationship using Bayesian or other approaches based on accrued real time data. The next patient is then randomized to a treatment group based on the utility-adaptive or response-adaptive randomization algorithm. We may allow the inferior treatment groups to be dropped when there are too many groups based on results from the analysis of the accrued data using Bayesian and/or frequentist approaches. It is expected that the predictive dose-response model in conjunction with a utility-adaptive randomization could lead to a design that assign more patients to the superior arms and consequently a more efficient design. We will illustrate this point further via computer trial simulations. In the next section, technical details for establishing dose-response relationship using CRM in conjunction with utility-adaptive randomization are provided.

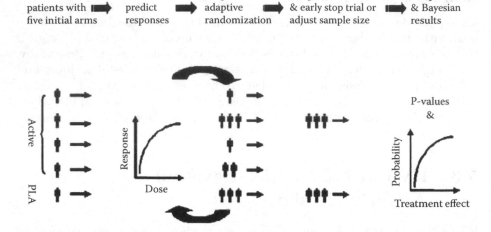

Figure 5.3.1: Bayesian adaptive trial.

Utility-based Unified CRM Adaptive Approach

The Utility-based unified CRM adaptive approach can be summarized by the following steps.

Step 1: Construct utility function based on trial objectives;

Step 2: Propose a probability model for dose response relationship;

Step 3: Construct prior probability distributions of the parameters in the response model;

Step 4: Form the likelihood function based on incremental information on treatment response during the trial;

Step 5: Reassess model parameters or calculate the posterior probability of the model parameters;

Step 6: Update the expected utility function based on dose response model;

Step 7: Determine next action or make adaptations such as changing the randomization or drop inferior treatment arms;

Step 8: Further collect trial data and repeat Steps 5 to 7 until stopping criteria are met.

Construction of Utility Function

Let $X = \{x_1, x_2, ...x_k\}$ be the action space where x_i is coded value for action of anything that would affect the outcomes or decision making, such as a treatment, a withdrawal of a treatment arm, a protocol amendment, stopping the trial, an investment of advertising for the prospective drug, or any combination of the above. x_i can be either a fixed dose or a variable of dose given to a patient. If action x_i is not taken, then $x_i = 0$. Let $y = \{y_1, y_2, ... y_m\}$ be the outcomes of interest, which can be efficacy or toxicity of a test drug, the cost of trial, etc. Each of these outcomes, y_i is a function of action $y_i(x)$, $x \in X$. The utility is defined as

$$U = \sum_{j=1}^{m} w_j = \sum_{j=1}^{m} w(y_j), \tag{5.1}$$

where U is normalized such that $0 \le U \le 1$ and w_j can are pre-specified weights.

Probability Model for Dose-Response

Each of the outcomes can be modeled by the following generalized probability model:

$$\Gamma_j(\mathbf{p}) = \sum_{i=1}^{k} a_{ji} x_i, \quad j = 1, ..., m \tag{5.2}$$

where

$$\mathbf{p} = \{p_1, ..., p_m\}, p_j = P(y_j \ge \tau_j),$$

and τ_j is a threshold for jth outcome. The link function, $\Gamma_j(.)$, is a generalized function of all the probabilities of the outcomes. For simplicity, we may consider

$$\Gamma_j(p_j) = \sum_{i=1}^{k} a_{ji} x_i, , \quad j = 1, ..., m, \tag{5.3}$$

and

$$p_j(\mathbf{x}, \mathbf{a}) = \Gamma_j^{-1}(\sum_{i=1}^{k} a_{ji} x_i), \quad j = 1, ..., m. \tag{5.4}$$

The essential difference between (5.4) and (5.5) is that the former models the outcomes jointly while the latter model each outcome independently. Therefore, for (5.5), Γ_j^{-1} is simply the inverse function of Γ_j. However, for (5.4), Γ_j^{-1} is not a simple inverse function and sometimes the explicit solution may not exist. Γ_j can be used to model the constraints between outcomes, e.g., the relationship between the two blood pressures. Using the link functions could reduce some of the irregular models in the modeling process when there are multiple outcome endpoints.

For a univariate case, logistic model is commonly used for monotonic response. However, for utility, we usually don't know whether it is monotonic or not. Therefore, we proposed the following model

$$p_j(\mathbf{x}, \mathbf{a}) = (a_{j1} \exp(a_{j2}x) + a_{j3} \exp(-a_{j4}x))^{-m}; \quad j = 1, ...m, \tag{5.5}$$

where a_{ji} and m are usually positive values and m is suggested to be 1. Note that when $a_{j1} = 1$, $a_{j2} = 0$, and $m = 1$, (5.5) degenerates to the common logistic model. When $a_{j1} = a_{j3} = 1$, $a_{j2} = 0$, and $a_{j4} = 2$, it reduces to the hyperbolic tangent model. Note that a_{ji} must be determined such that $0 \leq p_j(\mathbf{x}, \mathbf{a}) \leq 1$ for the dose range x under study. For convenience, we will refer to (5.5) as a hyper-logistic function.

The hyper-logistic function is useful especially in modeling utility index because it is not necessary monotonic. However, the range of parameters should be carefully determined before modeling. It is suggested that corresponding various shapes be examined. Some different shapes that generated by hyper-logistic function are presented in Figure 5.3.2.

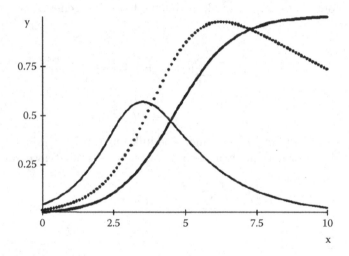

Figure 5.3.2: Curves of hyper-logistic function family.

A special case that is worth mentioning here is the following single utility index (or combined outcomes) model, where the probability is based on utility rather than each outcome

$$p = P(U \geq \tau). \tag{5.6}$$

Unlike the probability models defined based on individual outcomes such as single efficacy or safety outcome, the probability models defined based on utility are often single mode.

Prior Distribution of Parameter Tensor a

The Bayesian approach requires the specification of prior probability distribution of the unknown parameter tensor a_{ji}.

$$\mathbf{a} \sim g_{j0}(\mathbf{a}), \ j = 1, ...m, \tag{5.7}$$

where $g_{j0}(\mathbf{a})$ is the prior probability for the jth endpoint.

Likelihood Function

The next step is to construct the likelihood function. Given n observations with y_{ji} associated with endpoint j and dose x_{m_i}, the likelihood function can be written as

$$f_{jn}(\mathbf{r}\,|\mathbf{a}) = \prod_{i=1}^{n} \left[\Gamma_j^{-1}(a_{j\,m_i}x_{m_i})\right]^{r_{ji}} \left[1 - \Gamma_j^{-1}(a_{j\,m_i}x_{m_i})\right]^{1-r_{ji}}, \; j = 1, ...m,$$

(5.8)

where

$$r_{ji} = \begin{cases} 1, & \text{if } y_{ji} \geq \tau_j \\ 0, & \text{otherwise} \end{cases}, \; j = 1, ...m.$$

(5.9)

Assessment of Parameter a

The assessment of the parameters in the model can be carried out different ways: Bayesian, frequentist, or hybrid approach. Bayesian and hybrid approaches are to assess the probability distribution of the parameter, while frequentist approach is to provide a point estimate of the parameter.

Bayesian approach For Bayesian approach, the posterior probability can be obtained as follows

$$g_j(\mathbf{a}|\mathbf{r}) = \frac{f_{jn}(\mathbf{r}|\mathbf{a})g_{j0}(\mathbf{a})}{\int f_{jn}(\mathbf{r}|\mathbf{a})g_{j\,0}(\mathbf{a})\,d\mathbf{a}}, \; j = 1, ...m$$

(5.10)

We then update the probabilities of the outcome or the predictive probabilities

$$p_j = \int \Gamma_j^{-1}(\sum_{i=1}^{k} a_{ji}x_i)g_j(\mathbf{a}|\mathbf{r})\,d\mathbf{a}, \; j = 1, ...m$$

(5.11)

Note that Bayesian approach is computationally intensive. Alternatively, we may consider a frequentist approach to simplify the calculation, especially when limited knowledge about the prior is available and non-informative prior is to be used.

Maximum likelihood approach   The maximum likelihood estimate of the parameters are given by

$$a_{ji\ MLE} = \arg\max_{\mathbf{a}}\{f_{jn}(\mathbf{r}\,|\,\mathbf{a})\}, \ j = 1, ...m, \qquad (5.12)$$

where $a_{ji\ MLE}$ is the parameter set for the jth outcome. After having obtained $a_{ji\ MLE}$, we can update the probability using

$$p_j(\mathbf{x}, \mathbf{a}) = \Gamma_j^{-1}(\sum_{i=1}^{k} a_{ji\ MLE}\, x_i), \ j = 1, ...m. \qquad (5.13)$$

Least square approach   The least square approach minimizes the difference between predictive probability and the observed rate or probability, which is given below.

$$\mathbf{a}_{jLSE} = \arg\min_{\mathbf{a}}\{L_j(\mathbf{a}))\}, \ j = 1, ...m, \qquad (5.14)$$

where

$$L_j(\mathbf{a}) = \sum_{i=1}^{k} (p_j(x_i, \mathbf{a}) - \hat{p}_j(x_i, \mathbf{a}))^2 .$$

We then update the probability

$$p_j(\mathbf{x}, \mathbf{a}) = \Gamma_j^{-1}(\sum_{i=1}^{k} a_{ji\ LSE}\, x_i), \qquad (5.15)$$

where $a_{ji\ LSE}$, the component of $\mathbf{a}$, is the parameter set for the jth outcome.

Hybrid frequentist-Bayesian approach   Although Bayesian CRM allows the incorporation of prior knowledge about the parameters, some difficulties arise when it is used in a model with multiple parameters. There difficulties include (i) computational burden, (ii) numerical instability in evaluation posterior probability. A solution is to use frequentist approach to estimate all the parameters and use the Bayesian approach to re-estimate the posterior distribution of some parameters. This hybrid frequentist-Bayesian approach allows the incorporation of prior knowledge about parameter distribution but avoiding computational burden and numerical instability. Details regarding the hybrid method will be specified.

Determination of Next Action

As mentioned earlier, the actions or adaptations taken should be based on trial objectives or utility function. A typical action is a change of the randomization schedule. From the dose response model, since each dose associates with a probability of response, the expected utility function is then given by $\bar{U} = \sum_{j=1}^{m} p_j(\mathbf{x}, \mathbf{a})w_j$. Two approaches, deterministic and probabilistic approaches can be taken. The former refers to the optimal approach where actions can be taken to maximize the expected utility, while the latter is referred to adaptive randomization where treatment assignment to the next patient is not fully determined by the algorithm.

Optimal approach As mentioned earlier, in the optimal approach, the dose level assigned to the next patient is based on optimization of the expected utility, i.e.,

$$x_{n+1} = \arg\max_{x_i} \bar{U} = \sum_{j=1}^{m} p_j w_j$$

However, it is not feasible due to its difficulties in practice.

Utility-adaptive randomization approach Many of the response-adaptive randomizations (RAR) can be used to increase the expected response. However, these adaptive randomizations are difficult to apply directly to the case of the multiple endpoints. As an alternative, the following utility-adaptive randomization algorithm is proposed. This utility-adaptive randomization, which combines the idea from randomized-play-winner (Rosenberger and Lachin, 2002) and Lachin's urn models, is based on the following. The target randomization probability to x_i group is proportional to the current estimation of utility or response rate of the group, i.e., $U(x_i)/\sum_{i=1}^{k} U(x_i)$, where K is the number of groups. When a patient randomized into x_i group, the randomization probability to this group should be reduced. This leads to the following proposed randomization model:

Probability of randomizing a patient to group x_i is proportional to the corresponding posterior probability of the utility or response rate, i.e.,

$$\Re(x_i) = \frac{1}{c}\left(\frac{U(x_i)}{\sum_{i=1}^{k} U(x_i)} - \frac{n_i}{N}\right), \tag{5.16}$$

where the normalization factor

$$c = \sum_i \left(\frac{U(x_i)}{\sum_{i=1}^{k} U(x_i)} - \frac{n_i}{N}\right),$$

n_i is the number of patients that have been randomized to the x_i group, and N is the total estimated number of patients in the trial. We will refer to this model as the *utility-offset model*.

Rules for dropping losers   For ethical and economical reasons, we may consider to drop some inferior treatment groups. The issue is how to identify the inferior arms with certain statistical assurance. There are many possible rules for dropping an ineffective dose level. For example, just name a few, (i) maximum sample size ratio between groups that exceeds a threshold, R_n and the number of patients randomized exceeds a N_R, or (ii) the maximum utility difference, $U_{\max} - U_{\min} > \delta_u$ and its naive confidence interval width is less than a threshold, δ_{uw}. The naive confidence interval is calculated as if U_{max} and U_{min} are observed responses with the corresponding sample size at each dose level. Note that the normalized utility index U ranges from 0 to 1. Note that, optionally, we may also choose to retain the control group or all groups for the purpose of comparison between groups.

Stopping rule   Several stopping rules are available for stopping a trial. For example, we may stop the trial when

(i) General rule: total sample size exceeds N, a threshold, or

(ii) Utility rules: maximum utility difference $U_{max} - U_{min} > \delta_u$ and its naive confidence interval width is less than δ_{uw}, or

(iii) Futility Rules: $U_{max} - U_{min} < \delta_f$ and its naive confidence interval width is less than δ_{fw}.

5.3.1   Simulations

Design Settings

Without loss of generality, a total of five dose levels are chosen for the trial simulations. The response rates, $p(U > u)$, associated with each dose level are summarized in Table 5.3.1. These response rates are not chosen from the hyper-logistic model, but arbitrarily in the interest of reflecting common practices.

Table 5.3.1: Assumed Dose-Response Relationship for Simulations

Dose Level	1	2	3	4	5
Dose	20	40	70	95	120
Target Response Rate	0.02	0.07	0.37	0.73	0.52

Response Model

The probability model considered was $p(\mathbf{x}, \mathbf{a}) = P(U \geq u)$ under the hyper-logistic model with three parameters (a_1, a_3, a_4), i.e.,

$$p(\mathbf{x}, \mathbf{a}) = C\left(a_1 \, e^{0.03x} + a_3 e^{-a_4 x}\right)^{-1}, \tag{5.17}$$

where $a_1 \in [0.06, \, 0.1]$, $a_3 \in [150, \, 200]$. The use of scale factor C is a simple way to assure that $0 \leq p_j(\mathbf{x}, \mathbf{a}) \leq 1$ during in the simulation program.

Prior Distribution

Two non-informative priors for parameter a_4 were used for the trial simulations. They are defined over $[0.05, \, 0.1]$ and $[0.01, \, 0.1]$, respectively.

$$a_4 \sim g_0(a_4) = \begin{cases} \frac{1}{b-a}, & a \leq a_4 \leq b \\ 0, & \text{otherwise.} \end{cases} \tag{5.18}$$

Reassessment Method

In the simulations, the hybrid frequentist-Bayesian method was used. We first used the frequentist Least Squares method to estimate the 3 parameters a_i ($i = 1, 3, \, 4$), then use the estimated a_1, a_3, and the prior for a_4 in the model and Bayesian method to obtain the posterior probability distribution of parameter a_4 and the predictive probabilities.

Utility-Adaptive Randomization

Under the *utility-offset model* described earlier, the probability for randomizing a patient to the dose level x_i is given by

$$\Re(x_i) = \begin{cases} \frac{1}{K}, & \text{before an observed responder} \\ C\left(\frac{p(x_i)}{\sum_{i=1}^{k} p(x_i)} - \frac{n_i}{N}\right), & \text{after an observed responder,} \end{cases} \tag{5.19}$$

where $p(\mathbf{x}_i)$ is the response rate or the predictive probability in the Bayesian sense, n_i is the number of patients that have been randomized to the x_i group, N is the total estimated number of patients in the trial, and K is number of dose groups.

Rules of Dropping Losers and Stopping Rule

In the simulations, no losers were dropped. The trial was stopped when the subjects randomized reached the prespecified maximum number.

Simulation Results

Computer simulations were conducted to evaluate the operating characteristics. Four different sample sizes (i.e., N = 20, 30, 50, 100) and two different non-informative priors were used. The outcomes from a typical simulation are presented in Figure 5.3.3. It is shown that predicted response rates are still reasonably good even when the observed (simulated) response rates are showing the sine-shape. The average results from 1000 simulations per scenario are summarized in Table 5.3.2.

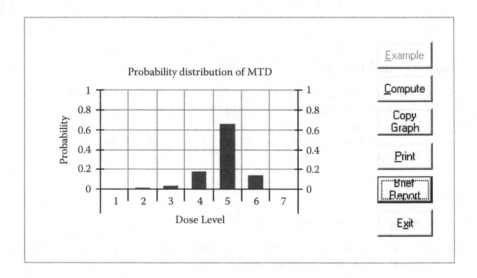

Figure 5.3.3: A typical example of simulation results.

We can see that number of patients randomized into each group is approximately proportional to the corresponding utility or rate in each dose group, which indicates that the utility-adaptive randomization is efficient in achieving the target patient allocations among treatment groups. Compared to traditional balanced designs with multiple arms, the adaptive design smartly allocates a majority of patients to the desirable dose levels. In all cases, the predicted rates are similar to the simulated rates. This is reasonable since non-informative priors were used. The precision of the predictive rate at each dose level is measured by its standard deviation:

$$\delta_p = \sqrt{\frac{1}{N_s} \sum_{i=1}^{N_s} [\hat{p}_i(x) - \bar{p}(x)]^2}, \tag{5.20}$$

Table 5.3.2: Comparisons of Simulation Results[#]

Scenario	Dose Level	1	2	3	4	5
	Target rate	0.02	0.07	0.37	0.73	0.52
$n^* = 100$	Simulated rate	0.02	0.07	0.36	0.73	0.52
	Predicted rate	0.02	0.07	0.41	0.68	0.43
	Standard deviation	0.00	0.01	0.08	0.07	0.03
	Number of subjects	1.71	4.78	25.2	41.8	26.6
$n^* = 50$	Simulated rate	0.02	0.07	0.36	0.73	0.52
	Predicted rate	0.02	0.07	0.40	0.65	0.41
	Standard deviation	0.00	0.02	0.11	0.09	0.04
	Number of subjects	1.02	2.48	12.6	20.5	13.4
$n^* = 30$	Simulated rate	0.02	0.05	0.36	0.73	0.51
	Predicted rate	0.02	0.07	0.40	0.63	0.40
	Standard deviation	0.00	0.02	0.13	0.11	0.05
	Number of subjects	1.00	1.62	7.50	11.9	8.00
$n^* = 20$	Simulated rate	0.02	0.06	0.34	0.72	0.51
	Predicted rate	0.02	0.07	0.37	0.58	0.38
	Standard deviation	0.00	0.02	0.15	0.14	0.06
	Number of subjects	1.00	1.03	4.68	7.60	5.68
$n^{**} = 50$	Simulated rate	0.02	0.07	0.36	0.73	0.51
	Predicted rate	0.02	0.07	0.41	0.65	0.41
	Standard deviation	0.00	0.02	0.11	0.09	0.04
	Number of subjects	1.02	2.53	12.7	20.5	13.3

From simulation software: ExpDesign Studio by www.CTriSoft.net
* Uniform prior over [0.05, 0.1]; ** uniform prior over [0.01, 0.1].

where N_s is the number of simulations, $\hat{p}_i(x)$ is the simulated response rate or predicted response rate, and $\bar{p}(x)$ is the mean response rate at dose level x. The hybrid method provides estimates with reasonable precision when there are 50 subjects (10 subjects per arm on average) or more. The precision reduces when sample size reduces, but the precision is not so bad even at only 20 patients. The relationships between number of subjects and precision for the most interested dose levels (level 3, 4, and 5) are presented in Figure 5.3.4.

The predicted response rates seem not sensitive to the non-informative priors. The simulation results for the two non-informative priors are very similar. Note that precision very much depends upon the number of parameters used in the response model. The more parameters, the less precision. In the simulations a three-parameter hyper-logistic model was used. If single parameter model were used, the precision of the predicted response rates would be greatly improved.

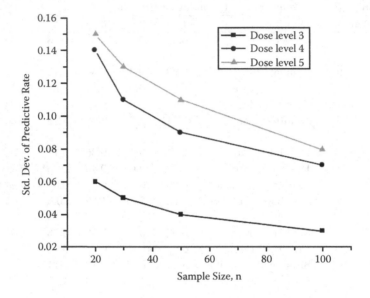

Figure 5.3.4: Relationship between sample size and standard deviation of predictive rate.

5.4   Design Selection and Sample Size

In most protocols of dose-escalation trials, little details regarding design selection and/or sample size calculation/justification are provided. Although many simulations have been performed to empirically compare the TER design and the CRM design and its various modifications, little or no empirical evidence is available regarding the relative performance between the TER trial design and the CRM design. In this section, some criteria for design selection and performance characteristics for sample size determination are proposed.

5.4.1   Criteria for design selection

For selecting an appropriate study design, two criteria based on a fixed sample size approach and a fixed probability of correctly identifying the MTD are commonly considered. For a fixed sample size, the optimal design can be chosen based on one of the following

(i)   Number of DLT expected;

(ii)   Bias and variability of the estimated MTD;

(iii)   Probability of observing DLT prior to MTD; and

(iv)   Probability of correctly identifying the MTD.

In other words, we may choose the design with the highest probability of correctly identifying the MTD. If it is undesirable to have patients experience the DLT, we may choose the design with the smallest number of DLT expected. In practice, we may compromise the above criteria for choosing the most appropriate design to meet our need.

On the other hand, for a fixed probability of correctly identifying the MTD, the optimal design can be chosen based on one of the following:

(i)   Number of patients expected;

(ii)   Number of DLT expected;

(iii)   Bias and variability of the estimated MTD; and

(iv)   Probability of observing DLT prior to MTD.

Thus, we may choose the design with the smallest number of patients expected. If it is desirable to minimize the exposure of patients prior to MTD, we may choose the design with the smallest probability of observing DLT prior to MTD. Similarly, we may compromise the above criteria for choosing the most appropriate design to meet our need.

Note that in some cases, the investigator may be interested in controlling potential overdoses. In this case, we may choose a design with minimum number of patients expected to expose to the dose beyond MTD.

5.4.2 Sample size justification

As indicated above, for most protocols of the dose-escalation trials, little or no details regarding sample size justification is provided. When conducting a clinical trial, Good Statistics Practice (GSP) are necessarily followed for Good Clinical Practice (GCP) in order to ensure the success of the intended clinical trial. Thus, it is suggested that statistical justification for the selected sample size be provided, which will give statistical assurance for achieving the study objectives of the intended trial. Unlike most clinical trials, the traditional pre-study power analysis for sample size calculation is not applicable for dose-escalation trials. For sample size justification of dose-escalation trials, the following performance characteristics are useful: (i) number of DLT expected prior to MTD, (ii) bias and variability of the estimated MTD, (iii) probability of observing DLT prior to MTD, and (iv) probability of correctly identifying the MTD. As an example, consider a dose-escalation trial for identifying MTD of a compound for treatment of a certain cancer. A simulation with 5,000 runs is planned for evaluation of the above performance characteristics. The simulation was conducted under the parameter specifications that

(i) The initial dose was chosen to be 0.3 mg/kg (e.g., one-tenth of LD_{10} in mice);

(ii) Dose range considered is from 0.3 mg/kg to 2.8 mg/kg (the MTD is assumed to be at 2.5 mg/kg);

(iii) Modified Fibonacci sequence is considered. That is, there are six dose levels, which are 0.3, 0.6, 1, 1.5, 2.1, and 2.8 mg/kg; and

(iv) DLT rate at MTD is assumed to be $1/3=33\%$.

For the algorithm-based trial design, the "3+3" TER design and the "3+3" STER design with maximum dose de-escalation allowed $= 1$ are considered. For the CRM method, CRM(n), where n is the number of patients per dose level, n=1, 2, and 3. A logistic toxicity model is assumed. Bayesian approach with a uniform prior is considered for estimation of the parameters of the toxicity model. For CRM(n), the dose escalation and stopping rules include

(i) Number of doses allowed to skip is 0, i.e., dose jump is not allowed;

(ii) Minimum number of patients per dose level before escalation is n;

(iii) Maximum number of patients at a dose level is 6.

Simulation results are summarized in Table 5.4.1.

As it can be seen from Table 5.4.1, the "3+3" TER without dose de-escalation and CRM(2) have smallest number of DLTs expected before reach the MTD. As expected, the "3+3" TER design and the "3+3" STER design underestimate the MTD with larger standard deviations as compared to the CRM(n) trial design. In terms of the probability of correctly identifying the MTD, CRM(n) with n=1 and n=2 are preferred. Sample sizes required for the trial designs under study range from 11 to 18. Based on the overall comparison in terms of the performance characteristics, CRM(n) with n=2 is recommended for the proposed study.

Table 5.4.1: Summary of Simulation Results

Design	#patients expected(N)	# of DLT Expected	Mean MTD(SD)	Prod. of selecting Correct MTD
"3 + 3" TER	15.96	2.8	1.26 (0.33)	0.526
"3 + 3" STER*	17.56	3.2	1.02 (0.30)	0.204
CRM(1)	10.60	3.4	1.51 (0.08)	0.984
CRM(2)	13.57	2.8	1.57 (0.20)	0.884
CRM(3)	16.37	2.7	1.63 (0.26)	0.784

* Allows dose de-escalation.

* CRM(n)=CRM with n patients per dose level; uniform prior was used.

5.5   Concluding Remarks

The proposed utility-adaptive randomization has the desirable property that the proportion of subjects assigned to the treatment is proportional to the response rate or the predictive probability. Assigning more patients to the superior groups allows a more precise evaluation of the superior groups with a relatively small number of patients. The hybrid CRM approach with hyper-logistic model gives reliable predictive results regarding dose response with minimum number of patients. It is important to choose proper ranges for the parameters of the hyper-logistic model, which can be managed when one becomes familiar with the curves of hyper-logistic function affected by its parameters. In the case of low response rates, the sample size is expected to increase accordingly. The hybrid approach allows the users to combine the computational simplicity and numerical stability of the frequentist method with the flexibility in priors and predictive nature of the Bayesian approach. The proposed method can be used in a phase II/III combined study to accelerate the drug development process. However, there are some practical issues such as *how to perform a thorough review when the trial is on-going?* which are necessarily considered for safety of the patients. Since the proposed Bayesian adaptive design is multiple-endpoint oriented, it can be used for various situations. For example, for ordinal responses (e.g., CTC grades), we can consider the different levels of responses as different endpoints, then model them separately, and calculate the expected utility based on the models. Alternatively, we can also form the utility first by assigning different weights to the response levels and then model the utility.

Chapter 6

Adaptive Group Sequential Design

In clinical trials, it is not uncommon to perform data safety monitoring and/or interim analyses based on accrued data up to a certain time point during the conduct of a clinical trial. The purpose is not only to monitor the progress and integrity of the trial, but also to take action regarding early termination (if there is evidence that the trial will put subjects at an unreasonable risk or the treatment is ineffective) or modifications to the study design in compliance with ICH GCP for data standards and data quality. In most clinical trials, the primary reasons for conducting interim analyses of accrued data are probably due to (Jennison and Turnbull, 2000): (i) ethical consideration, (ii) administrative reasons, and (iii) economic constraints. In practice, since clinical trials involve human subjects, it is ethical to monitor the trials to ensure that individual subjects are not exposed to unsafe or ineffective treatment regimens. When the trails are found to be negative (i.e., the treatment appears to be ineffective), there is an ethical imperative to terminate the trials early. Ethical consideration indicates that clinical data should be evaluated in terms of safety and efficacy of the treatment under study based on accumulated data in conjunction with updated clinical information from literature and/or other clinical trials.

From an administrative point of view, interim analyses are necessarily conducted to ensure that the clinical trials are being executed as planned. For example, it is always a concern whether subjects who meet the eligibility criteria are from the correct patient population (which is representative of the target patient population). Also, it is important to assure that the trial procedures, dose/dose regimen and treatment duration are adhered to in the study protocol. An early examination of interim results can reveal the problems (such as protocol deviations and/or protocol violations) of the trials early. Immediate actions can be taken to remedy issues and problems detected by interim analyses. An early interim analysis can also verify critical assumptions made at the planning stage of the trials. If serious violations of the critical assumptions are found, modifications or adjustment must be made to ensure the quality and integrity of the trials.

The remainder of this chapter is organized as follows. In the next section, basic concepts of sequential methods in clinical trials are introduced. In Section 6.2, a unified approach for group sequential designs for normal, binary, and survival endpoints is introduced. In Section 6.3, the boundary function proposed by Wang and Tsiatis (1987) is considered for construction of the stopping boundaries based on equal information intervals. Also included in this section is the discussion of the use of unequal information intervals under a two-stage design which is of practical interest in clinical trials. Section 6.4 introduces a more flexible (adaptive) design, i.e., error-spending approach, where the information intervals and number of analyses are not pre-determined, but the error-spending function is pre-determined. The relationship between error-spending function and Wang and Tsiatis' boundary function is also discussed in this section. A proposed approach for formulating the group sequential design based on independent p-values from the sub-samples from different stages is described in Section 6.5. The formulation is valid regardless of the methods used for calculation of the p-values. Trial monitoring and conditional powers for assessment of futility for comparing means and comparing proportions are derived in Sections 6.7 and 6.8, respectively. Practical issues are given in the last section.

6.1   Sequential Methods

As pointed out by Jennison and Turnbull (2000), the concept of sequential statistical methods was originally motivated for obtaining clinical benefits under certain economic constraints. For a trial with a positive result, early stopping means that a new product can be exploited sooner. If a negative result is indicated, early stopping ensures that resources are not wasted. Sequential methods typically lead to savings in sample size, time, and cost when compared with the standard fixed sample procedures. Interim analyses enable management to make appropriate decisions regarding the allocation of limited resources for continued development of the promising treatment.

In clinical trials, sequential methods are used when there are formal interim analyses. An interim analysis is an analysis intended to assess treatment effect with respect to efficacy or safety at any time prior to the completion of a clinical trail. Because interim analysis results may introduce bias to subsequent clinical evaluation of the subjects who enter the trial, all interim analyses should be carefully planned in advance and described in the study protocol. Under special circumstances, there may be a need for an interim analysis that was not planned originally. In this case, a protocol amendment describing the rationale for such an interim analysis should be implemented prior to any clinical data are unblinded. For many clinical trials of investigational products, especially those that have public attention for major health significance, an external independent group or Data Monitoring Committee (DMC) should be formed to perform clinical data monitoring for safety and interim analysis for efficacy. The U.S. FDA requires that the role/responsibility and function/activities of a DMC be clearly stated in the study protocol to maintain the integrity of the clinical trial (FDA, 2000, 2005c; Offen, 2003).

Basic Concepts

A (fully) sequential test is referred to as a test conducted based on accrued data after every new observation is obtained. A group sequential test, as opposed to a fully sequential test, is referred to as a test performed based on accrued data at some pre-specified intervals rather than after every new observation is obtained (Jennison and Turnbull, 2000).

Error-inflation For a conventional single-stage trial with one-sided $\alpha = 0.025$, the null hypothesis (H_0) is rejected if the statistic $z \geq 1.96$. For a sequential trial with K analyses, if at the k-th analysis $(k = 1, 2, \ldots, K)$, if the absolute value of Z_k is sufficiently large, we will reject H_0 and stop the trial. It is not appropriate to simply apply a level-α one-sided test at each analysis since the multiple tests would lead to an inflation of the type I error rate. In fact, the actual α level is given by $1 - (1 - \alpha^k)$. Thus, for $K = 5$, the actual α level is 0.071, nearly 3 times as big as that of the 0.025 significance level applied at each individual analysis.

Stopping boundary Stopping boundaries consist of a set of critical values that the test statistics calculated from actual data will be comparing with to determine whether the trial should be terminated or continue. An example, Figure 6.1.1, provides a set of critical values as boundaries for stopping. In other words, if the observed sample mean at a given stage falls outside the boundaries, we will terminate the trial; otherwise, the trial continues.

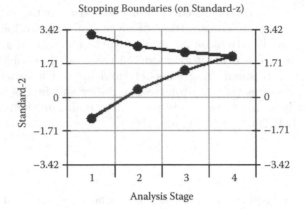

Figure 6.1.1: Stopping boundaries.

Boundary scales   Many different scales can be used to construct the stopping boundaries. The four commonly used scales are the standardized z-statistic, the sample-mean scale, the error-spending scale, and the sum-mean scale. In principle, these scales are equivalent to one another after appropriate transformation. Among the four scales, sample-mean scale and error-spending scales have most intuitive interpretations. As an example, consider the hypothesis for testing difference between two-sample independent means. These scales are defined as follows:

- Sample-mean scale: $\theta_k = \bar{x}_{Ak} - \bar{x}_{Bk}$.

- Standardized z-statistic: $Z_k = \theta_k \sqrt{I_k}$, where $I_k = \frac{n_k}{2\sigma^2}$ is the information level.

- Sum-mean scale: $D_k = \sum_{i=1}^{k} x_{Ai} - \sum_{i=1}^{k} x_{Bi}$.

- Error-spending scale: $\alpha(s_k)$, which is also known as probability scale.

When the number of interim analyses increases, there are too many possible designs with desired α and power. Hence, in practice, it is difficult to select a most appropriate design that can fit our need. Thus, it is suggested using a simple function to define the preferred stopping boundaries. Such a function with a few parameters such as the O'Brien-Fleming, Pocock, Lan-DeMets-Kim, or Wang-Tsiatis's boundary functions are useful.

Optimal/flexible multiple-stage designs In early phase cancer trials, it is undesirable to stop a study early when the test drug is promising. On the other hand, it is desirable to terminate the study as early as possible when the test treatment is not effective due to ethical considerations. For this purpose, an optimal or flexible multiple-stage design is often employed to determine whether the test treatment holds sufficient promise to warrant further testing. In practice, optimal or flexible multiple-stage designs are commonly employed in phase II cancer trials with single arm. These multiple-stage designs include optimal multiple-stage designs such as minimax design and Simon's optimal two-stage design (Simon, 1989; Ensign et al., 1994) and flexible multiple-stage designs (see, e.g., Chen, 1997; Chen and Ng, 1998; Sargent and Goldberg, 2001).

The concept of an optimal two-stage design is to permit early stopping when a moderately long sequence of initial failures occurs, denoted by the number of subjects studied in the first and second stage by n_1 and n_2, respectively. Under a two-stage design, n_1 patients are treated at the first stage. If there are fewer than r_1 responses, then stop the trial. Otherwise, stage 2 is implemented by including the other n_2 patients. A decision regarding whether the test treatment is promising is then made based on the response rate of the $N = n_1 + n_2$ subjects. Let p_0 be the undesirable response rate and p_1 be the desirable response rate ($p_1 > p_0$). If the response rate of a test treatment is at the undesirable level, one may reject it as an ineffective compound with a high probability, and if its response rate is at the desirable level, one may not reject it as a promising compound with a high probability. As a result, under a two-stage trial design, it is of interest to test the following hypotheses:

$$H_0 : p \leq p_0 \quad \text{vs.} \quad H_a : p \geq p_1.$$

Rejection of H_0 (or H_a) means that further (or not further) study if the test treatment should be carried out. Note that under the above hypotheses, the usual type I error is the false positive in accepting an ineffective drug and the type II error is the false negative in rejecting a promising compound. An alternative to the optimal two-stage design described above is so-called flexible two-stage design (Chen and Ng, 1998). The flexible two-stage design simply assumes that the sample sizes are uniformly distributed on a set of k consecutive possible values.

For comparison of multiple arms, Sargent and Goldberg (2001) proposed a flexible optimal design that allows clinical scientists to select the treatment to proceed for further testing based on other factors when the difference in the observed response rates between treatment arms falls into the interval of $[-\delta, \delta]$, where δ is a pre-specified quantity. The proposed rule is that if the observed difference in the response rates of the treatments is larger than δ, then the treatment with the highest observed response rate is selected. On the other hand, if the observed difference is less than or equal to δ, other factors may be considered in the selection. It should be noted that under this framework, it is not essential that the very best treatment is definitely selected; rather it is important that a substantially inferior treatment is not selected when a superior treatment exists.

Remarks Note that in a classic design with a fixed sample size, either a one-sided α of 0.025 or a two-sided α of 0.05 can be used because they will lead to the same results. However, in group sequential trials, two-sided tests should not be used based on the following reasons. For a trial that is designed to allow early stopping for efficacy, when the test drug is significantly worse than the control, the trial may continue to claim efficacy instead of stopping. This is due to the difference in continuation region between a one-sided and a two-sided test, which will have an impact on the differences in the consequent stopping boundaries between the one-sided and the two-sided test. As a result, it is suggested that the relative merits and disadvantages for the use of a one-sided test and a two-sided test should be carefully evaluated. It should be noted that if a two-sided test is used, the significance level α could be inflated (for futility design) or deflated (for efficacy design).

6.2 General Approach for Group Sequential Design

Lan et al. (1992) introduced a unified approach for group sequential trial design. This unified approach is briefly described below. Consider a group sequential study consisting of up to K analyses. Thus, we have a sequence of test statistics $\{Z_1, \ldots, Z_K\}$. Assuming that these statistics follow a joint canonical distribution with information levels $\{I_1, \ldots, I_k\}$ for the parameter. Thus, we have

$$Z_k \sim N(\theta\sqrt{I_k}, 1), 1, \ldots, K,$$

where $Cov(Z_{k_1}, Z_{k_2}) = \sqrt{I_{k_1} I_{k_2}}$, $1 \leq k_1 \leq k_2 \leq K$.

Table 6.2.1 provides formulas for sample size calculations for different types of study endpoints in clinical trials, while Table 6.2.2 summarizes unified formulation for different types of study endpoints under a group sequential design. As an example, for the logrank test in a time-to-event analysis, the information can be expressed as

$$I_k = \frac{r}{(1+r)^2} d_k = \frac{r}{(1+r)^2} \frac{N_k}{\sigma^2},$$

where d_k is the expected number of deaths, N_k is the expected number of patients, and r is the sample size ratio.

Let T_0 and T_{max} be the accrual time and the total follow-up time, respectively. Then, under the condition of exponential survival distribution, we have

$$d_{ik} = \frac{N_{ik}}{T_o}\left(T_o - \frac{1}{\lambda_i e^{\lambda_i T}}\left(e^{\lambda_i T_o} - 1\right)\right), \quad T > T_o; \quad i = 1,2; \quad k = 1,...,K,$$

where d_{ik} is the number of deaths in group i at stage k, and N_{ik} is the number of patients in group i at stage k.

$$\sigma^2 = \frac{N_{1k} + N_{2k}}{d_{1k} + d_{2k}} = \frac{1+r}{\xi_1 + r\xi_2},$$

where

$$\xi_i = 1 - \frac{e^{\lambda_i T_o} - 1}{T_o \lambda_i e^{-\lambda_i T}}.$$

Note that in practice, we may first choose c and α in the stopping boundaries using the conditional probabilities and then perform sample size calculation based on the determined boundaries and the corresponding conditional probabilities for achieving the desired power.

Table 6.2.1: Sample Sizes for Different Types of Endpoints

Endpoint	Sample size	Variance
One mean	$n = \frac{(z_{1-a}+z_{1-\beta})^2 \sigma^2}{\varepsilon^2}$;	
Two means	$n_1 = \frac{(z_{1-a}+z_{1-\beta})^2 \sigma^2}{(1+1/r)^{-1}\varepsilon^2}$;	
One proportion	$n = \frac{(z_{1-a}+z_{1-\beta})^2 \sigma^2}{\varepsilon^2}$;	$\sigma^2 = p(1-p)$
Two proportions	$n_1 = \frac{(z_{1-a}+z_{1-\beta})^2 \sigma^2}{(1+1/r)^{-1}\varepsilon^2}$;	$\sigma^2 = \bar{p}(1-\bar{p})$; $\bar{p} = \frac{n_1 p_1 + n_2 p_2}{n_1 + n_2}$.
One survival curve	$n = \frac{(z_{1-a}+z_{1-\beta})^2 \sigma^2}{\varepsilon^2}$;	$\sigma^2 = \lambda_0^2 \left(1 - \frac{e^{\lambda_0 T_0} - 1}{T_0 \lambda_0 e^{\lambda_0 T_s}}\right)^{-1}$
Two survival curves	$n_1 = \frac{(z_{1-a}+z_{1-\beta})^2 \sigma^2}{(1+1/r)^{-1}\varepsilon^2}$;	$\sigma^2 = \frac{r\sigma_1^2 + \sigma_2^2}{1+r}$, $\sigma_i^2 = \lambda_i^2 \left(1 - \frac{e^{\lambda_i T_0} - 1}{T_0 \lambda_i e^{\lambda_i T_s}}\right)^{-1}$

Note: $r = \frac{n_2}{n_1}$. λ_0 = expected hazard rate, T_0 = uniform patient accrual time and T_s = trial duration. Logrank-test is used for comparison of the two survival curves.

Table 6.2.2: Unified Formulation for Sequential Design

Single mean	$Z_k = (\bar{x}_k - \mu_0)\sqrt{I_k}$	$I_k = \frac{n_k}{\sigma^2}$
Paired means	$Z_k = \bar{d}_k \sqrt{I_k}$	$I_k = \frac{n_k}{\sigma^2}$
Two means	$Z_k = (\bar{x}_{Ak} - \bar{x}_{Bk})\sqrt{I_k}$	$I_k = \left(\frac{\sigma_A^2}{n_{Ak}} + \frac{\sigma_B^2}{n_{Bk}} \right)^{-1}$
One proportion	$Z_k = (p_k - p_0)\sqrt{I_k}$	$I_k = \frac{n_k}{\sigma^2},\ \sigma^2 = \bar{p}(1-\bar{p})$
Two proportions	$Z_k = (p_{Ak} - p_{Bk})\sqrt{I_k}$	$I_k = \frac{1}{\sigma^2} \left(\frac{1}{n_{Ak}} + \frac{1}{n_{Bk}} \right)^{-1},$ $\sigma^2 = \bar{p}(1-\bar{p})$
One survival curve	$Z_k = S_k/\sqrt{I_k}$	$I_k = d_k = \frac{N_k}{\sigma^2},$ σ^2 is given in (6.2.1)
Two survival curves	$Z_k = S_k/\sqrt{I_k}$	$I_k = \frac{r\,d_k}{(1+r)^2} = \frac{r\,N_k}{(1+r)^2\sigma^2},$ σ^2 is given in (6.2.1)

6.3 Early Stopping Boundaries

In clinical trials, it is desirable to stop the trial early if the treatment under investigation is ineffective. On the other hand, if a strong (or highly significant) evidence of efficacy is observed, we may also terminate the trial early. In what follows, we will discuss boundaries for early stopping of a given trial due to (i) efficacy, (ii) futility, and (iii) efficacy or futility assuming that there are a total of K analyses in the trial.

Early Efficacy Stopping

For the case of early stopping for efficacy, we consider testing the one-sided null hypothesis that $H_0 : \mu_A \leq \mu_B$, where μ_A and μ_B could be means, proportions or hazard rates for treatment groups A and B, respectively. The decision rules for early stopping for efficacy are then given by

$$\begin{cases} \text{If } Z_k < \alpha_k, & \text{continue on next stage;} \\ \text{If } Z_k \geq \alpha_k, & \text{stop and reject } H_0, k = 1, ...K - 1, \end{cases}$$

and

$$\begin{cases} \text{If } Z_K < \alpha_K, & \text{stop and accept } H_0; \\ \text{If } Z_K \geq \alpha_K, & \text{stop and reject } H_0. \end{cases}$$

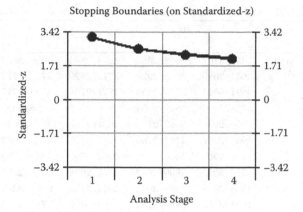

Figure 6.3.1: Stopping boundary for efficacy.

In addition to Pocock's test and O'Brien and Fleming's test, Wang and Tsiatis (1987) proposed a family of two-sided tests indexed by the parameter of Δ, which is also based on the standardized test statistic Z_k. Wang and Tsiatis' test includes Pocock's and O'Brien-Fleming's boundaries as special cases. As a result, in this section, we will simply focus on the method proposed by Wang and Tsiatis (1987). Wang and Tsiatis' boundary function is given by

$$a_k > \alpha_K \left(\frac{k}{K} \right)^{\Delta-1/2},\qquad(6.1)$$

where c is function of $K, \alpha,$ and Δ.

Table 6.3.1A: Final Efficacy Stopping Boundary α_K

			K		
Δ	1	2	3	4	5
0	1.9599	1.9768	2.0043	2.0242	2.0396
0.1		1.9936	2.0258	2.0503	2.0687
0.2		2.0212	2.0595	2.0870	2.1085
0.3		2.0595	2.1115	2.1452	2.1697
0.4		2.1115	2.1850	2.2325	2.2662
0.5		2.1774	2.2891	2.3611	2.4132
0.6		2.2631	2.4270	2.5403	2.6245
0.7		2.3642	2.6061	2.7807	2.9185
0.8		2.4867	2.8297	3.0900	3.3074
0.9		2.6306	3.1022	3.4820	3.8066
1.0		2.7960	3.4268	3.9566	4.4252

Note: Equal info intervals, one-sided $\alpha = 0.025$

Table 6.3.1B: Maximum Sample Size and Expected Sample Size Under Ha

Δ	1	2	3	4	5
			K		
0	3592	3616/3161	3652/2986	3674/2884	3689/2828
0.1		3644/3080	3685/2920	3713/2829	3732/2774
0.2		3691/3014	3739/2855	3771/2768	3794/2717
0.3		3758/2966	3829/2804	3870/2720	3898/2669
0.4		3850/2941	3962/2773	4031/2695	4078/2649
0.5		3968/2937	4161/2780	4285/2715	4374/2682
0.6		4128/2965	4436/2828	4662/2792	4834/2785
0.7		4316/3012	4809/2923	5195/2933	5520/2975
0.8		4548/3088	5288/3063	5914/3135	6487/3249
0.9		4821/3188	5881/3242	6860/3400	7788/3593
1.0		5130/3307	6586/3454	8011/3696	9427/3974

Note: Equal info intervals, one-sided $\alpha = 0.025$, power=85%
and effect size $= 0.01$.

Note that sample sizes N_0 in Table 6.3.1B (also, Table 6.3.2B, 6.3.3B) are generated using ExpDesign Studio® based on effect size $\delta_0 = 0.1$. Therefore, for an effect size δ, the sample size is given by $N = N_0 \left(\frac{0.1}{\delta}\right)^2$.

Example 6.3.1 (normal endpoint) Suppose that an investigator is interested in conducting a clinical trial with five analyses for comparing a test drug (T) with a placebo (P). Based on information obtained from a pilot study, data from the test drug and the placebo seem to have a common variance, i.e., $\sigma^2 = \sigma_1^2 = \sigma_2^2 = 4$ with $\mu_T - \mu_P = 1$. Assuming these observed values are true, it is desirable to select a maximum sample size such that there is a 85% power $(1 - \beta = 0.85)$ for detecting such a difference between the test drug and the placebo at the 2.5% (one-sided $\alpha = 0.025$) level of significance. The Wang and Tsiatis' stopping boundary with $\Delta = 0.3$ is used.

The stopping boundaries are given in Table 6.3.1A. From Table 6.3.1A, $\alpha_5 = 2.1697$. Since the effect size $\delta = \frac{\mu_T - \mu_P}{\sigma} = 0.5$, the required sample size for a classic design when there are no planned interim analyses is

$$N_{\text{fixed}} = 3592 \left(\frac{0.1}{0.5}\right)^2 = 144.$$

The maximum sample is given by

$$N_{\text{max}} = 3898 \left(\frac{0.1}{0.5}\right)^2 = 156,$$

while the expected sample size under the alternative hypothesis is

$$N = 2669 \left(\frac{0.1}{0.5}\right)^2 = 107.$$

Hence, the sample size required for each interim analysis is $156/5 = 31$.

Early Futility Stopping

For the case of early stopping for futility, similarly, we consider testing the one-sided null hypothesis that $Ho : \mu_A \leq \mu_B$, where μ_A and μ_B could be means, proportions or hazard rates for treatment groups A and B, respectively. The decision rules for early stopping for futility are then given by

$$\begin{cases} \text{If } Z_k < \beta_k, & \text{stop and accept } H_0; \\ \text{If } Z_k \geq \beta_k, & \text{continue on next stage, } k = 1, ...K - 1, \end{cases}$$

and

$$\begin{cases} \text{If } Z_K < \beta_K, \text{ stop and accept } H_0; \\ \text{If } Z_K \geq \beta_K, \text{ stop and reject } H_0. \end{cases}$$

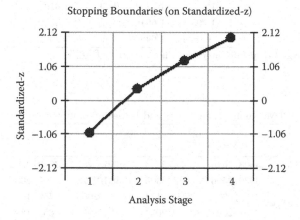

Figure 6.3.2: Stopping boundary for futility.

We propose an inner futility stopping boundary that is symmetric to the Wang and Tsiatis' efficacy stopping boundary on the z-scale and triangular boundary, which are given below, respectively

- Symmetric boundary:

$$\beta_k > 2\beta_K \sqrt{\frac{k}{K}} - \beta_K \left(\frac{k}{K}\right)^{\Delta - 1/2}. \tag{6.2}$$

- Triangular boundary:

$$\beta_k = \beta_K \frac{k - k_0}{K - k_0}, \text{where } k_0 = \left[\frac{K}{2}\right] + 1. \tag{6.3}$$

where $[x]$ is the integer part of x.

Table 6.3.2A: Final Symmetric Futility Stopping Boundary β_K

			K		
Δ	1	2	3	4	5
0	1.9599	1.9546	1.9431	1.9316	1.9224
0.1		1.9500	1.9339	1.9201	1.9098
0.2		1.9419	1.9224	1.9063	1.8926
0.3		1.9316	1.9063	1.8857	1.8696
0.4		1.9155	1.8834	1.8581	1.8374
0.5		1.8972	1.8535	1.8202	1.7938
0.6		1.8765	1.8191	1.7754	1.7398
0.7		1.8512	1.7777	1.7238	1.6790
0.8		1.8237	1.7364	1.6698	1.6169
0.9		1.7950	1.6916	1.6169	1.5572
1.0		1.7651	1.6480	1.5641	1.4998

Note: Equal info intervals, one-sided $\alpha = 0.025$

Table 6.3.2B: Maximum Sample Size and Expected Sample Size Under H_0

			K		
Δ	1	2	3	4	5
0	3592	3608/2616	3636/2433	3656/2287	3672/2202
0.1		3626/2496	3658/2305	3683/2178	3705/2096
0.2		3655/2396	3700/2174	3734/2053	3759/1974
0.3		3701/2321	3770/2054	3817/1924	3855/1845
0.4		3761/2267	3874/1960	3956/1815	4020/1728
0.5		3845/2241	4024/1901	4165/1742	4285/1648
0.6		3950/2238	4223/1880	4454/1713	4662/1618
0.7		4073/2254	4459/1889	4805/1723	5131/1632
0.8		4207/2285	4726/1923	5196/1761	5651/1675
0.9		4352/2327	4999/1971	5594/1813	6167/1732
1.0		4500/2376	5266/2026	5963/1868	6632/1788

Note: Equal info intervals, one-sided $\alpha = 0.025$ and $\delta = 0.1$.Power = 85%

Example 6.3.2 (binary endpoint) Suppose that an investigator is interested in conducting a group sequential trial comparing a test drug with a placebo. The primary efficacy study endpoint is a binary response. Based on information obtained in a pilot study, the response rates for the test drug and the placebo are given by 20% ($p_1 = 0.20$) and 30% ($p_2 = 0.30$), respectively. Suppose that a total of 2 ($K = 2$) analyses are planned. It is desirable to select a maximum sample size in order to have an 85% ($1 - \beta = 0.85$) power at the 2.5% (one-sided $\alpha = 0.025$) level of significance. The effect size

$$\delta = \frac{p_2 - p_1}{\sqrt{(\bar{p}(1 - \bar{p})}} = \frac{0.3 - 0.2}{\sqrt{0.25(1 - 0.25)}} = 0.23094.$$

If a symmetric inner boundary boundaries are used with $\Delta = 0.6$, which is an optimal design with the minimum expected sample size under the null hypothesis. From table 6.3.2A, $\beta_2 = 1.8765$, and from (6.2), we have

$$\begin{aligned}
\beta_1 &= 2\beta_K\sqrt{\frac{k}{K}} - \beta_K(\frac{k}{K})^{\Delta - 1/2} \\
&= 2(1.8765)\sqrt{1/2} - 1.8765\,(1/2)^{0.6 - 0.5} \\
&= 0.902\,94.
\end{aligned}$$

From Table 6.3.2B, the sample size needed for a fixed sample size design is

$$N_{\text{fixed}} = 3592\left(\frac{0.1}{0.23094}\right)^2 = 674.$$

The maximum sample size and the expected sample size under the null hypothesis are

$$N_{\max} = 3950\left(\frac{0.1}{0.23094}\right)^2 = 742$$

and

$$N_{\exp} = 2238\left(\frac{0.1}{0.23094}\right)^2 = 420.$$

Early Efficacy-Futility Stopping

For the case of early stopping for efficacy or futility, similarly, we consider testing the one-sided null hypothesis that $Ho : \mu_A \leq \mu_B$, where μ_A and μ_B could be means, proportions or hazard rates for treatment groups A and B, respectively. The decision rules for early stopping for efficacy or futility are then given by

$$\begin{cases} \text{If } Z_k < \beta_k, \ (k = 1, ...K), & \text{stop and accept } H_0; \\ \text{If } Z_k \geq \alpha_k, \ (k = 1, ...K), & \text{stop and reject } H_0. \end{cases}$$

The stopping boundaries are the combination of the previous efficacy and futility stopping boundaries, i.e.,

Symmetric boundary

$$\begin{cases} a_k = \alpha_K (k/K)^{\Delta-1/2} \\ \beta_k = 2\beta_K \sqrt{\frac{k}{K}} - \beta_K (\frac{k}{K})^{\Delta-1/2} \end{cases} \tag{6.4}$$

Triangle boundary

$$\begin{cases} a_k = \alpha_K (k/K)^{\Delta-1/2} \\ \beta_k = \beta_K \frac{k-k_0}{K-k_0}, \end{cases} \tag{6.5}$$

where the starting inner boundary is given by $k_0 = \left[\frac{K}{2}\right] + 1$.

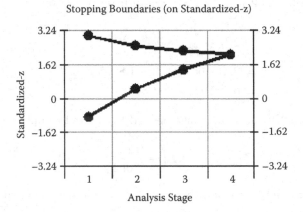

Figure 6.3.3: Stopping boundary for efficacy or futility.

Table 6.3.3A: Final Stopping Boundaries $\alpha_K = \beta_K$

Δ	K				
	1	2	3	4	5
0	1.9599	1.9730	1.9902	2.0028	2.0143
0.1		1.9856	2.0074	2.0235	2.0373
0.2		2.0074	2.0361	2.0568	2.0717
0.3		2.0396	2.0821	2.1096	2.1303
0.4		2.0866	2.1521	2.1946	2.2256
0.5		2.1487	2.2532	2.3301	2.3737
0.6		2.2290	2.3898	2.5035	2.5896
0.7		2.3301	2.5678	2.7458	2.8871
0.8		2.4530	2.7929	3.0593	3.2798
0.9		2.6000	3.0685	3.4475	3.7759
1.0		2.7722	3.3947	3.9183	4.3823

Note: Equal info intervals, one-sided $\alpha = 0.025$.

Table 6.3.3B: Maximum Sample Size and Expected Sample Size Under H_0 and H_a

Δ	K 1	2	3	4	5
0	3592	3636/2722/3142	3698/2558/2942	3744/2420/2826	3785/2346/2764
0.1		3680/2615/3050	3758/2449/2868	3818/2333/2760	3868/2260/2698
0.2		3755/2534/2974	3860/2342/2793	3937/2236/2692	3995/2167/2628
0.3		3868/2484/2918	4024/2251/2728	4128/2140/2628	4207/2073/2567
0.4		4037/2472/2893	4280/2193/2689	4442/2067/2587	4562/1994/2527
0.5		4265/2497/2897	4662/2181/2687	4931/2034/2584	5136/1950/2527
0.6		4573/2568/2937	5209/2226/2726	5675/2059/2630	6038/1959/2578
0.7		4984/2695/3017	5985/2348/2816	6775/2164/2724	7427/2047/2677
0.8		5525/2891/3143	7078/2580/2967	8402/2397/2879	9574/2272/2830
0.9		6238/3180/3327	8619/2972/3207	10805/2835/3131	12885/2736/3083
1.0		6238/3180/3327	10784/3591/3591	14358/3590/3590	17953/3591/3591

Note: Equal info intervals, one-sided $\alpha = 0.025$, $\delta = 0.1$, power $= 85.\%$

Example 6.3.3 (survival endpoint) Suppose that an investigator is interested in conducting a survival trial with 3 ($K = 3$) analyses at the 2.5% level of significance (one-sided $\alpha = 0.025$) with an 85% ($1 - \beta = 0.85$) power. Assume that median survival time is 0.990 year ($\lambda_1 = 0.7$/Year) for group 1, 0.693 year ($\lambda_2 = 1$/Year) for group 2. $T_0 = 1$ year and study duration $T_s = 2$ years. Using

$$\sigma_i^2 = \lambda_i^2 \left(1 - \frac{e^{\lambda_i T_0} - 1}{T_0 \lambda_i e^{\lambda_i T_s}} \right)^{-1},$$

we obtain $\sigma_1^2 = 0.762\,2$, and $\sigma_2^2 = 1.303$. Note that

$$\delta = \frac{\lambda_2 - \lambda_1}{\sigma} = \frac{1 - 0.7}{\sqrt{0.762\,2 + 1.303}} = 0.208\,76.$$

The stopping boundaries ($\Delta = 0.1$) are given by $\alpha_3 = \beta_3 = 2.0074$ (Table 6.3.3A). Thus, we have

$$\alpha_1 = 3.115\,2, \quad \alpha_2 = 2.360\,9;$$
$$\beta_1 = -0.797\,23, \beta_2 = 0.917\,21.$$

Thus,

$$N_{\text{fixed}} = \frac{(z_{\alpha/2} + z_\beta)^2 \left(\sigma_1^2 + \sigma_2^2 \right)}{(\lambda_2 - \lambda_1)^2}$$
$$= \frac{(1.96 + 1.0364)^2 (0.762\,2 + 1.303)}{(1 - 0.7)^2}$$
$$= 206.$$

The maximum sample size is given by

$$N_{\max} = 3758 \left(\frac{0.1}{0.20876} \right)^2 = 862.$$

The expected sample size under the null hypothesis is given by

$$\bar{N}_o = 2449 \left(\frac{0.1}{0.20876} \right)^2 = 562.$$

The expected sample size under the alternative hypothesis is given by

$$\bar{N}_a = 2868 \left(\frac{0.1}{0.20876} \right)^2 = 658.$$

6.4 Alpha Spending Function

Lan and DeMets (1983) proposed to distribute (or spend) the total probability of false positive risk as a continuous function of the information time in group sequential procedures for interim analyses. If the total information scheduled to accumulate over the maximum duration T is known, the boundaries can be computed as a continuous function of the information time. This continuous function of the information time is referred to as the alpha spending function, denoted by $\alpha(s)$. The alpha spending function is an increasing function of information time. It is 0 when the information time is 0; and is equal to the overall significance level when information time is 1. In other words, $\alpha(0) = 0$ and $\alpha(1) = \alpha$. Let s_1 and s_2 be two information times, $0 < s_1 < s_2 \leq 1$. Also, denote $\alpha(s_1)$ and $\alpha(s_2)$ as their corresponding value of alpha spending function at s_1 and s_2. Then,

$$0 < \alpha(s_1) < \alpha(s_2) \leq \alpha.$$

$\alpha(s_1)$ is the probability of type I error one wishes to spend at information time s_1. For a given alpha spending function $\alpha(s)$ and a series of standardized test statistic $Z_k, k = 1, ..., K$. The corresponding boundaries $c_k, k = 1, ..., K$ are chosen such that under the null hypothesis

$$P(Z_1 < c_1, ..., Z_{k-1} < c_{k-1}, Z_k \geq c_k)$$
$$= \alpha \left(\frac{k}{K} \right) - \alpha \left(\frac{k-1}{K} \right).$$

Some commonly used alpha-spending functions are summarized in the following table.

Table 6.4.1: Error Spending Functions

O'Brien-Fleming	$\alpha_1(s) = 2\{1 - \Phi(z_\alpha / \sqrt{2})$
Pocock	$\alpha_2(s) = \alpha \log \left[1 + (e - 1)s \right]$
Lan-DeMets-Kim	$\alpha_3(s) = \alpha s^\theta, \theta > 0$
Hwang-Shih	$\alpha_4(s) = \alpha[(1 - e^{\zeta s})/(1 - e^{-\zeta})], \zeta \neq 0$

We now introduce the procedure for sample size calculation based on Lan-DeMets' alpha spending function, i.e.,

$$\alpha(s) = \alpha s^{\theta}, \theta > 0.$$

Although alpha spending function does not require a fixed maximum number and equal spaced interim analyses, it is necessary to make those assumptions in order to calculate the sample size under the alternative hypothesis. The sample size calculation can be performed using computer simulations. As an example, in order to achieve a 90% power at the one-sided 2.5% level of significance, it is necessary to have $n_{\text{fixed}} = 84$ subjects per treatment group for classic design. The maximum sample size needed for achieving the desired power with five interim analyses using the Lan-DeMets type alpha spending function with $\delta = 2$ can be calculated as 92 subjects.

6.5 Group Sequential Design Based on Independent P-values

In this section, we discuss n-stage adaptive design based on individual p-values from each stage proposed by Chang (Chang, 2005). In an adaptive group sequential design with K stages, a hypothesis test is performed at each stage, followed by certain actions according to the outcomes. Such actions could be early stopping for efficacy or futility, sample size re-estimation, modification of randomization, or other adaptations. At the kth stage, a typical set of hypotheses for the treatment difference is given by

$$H_{0k}: \eta_{k1} \geq \eta_{k2} \quad \text{vs.} \quad H_{ak}: \eta_{k1} < \eta_{k2}, \tag{6.7}$$

where η_{k1} and η_{k2} are the treatment response such as mean, proportion or survival at the kth stage. We denote the test statistic for H_{0k} and the corresponding p-value by T_k and p_k, respectively.

The global test for the null hypothesis of no treatment effect can be written as an intersection of the individual hypotheses at different stages.

$$H_0: H_{01} \cap ... \cap H_{0K}, \tag{6.8}$$

Note that a one-sided test is assumed in this chapter. At the kth stage, the decision rules are given by

$$\begin{cases} \text{Stop for efficacy} & \text{if } T_k \leq \alpha_k, \\ \text{Stop for futility} & \text{if } T_k > \beta_k, \\ \text{Continue with adaptations} & \text{if } \alpha_k < T_k \leq \beta_k, \end{cases} \tag{6.9}$$

where $\alpha_k < \beta_k$ ($k = 1, ..., K - 1$), and $\alpha_K = \beta_K$. For convenience's sake, α_k and β_k are referred to as the efficacy and futility boundaries, respectively.

To reach the kth-stage, a trial has to pass all stages up to the $(k-1)^{th}$ stages, i.e.,

$$0 \le \alpha_i < T_i \le \beta_i \le 1 (i = 1, ..., k-1).$$

Therefore, the cumulative distribution function of T_k is given by

$$
\begin{aligned}
\varphi_k(t) &= \Pr(T_k < t, \alpha_1 < t_1 \le \beta_1, ..., \alpha_{k-1} < t_{k-1} \le \beta_{k-1}) \\
&= \int_{\alpha_1}^{\beta_1} \cdots \int_{\alpha_{k-1}}^{\beta_{k-1}} \int_0^t f_{T_1...T_k} \, dt_k \, dt_{k-1}...dt_1,
\end{aligned}
\tag{6.10}
$$

where $f_{T_1...T_k}$ is the joint probability density function of $T_1, ...,$ and T_k, and t_i is realization of T_i.

The joint probability density function $f_{T_1...T_k}$ in (6.5) can be any density functions. However, it is desirable to choose T_i such that $f_{T_1...T_k}$ has a simple form. Note that when $\eta_{k1} = \eta_{k2}$, the p-value p_k from the sub-sample at the kth stage is uniformly distributed on [0,1] under H_0 and p_k ($k = 1, ..., K$) are mutually independent. These two desirable properties can be used to construct test statistics for adaptive designs.

The simplest form of the test statistic at the kth stage is given by

$$T_k = p_k, \quad k = 1, ..., K, \tag{6.11}$$

Due to independence of p_k, $f_{T_1...T_k} = 1$ under H_0 and

$$\varphi_k(t) = t \prod_{i=1}^{k-1} L_i. \tag{6.12}$$

where $L_i = (\beta_i - \alpha_i)$. For convenience's sake, when the upper bound exceeds the lower bound, define $\prod_{i=1}^K (\cdot) = 1$. It is obvious that the error rate (α spent) at the kth stage is given by

$$\pi_k = \varphi_k(\alpha_k). \tag{6.13}$$

When the efficacy is claimed at a certain stage, the trial is stopped. Therefore, the type I errors at different stages are mutually exclusive. Hence, the experiment-wise type I error rate can be written as

$$\alpha = \sum_{k=1}^K \pi_k. \tag{6.14}$$

From (6.14), the experiment-wise type I error rate is given by

$$\alpha = \sum_{k=1}^K \alpha_k \prod_{i=1}^{k-1} L_i. \tag{6.15}$$

Note that (6.15) is the necessary and sufficient condition for determination of the stopping boundaries (α_i, β_i).

6.6 Calculation of Stopping Boundaries

Two-Stage Design

For a two-stage design, (6.15) becomes

$$\alpha = \alpha_1 + \alpha_2(\beta_1 - \alpha_1). \qquad (6.16)$$

For convenience's sake, a table of stopping boundaries is constructed using (6.16) (Table 6.6.1). The adjusted p-value is given by

$$p(t, k) = \begin{cases} t & \text{if } k = 1, \\ \alpha_1 + (\beta_1 - \alpha_1)t & \text{if } k = 2. \end{cases} \qquad (6.17)$$

Table 6.6.1: Stopping Boundaries for Two-Stage Designs

β_1	α_1	0.000	0.005	0.010	0.015	0.020
0.15		0.1667	0.1379	0.1071	0.0741	0.0385
0.20		0.1250	0.1026	0.0789	0.0541	0.0278
0.25		0.1000	0.0816	0.0625	0.0426	0.0217
0.30		0.0833	0.0678	0.0517	0.0351	0.0179
0.35	α_2	0.0714	0.0580	0.0441	0.0299	0.0152
0.40		0.0625	0.0506	0.0385	0.026	0.0132
0.50		0.0500	0.0404	0.0306	0.0206	0.0104
0.80		0.0312	0.0252	0.0190	0.0127	0.0064
1.00		0.0250	0.0201	0.0152	0.0102	0.0051

Note: One-sided $\alpha = 0.025$.

K-Stage Design

For K-stage designs, it is convenient to define a function for L_i and α_i. Such functions could be of the form

$$L_k = b\left(\frac{1}{k} - \frac{1}{K}\right), \qquad (6.18)$$

and

$$a_k = c\,k^\theta \alpha, \qquad (6.19)$$

where b, c and θ are constants. Because of the equality $L_k^* = \beta_k - \alpha_k$, the futility boundaries become

$$\beta_k = b\left(\frac{1}{k} - \frac{1}{K}\right) + ck^{\theta}\alpha. \tag{6.20}$$

Note that the coefficient b is used to determine how fast the continuation band shrinks when a trial proceeds from one stage to another. θ is used to determine the curvity of the stopping boundaries α_k and β_k. Substituting (6.18) and (6.19) into (6.16) and solving it for constant c, leads to

$$c = \left[\sum_{k=1}^{K}\left\{b^{k-1}k^{\theta}\prod_{i=1}^{k-1}(\frac{1}{i} - \frac{1}{K})\right\}\right]^{-1} \tag{6.21}$$

When K, b and θ are pre-determined, (6.21) can be used to obtain c. Then, (6.19) and (6.20) can be used to obtain the stopping boundaries α_k and β_k. For convenience, constant c is tabulated for different b, θ and K (Table 6.6.2).

Note that when $\theta < 0$, $\theta > 0$, and $\theta = 0$, the efficacy stopping boundaries are a monotonically decreasing function of k, an increasing function of k, and a constant, respectively. When the constant b increases, the continuation-band bound by the futility and efficacy stopping boundaries will shrink faster. It is suggested that b should be small enough such that all $\beta_k < 1$. Also, it should be noted that $L_K = 0$.

Table 6.6.2: Constant c in (6.21)

b	θ	K 2	3	4	5	6
0.25	-0.5	0.9188	0.8914	0.8776	0.8693	0.8638
	0.0	0.8889	0.8521	0.8337	0.8227	0.8154
	0.5	0.8498	0.8015	0.7776	0.7635	0.7540
	1.0	0.8000	0.7385	0.7087	0.6911	0.6795
0.50	-0.5	0.8498	0.7989	0.7733	0.7578	0.7475
	0.0	0.8000	0.7347	0.7023	0.6830	0.6702
	0.5	0.7388	0.6581	0.6190	0.5960	0.5808
	1.0	0.6667	0.5714	0.5267	0.5009	0.4840
0.75	-0.5	0.7904	0.7196	0.6840	0.6626	0.6483
	0.0	0.7273	0.6400	0.5972	0.5718	0.5549
	0.5	0.6535	0.5509	0.5022	0.4738	0.4553
	1.0	0.5714	0.4571	0.4052	0.3757	0.3567
1.00	-0.5	0.7388	0.6512	0.6074	0.5811	0.5635
	0.0	0.6667	0.5625	0.5120	0.4823	0.4627
	0.5	0.5858	0.4683	0.4138	0.3825	0.3622
	1.0	0.5000	0.3750	0.3200	0.2894	0.2699

Trial Examples

To illustrate the group sequential methods described in the previous section, in what follows, two examples concerning clinical trials with group sequential designs are given. For illustration purposes, these two examples have been modified slightly from actual trials.

Example 6.6.1 Consider a two-arm comparative oncology trial comparing a test treatment with a control. Suppose that the primary efficacy endpoint of interest is time to disease progression (TTP). Based on data from previous studies, the median time for TTP is estimated to be 8 months (hazard rate = 0.08664) for the control group, and 10.5 months (hazard rate = 0.06601) for the test treatment group. Assume that there is a uniform enrollment with an accrual period of 9 months, and the total study duration is expected to be 24 months. The logrank test will be used for the analysis. Sample size calculation will be performed under the assumption of an exponential survival distribution.

Assuming that the median time for TTP for the treatment group is 10.5 months, the classic design requires a sample size of 290 per treatment group in order to achieve an 80% power at the $\alpha = 0.025$ level of significance (based on a one-sided test). Suppose that an adaptive group sequential design is considered in order to improve efficiency and allow some flexibility of the trial. Under an adaptive group sequential design with an interim analysis, a sample size of 175 patients per treatment group is needed for controlling the overall type I error rate at 0.025 and for achieving the desired power of 80%. The interim analysis allows for early stopping for efficacy with stopping boundaries $\alpha_1 = 0.01$, $\beta_1 = 0.25$, and $\alpha_2 = 0.0625$ from Table 6.6.1). The maximum sample size allowed for adjustment is $n_{\max} = 350$. Note that the simulation results are summarized in Table 6.6.3, where EESP and EFSP stand for early efficacy stopping probability and early futility stopping probability, respectively.

Table 6.6.3: Operating Characteristics of Adaptive Methods

| Median time | | | | Expected | |
Test	Control	EESP	EFSP	N	Power (%)
0	0	0.010	0.750	216	2.5
10.5	8	0.440	0.067	254	79

Note: 1,000,000 simulation runs.

Note that power is the probability of rejecting the null hypothesis. Therefore, when the null hypothesis is true, the power is equal to the type I error rate α. From Table 6.6.3, it can be seen that the one-sided α is controlled at the 0.025 level as expected. The expected sample sizes under both hypothesis conditions are smaller than the sample size for the classic design (290/group). The power under the alternative hypothesis is 79%.

To demonstrate the calculation of the adjusted p-value, assume that (i) naive p-values from the logrank test (or other tests) are $p_1 = 0.1$ and $p_2 = 0.07$, and (ii) the trial stops at stage 2. Therefore, $t = p_2 = 0.07 > \alpha_2 = 0.0625$, and we fail to reject the null hypothesis of no treatment difference.

Example 6.6.2 Consider a phase III, randomized, placebo-controlled, parallel group study for evaluation of the effectiveness of a test treatment in adult asthmatics. Efficacy will be assessed based on the forced expiratory volume in one second (FEV1). The primary endpoint is the change in FEV1 from baseline. Based on data from phase II studies and other resources, the difference in FEV1 change from baseline between the test drug and the control is estimated to be $\delta = 8.18\%$ with a standard deviation σ of 18.26%. The classic design requires 87 subjects per group for achieving an 85% power at the significance level of $\alpha = 0.025$ (based on a one-sided test). Alternatively, a 4-stage adaptive group sequential design is considered for allowing comparisons at various stages. The details of the design and the corresponding operating characteristics are given in Table 6.6.4 and Table 6.6.5, respectively.

Table 6.6.4: Four-Stage Adaptive Design Specifications

Design	Scenario	Stage k 1	2	3	4
	α_i	0.01317	0.02634	0.03950	0.05267
	β_i	0.38817	0.15134	0.08117	0.05267
GSD	N	60	120	170	220
	α_i	0.00800	0.01600	0.02400	0.03200
	β_i	0.78200	0.28200	0.11533	0.03200
GSD	N	50	95	135	180

Note: For design 1 and 2, b=0.5, $\theta = 1$, and c = 0.5267.
For design 3 and 4, b=0.5, $\theta = 1$, and c = 0.5267.
In design 2 and 4, sample size adjustment is allowed with $N_{max} = 300$.

Note that the two sequential designs and the classic design have the same expected sample size under the alternative hypothesis condition. The two sequential designs have an increase in power as compared to the classic design.

Table 6.6.5: Operating Characteristics of Various Designs

Design	Scenario	Expected N	Range of N	Power (%)
Classic	H_o	87	87-87	2.5
	H_a	87		85
GSD 1	H_o	85	60-220	2.5
	H_a	87		94
GSD 2	H_o	92	50-180	2.5
	H_a	87		89

Note: 500,000 and 100,000 simulation runs for each H_0 and H_a scenarios, respectively.

6.7 Group Sequential Trial Monitoring

Data Monitoring Committee

As indicated in Offen (2003), the stopping rule can only serve as a guide for stopping a trial. For clinical trials with group sequential design, a Data Monitoring Committee (DMC) is usually formed. The DMC will usually evaluate all aspects of clinical trial including integrity, quality, benefits and the associated risks before a decision regarding the termination of the trial can be reached (Ellenberg, Fleming and DeMets, 2002). In practice, it is recognized that although all aspects of the conduct of the clinical trial adhered exactly to the conditions stipulated during the design phase, the stopping rule chosen at the design phase may not be used directly because there are usually complicated factors that must be dealt with before such a decision can be made. It what follows, the rationales of why we need to closely monitor a group sequential trial are briefly outlined.

DMC meetings are typically scheduled based on the availability of its members, which may be different from the schedules as specified at the design phase. In addition, the enrollment may be different from the assumption made at the design phase. The deviation of the analysis schedule will affect the stopping boundaries. Therefore, the boundaries should be recalculated based on the actual schedules.

In practice, the variability of the response variable is usually unknown. At interim analysis, an estimate of the variability can be obtained based on the actual data collected for the interim analysis. However, the estimate may be different from the initial guess of the variability at the design phase. The deviation of the variability will certainly affect the stopping boundaries. In this case, it is of interest to study the likelihood of success of the trial based on current available information such as conditional and predictive power and repeated confidence intervals. Similarly, the estimation of treatment difference in response could be different from the original expectation in the design phase.

This could lead to the use of an adaptive design or sample size re-estimation (Jennison and Turnbull, 2000).

In general, efficacy is not the only factor that will affect DMC's recommendation regarding the stop or continue of the trial. Safety factors are critical for DMC to make an appropriate recommendation to stop or continue the trial. The term benefit-risk ratio is probably the most commonly used composite criterion in assisting the decision making. In this respect, it is desirable to know the likelihood of success of the trial based on the conditional power or the predictive power.

In many clinical trials, the company may need to make critical decisions on their spending during the conduct of the trials due to some financial constraints. In this situation, the concept of benefit-risk ratio is also helpful but viewed from the financial perspective. In practice, the conditional and/or predictive powers are tools for the decision making. In group sequential trials, the simplest tool that is commonly used for determining whether or not to continue or terminate a trial is the use of sequential stopping boundaries. The original methodology for group sequential boundaries required that the number and timing of interim analyses be specified in advance in the study protocol. Whitehead (1983, 1994) introduced another type of stopping boundary method (the Whitehead triangle boundaries). This method permits unlimited analyses as the trial progresses. This method is referred to as a continuous monitoring procedure. In general, group sequential methods allow for symmetric or asymmetric boundaries. Symmetric boundaries would demand the same level of evidence to terminate the trial early and claim either lack of a beneficial effect or establishment of a harmful effect. Asymmetric boundaries might allow for less evidence for negative harmful trend before an early termination is recommended. For example, the O'Brien-Fleming sequential boundary might be used for monitoring beneficial effects, while a Pocock-type sequential boundary could provide guidance for safety monitoring.

A practical and yet complicated method is to use the operating characteristics desired for the design which typically include false positive error rate, the power curve , the sample size distribution or information levels, the estimates of treatment effect that would correspond to early stopping, the naive confidence interval, repeated confidence intervals, the curtailment (conditional power and predictive powers), and the futility index. Both the *conditional power* and the predictive power are the likelihood of rejecting the alternative hypothesis conditioning on the current data. The difference is that the *conditional power* is based on a frequentist approach, and the *predictive power* is a Bayesian approach. *Futility index* is a measure of the likelihood of failure to reject Ho at k analysis given that H_a is true. The defining property of a (1-α)-level sequence of repeated confidence interval (RCI) for θ is

$$\Pr\left\{\theta \in I_k \text{ for } all \ k = 1, ..., K\right\} = 1 - \alpha.$$

Here each I_k (k = 1,..., K) is an interval computed from the information available at analysis k. The calculation of the RCI at analysis k is similar to the naive confidence interval but $z_{1-\alpha}$ is replaced with α_k, the stopping boundary on the standard z-statistic. For example, $CI = d \pm z_{1-\alpha}\sigma$; $RCI = d \pm \alpha_k\sigma$(Jennison and Turnbull, 2000)

The conditional power method can be used to assess whether an early trend is sufficiently unfavorable so that reversal to a significant positive trend is very unlikely or nearly impossible. The futility index can also be used to monitor a trial. Prematurely terminating a trial with a very small futility index might be inappropriate. It is the same for continuing a trial with very high futility index.

Principles for Monitoring a Sequential Trial

Ellenberg, Fleming and DeMets (2002) shared their experiences on DMC and provided the following useful principles for monitoring a sequential trial.

Short-term vs. long-term treatment effects When early data from the clinical trial appear to provide compelling evidence for short-term treatment effects, and yet the duration of patient follow-up is insufficient to assess long-term treatment efficacy and safety, early termination may not be warranted and perhaps could even raise ethical issues. The relative importance of short-term and long-term results depends on the clinical setting.

Early termination philosophies Three issues should be addressed. First, what magnitude of estimated treatment difference, and over what period of time, would be necessary before a beneficial trend would be sufficiently convincing to warrant early termination? Second, should the same level of evidence be required for a negative trend as for a positive trend before recommending early termination? Third, for a trial with no apparent trend, should the study continue to the scheduled termination?

Responding to early beneficial trends Determination of optimal length of follow-up can be difficult in a clinical trial having an early beneficial trend. Ideally, evaluating the duration of treatment benefit while continuing to assess possible side-effects over a longer period of time would provide the maximum information for clinical use. However, for patients with life-threatening diseases such as heart failure, cancer, or advanced HIV/AIDS, strong evidence of substantial short-term therapeutic benefits may be compelling even if it is unknown whether these benefits are sustained over the long term. Under these circumstances, early termination might be justified to take advantage of this important short-term benefit, with some plan for continued follow-up implementation to identify any serious long-term toxicity.

Responding to early unfavorable trends   When an unfavorable trend emerges, three criteria should be considered by a DMC as it wrestles with the question of whether trial modification or termination should be recommended: (i) Are the trends sufficiently unfavorable that there is very little chance of establishing a significant beneficial effect by the completion of the trial? (ii) Have the negative trends ruled out the smallest treatment effect of clinical interest? (iii) Are the negative trends sufficiently strong to conclude a harmful effect?

While the conditional power argument only allows a statement of failure to establish benefit, the symmetric or asymmetric boundary approach allows the researchers to rule out beneficial for a treatment or, with more extreme results, to establish harm. When early trends are unfavorable in a clinical trial that is properly powered, stochastic curtailment criteria would generally yield monitoring criteria for termination that would be similar to the symmetric lower boundary for lack of benefit. However, in underpowered trials having unfavorable trends, the stochastic curtailment criteria for early termination generally would be satisfied earlier than criteria based on the group sequential lower boundary for lack of benefit. Most trials comparing a new intervention to a standard of care or a control regimen do not set out to establish that the new intervention is inferior to the control. However, some circumstances may in fact lead to such a consideration.

Responding to unexpected safety concerns   Statistical methods are least helpful when an unexpected and worrying toxicity profile begins to emerge. In this situation there can be no pre-specified statistical plan, since the outcome being assessed was unanticipated.

Responding when there are no apparent trends   In some trials, no apparent trends of either beneficial or harmful effects emerge as the trial progresses to its planned conclusion. In such instances, a decision must be made as to whether the investment in participant, physician, and fiscal resources, as well as the burden of the trial to patients, remains viable and compelling.

6.8   Conditional Power

Conditional power at a given interim analysis in group sequential trials is defined as the power of rejecting the null hypothesis at the end of the trial conditional on the observed data accumulated up to the time point of the planned interim analysis. For many repeated significance tests such as Pocock's test, O'Brien and Fleming's test, and Wang and Tsiatis' test, the trial can only be terminated under the alternative hypothesis. In practice, this is usually true if the test treatment demonstrates substantial evidence of efficacy. However, it should be noted that if the trial indicates a strong evidence of futility (lack of efficacy) during the interim analysis, it is unethical to continue the trial. Hence, the trial may also be terminated under the null hypothesis. However, except for the inner wedge test, most repeated significance tests are designed for early stop under the alternative hypothesis. In such a situation, the analysis of conditional power (or equivalently futility analysis) can be used as a quantitative method for determining whether the trial should be terminated prematurely.

Comparing Means

Let x_{ij} be the observation from the jth subject $(j = 1, ..., n_i)$ in the ith treatment group $(i = 1, 2)$. $x_{ij}, j = 1, ..., n_i$, are assumed to be independent and identically distributed normal random variables with mean μ_i and variance σ_i^2. At the time of interim analysis, it is assumed that the first m_i of n_i subjects in the ith treatment group have already been observed. The investigator may want to evaluate the power for rejection of the null hypothesis based on the observed data and appropriate assumption under the alternative hypothesis. More specifically, define

$$\bar{x}_{a,i} = \frac{1}{m_i} \sum_{j=1}^{m_i} x_{ij} \quad and \quad \bar{x}_{b,i} = \frac{1}{n_i - m_i} \sum_{j=m_i+1}^{n_i} x_{ij}.$$

At the end of the trial, the following Z test statistic is calculated:

$$\begin{aligned} Z &= \frac{\bar{x}_1 - \bar{x}_2}{\sqrt{s_1^2/n_1 + s_2^2/n_2}} \\ &\approx \frac{\bar{x}_1 - \bar{x}_2}{\sqrt{\sigma_1^2/n_1 + \sigma_2^2/n_2}} \\ &= \frac{(m_1\bar{x}_{a,1} + (n_1 - m_1)\bar{x}_{b,1})/n_1 - (m_2\bar{x}_{a,2} + (n_2 - m_2)\bar{x}_{b,2})/n_2}{\sqrt{\sigma_1^2/n_1 + \sigma_2^2/n_2}}. \end{aligned}$$

Under the alternative hypothesis, we assume $\mu_1 > \mu_2$. Hence, the power for rejecting the null hypothesis can be approximated by

$$\begin{aligned} 1 - \beta &= P(Z > z_{\alpha/2}) \\ &= P\left(\frac{\frac{(n_1-m_1)(\bar{x}_{b,1}-\mu_1)}{n_1} - \frac{(n_2-m_2)(\bar{x}_{b,2}-\mu_2)}{n_2}}{\sqrt{\frac{(n_1-m_1)\sigma_1^2}{n_1^2} + \frac{(n_2-m_2)\sigma_2^2}{n_2^2}}} > \tau \right) \\ &= 1 - \Phi(\tau), \end{aligned}$$

where

$$\tau = \left[z_{\alpha/2}\sqrt{\sigma_1^2/n_1 + \sigma_2^2/n_2} - (\mu_1 - \mu_2) \right.$$

$$\left. - \left(\frac{m_1}{n_1}(\bar{x}_{a,1} - \mu_1) - \frac{m_2}{n_2}(\bar{x}_{a,2} - \mu_2) \right) \right]$$

$$\left[\frac{(n_1 - m_1)\sigma_1^2}{n_1^2} + \frac{(n_2 - m_2)\sigma_2^2}{n_2^2} \right]^{-1/2}.$$

As it can be seen from the above, the conditional power depends not only upon the assumed alternative hypothesis (μ_1, μ_2) but also upon the observed values $(\bar{x}_{a,1}, \bar{x}_{a,2})$ and the amount of information that has been accumulated (m_i/n_i) at the time of interim analysis.

Comparing Proportions

When the responses are binary, similar formulas can also be obtained. Let x_{ij} be the binary response observed from the jth subject $(j = 1, ..., n_i)$ in the ith treatment group $(i = 1, 2)$. Again, $x_{ij}, j = 1, ..., n_i$, are assumed to be independent and identically distributed binary variables with mean p_i. At the time of interim analysis, it is also assumed that the first m_i of n_i subjects in the ith treatment group have been observed. Define

$$\bar{x}_{a,i} = \frac{1}{m_i} \sum_{j=1}^{m_i} x_{ij} \quad and \quad \bar{x}_{b,i} = \frac{1}{n_i - m_i} \sum_{j=m_i+1}^{n_i} x_{ij}.$$

At the end of the trial, the following Z test statistic is calculated:

$$Z = \frac{\bar{x}_1 - \bar{x}_2}{\sqrt{\bar{x}_1(1 - \bar{x}_1)/n_1 + \bar{x}_2(1 - \bar{x}_2)/n_2}}$$

$$\approx \frac{\bar{x}_1 - \bar{x}_2}{\sqrt{p_1(1 - p_1)/n_1 + p_2(1 - p_2)/n_2}}$$

$$= \frac{(m_1\bar{x}_{a,1} + (n_1 - m_1)\bar{x}_{b,1})/n_1 - (m_2\bar{x}_{a,2} + (n_2 - m_2)\bar{x}_{b,2})/n_2}{\sqrt{p_1(1 - p_1)/n_1 + p_2(1 - p_2)/n_2}}.$$

Under the alternative hypothesis, we assume $p_1 > p_2$. Hence, the power for rejecting the null hypothesis can be approximated by

$$1 - \beta = P(Z > z_{\alpha/2})$$

$$= P\left(\frac{\frac{(n_1-m_1)(\bar{x}_{b,1}-\mu_1)}{n_1} - \frac{(n_2-m_2)(\bar{x}_{b,2}-\mu_2)}{n_2}}{\sqrt{\frac{(n_1-m_1)p_1(1-p_1)}{n_1^2} + \frac{(n_2-m_2)p_2(1-p_2)}{n_2^2}}} > \tau \right)$$

$$= 1 - \Phi(\tau),$$

where

$$\tau = \left[z_{\alpha/2} \sqrt{p_1(1-p_1)/n_1 + p_2(1-p_2)/n_2} - (\mu_1 - \mu_2) \right.$$
$$\left. - \left(\frac{m_1}{n_1}(\bar{x}_{a,1} - \mu_1) - \frac{m_2}{n_2}(\bar{x}_{a,2} - \mu_2) \right) \right]$$
$$\left[\frac{(n_1 - m_1)p_1(1-p_1)}{n_1^2} + \frac{(n_2 - m_2)p_2(1-p_2)}{n_2^2} \right]^{-1/2}.$$

Similarly, the conditional power depends not only upon the assumed alternative hypothesis (p_1, p_2) but also upon the observed values $(\bar{x}_{a,1}, \bar{x}_{a,2})$ and the amount of information that has been accumulated (m_i/n_i) at the time of interim analysis.

6.9 Practical Issues

The group sequential procedures for interim analyses are basically in the context of hypothesis testing, which is aimed at pragmatic study objectives, i.e., which treatment is better. However, most new treatments such as cancer drugs are very expensive or very toxic or both. As a result, only if the degree of the benefit provided by the new treatment exceeds some minimum clinically significant requirement, it will then be considered for the treatment of the intended medical conditions. Therefore, an adequate well-controlled trial should be able to provide not only the qualitative evidence whether the experimental treatment is effective but also the quantitative evidence from the unbiased estimation of the size of the effectiveness or safety over placebo given by the experimental therapy. For a fixed sample design without interim analyses for early termination, it is possible to achieve both qualitative and quantitative goals with respect to the treatment effect. However, with group sequential procedure the size of benefit of the experimental treatment by the maximum likelihood method is usually overestimated because of the choice of stopping rule. Jennison and Turnbull (1990) pointed out that the sample mean might not be even contained in the final confidence interval. As a result, estimation of the size of treatment effect has received a lot of attention. Various estimation procedures have been proposed such as modified maximum likelihood estimator (MLE), median unbiased estimator (MUE), and the midpoint of the equal-tailed 90% confidence interval. For more details, see Cox (1952), Tsiatis et al., (1984), Kim and DeMets (1987), Kim (1989), Chang and O'Brien (1986), Chang et al. (1989), Chang (1989), Hughes and Pocock (1988), and Pocock and Hughes (1989).

The estimation procedures proposed in the above literature require extensive computation. On the other hand, simulation results (Kim, 1989; Hughes and Pocock, 1988) showed that the alpha spending function corresponding to the O'Brien-Fleming group sequential procedure is very concave and allocates only a very small amount of total nominal significance level to early stages of interim analyses, and hence, the bias, variance, and mean square error of the point estimator following O'Brien-Fleming procedure are also the smallest. Current researches mainly focus upon the estimation of the size of the treatment effect for the primary clinical endpoints on which the group sequential procedure is based. However, there are many other secondary efficacy and safety endpoints to be evaluated in the same trial. The impact of early termination of the trial based on the results from primary clinical endpoints on the statistical inference for these secondary clinical endpoints is unclear. In addition, group sequential methods and their followed estimation procedures so far are only concentrated on the population average. On the other hand, inference of variability is sometimes also of vital importance for certain classes of drug products and diseases. Research on estimation of variability following early termination is still lacking. Other areas of interest for interim analyses include clinical trials with more than two treatments and bioequivalence assessment. For group sequential procedures for the trials with multiple treatments, see Hughes (1993) and Proschan et al. (1994). For group sequential bioequivalence testing procedure, see Gould (1995).

Chapter 7

Statistical Tests for Seamless Adaptive Designs

A seamless phase II/III trial design is referred to a program that addresses within a single trial the objectives that are normally achieved through separate trials in phases IIb and III (Gallo et al., 2006). An seamless phase II/III adaptive design is a combination of phase II and phase III, which aims at achieving the primary objectives normally achieved through the conduct of separate phase II and phases III trials, and would use data from patients enrolled before and after the adaptation in the final analysis (Maca et al, 2006). In a seamless design, there is usually a so-called learning phase that serves the same purpose as a traditional phase II trial, and a confirmatory phase that serves the same objective as a traditional phase III study. Compared to traditional designs, a seamless design can not only reduce sample size but also shorten the time to bring a positive drug candidate to the marketplace. In this chapter, for illustration purpose, we will discuss different seamless designs and their utilities, through real examples. We will also discuss the issues that are commonly encountered followed by some recommendations for assuring the validity and integrity of a clinical trial with seamless design.

7.1 Why a Seamless Design Efficient

The use of a seamless design enjoys the following advantages. There are opportunities for savings when (i) a drug is not working through early stopping for futility and when (ii) a drug has a dramatic effect by early stopping for efficacy. A seamless design is efficient because there is no lead time between the learning and confirmatory phases. In addition, the data collected at the learning phase are combined with those data obtained at the confirmatory phase for final analysis.

The most notable difference between an seamless phase II/III adaptive design and the traditional approach that have separate phase II and phase III trials are the control of the overall type I error rate (alpha) and the corresponding power for correctly detecting a clinically meaningful difference. In the traditional approach, the actual α is equal to $\alpha_{II}\alpha_{III}$, where α_{II} and α_{III} are the type I error rates controlled at phase II and phase III, respectively. If two phase III trials are required, then

$$\alpha = \alpha_{II}\alpha_{III}\alpha_{III}.$$

In a seamless adaptive phase II/III design, actual $\alpha = \alpha_{III}$. If two phase III studies are required, then $\alpha = \alpha_{III}\alpha_{III}$. Thus, the α for a seamless design is actually $1/\alpha_{II}$ times larger than the traditional design. Similarly, we can steal power (permissible) by using a seamless design. Here *power* is referred to the probability of correctly detecting a *true* but not *hypothetical* treatment difference. In a classic design, the actual power is given by

$$power = power_{II} * power_{III},$$

while in a seamless adaptive phase II/III design, actual power is

$$power = power_{III},$$

which is $1/power_{II}$ times larger than the traditional design.

7.2   Step-wise Test and Adaptive Procedures

Consider a clinical trial with K stages. At each stage, a hypotheses testing is performed followed by some actions that are dependent of the analysis results. In practice, three possible actions are often considered. They are (i) an early futility stopping, (ii) an early stopping due to efficacy, or (iii) dropping the losers (i.e., inferior arms including pre-determined sub-populations are dropped after the review of analysis results at each stage). In practice, the objective of the trial (e.g., testing for efficacy of the experimental drug) can be formulated as a global hypotheses testing problem. In other words, the null hypothesis is the intersection of individual null hypotheses at each stage, that is

$$H_0 : H_{01} \cap ... \cap H_{0K}, \tag{7.1}$$

where H_{0k} $(k = 1, ..., K)$ is the null hypothesis at the kth stage. Note that the H_{0k} have some restrictions, that is, the rejection of any H_{0k} $(k = 1, ..., K)$ will lead to the common clinical implication of the efficacious of the study medication. Otherwise, the global hypothesis can not be interpreted. The following step-wise test procedure is often employed. Let T_k be the test statistic associated with H_{0k}. Note that for convenience sake, we will only consider one-sided test throughout this chapter.

Stopping Rules

To test (7.1), first, we need specify stopping rules at each stage. The stopping rules considered here are given by

$$\begin{cases} \text{Stop for efficacy} & \text{if } T_k \leq \alpha_k, \\ \text{Stop for futility} & \text{if } T_k > \beta_k, \\ \text{Drop losers and continue} & \text{if } \alpha_k < T_k \leq \beta_k, \end{cases} \qquad (7.2)$$

where $\alpha_k < \beta_k$ $(k = 1, ..., K - 1)$, and $\alpha_K = \beta_K$. For convenience's sake, we denote α_k and β_k as the efficacy and futility boundaries, respectively. The test statistic is defined as

$$T_k = \Pi_{i=1}^{k} p_i, \quad k = 1, ..., K, \qquad (7.3)$$

where p_i is the naive p-value for testing H_{0k} based on sub-sample collected at the kth stage. It is assumed that p_k is uniformly distributed under the null hypothesis H_{0k}.

7.3 Contrast Test and Naive P-value

In clinical trials with M arms, the following general one-sided contrast hypotheses testing is often considered:

$$H_0 : L(u) \leq 0 \text{ vs. } H_a : L(u) = \varepsilon > 0, \qquad (7.4)$$

where

$$L(u) = \sum_{i=1}^{M} c_i u_i$$

is a linear combination of u_i, $i = 1, ..., M$, in which c_i are the contrast coefficients satisfying

$$\sum_{i=1}^{M} c_i = 0,$$

and ε is a pre-specified constant. In practice, u_i can be the mean, proportion, or hazard rate for the ith group depending on the study endpoint. Under the null hypothesis of (7.4), a contrast test can be obtained as follows

$$Z = \frac{L(\hat{u}; H)}{\sqrt{varL(\hat{u})}}, \qquad (7.5)$$

where $\hat{u}$ is an unbiased estimator of u, where $u = (u_i)$ and

$$\hat{u}_i = \sum_{j=1}^{n_{ij}} \frac{x_{ij}}{n_{ij}}.$$

Let

$$\varepsilon = E(L(\hat{u})), \quad v^2 = \mathrm{var}(L(\hat{u})), \tag{7.6}$$

where homogeneous variance assumption under H_0 and H_a is assumed. It is also assumed that u_i, $i = 1, ..., M$ are mutually independent. Without loss of generality, assume that $c_i u_i > 0$ as an indication of efficacy. Then, for a superiority design, if the null hypothesis H_0 given in (7.4) is rejected for some c_i satisfying $\sum_{i=1}^{M} c_i = 0$, then there is a difference among u_i, $i = 1, ..., M$.

Let $\hat{u}$ be the mean for a normal endpoint (proportion for a binary endpoint, or MLE of the hazard rate for a survival endpoint). Then, by the *Central Limit Theorem*, the asymptotic distribution of the test statistic and the pivotal statistic can be obtained as follows:

$$Z = \frac{L(\hat{u}|H_0)}{v} \sim N(0, 1), \tag{7.7}$$

and

$$Z = \frac{L(\hat{u}|H_a)}{v} \sim N(\frac{\varepsilon}{v}, 1), \tag{7.8}$$

where

$$v^2 = \sum_{i=1}^{M} c_i^2 var(\hat{u}_i) = \sigma^2 \sum_{i=1}^{M} \frac{c_i^2}{n_i} = \frac{\theta^2}{n}, \tag{7.9}$$

and

$$\theta^2 = \sigma^2 \sum_{i=1}^{M} \frac{c_i^2}{f_i}, \tag{7.10}$$

in which n_i is the sample size for the ith arm, $f_i = \frac{n_i}{n}$ is the size fraction, $n = \sum_{i=0}^{k} n_i$, and σ^2 is the variance of the response under H_0. Thus, the power is given by

$$\mathrm{power} = \Phi_0 \left(\frac{\varepsilon \sqrt{n} - \theta z_{1-\alpha}}{\theta} \right), \tag{7.11}$$

where Φ_0 is cumulative distribution function of $N(0, 1)$. Thus, the sample size required for achieving a desired power can obtained as

$$n = \frac{(z_{1-\alpha} + z_{1-\beta})^2 \theta^2}{\varepsilon^2}. \tag{7.12}$$

It can be seen from above that (7.11) and (7.12) include the commonly employed one-arm or two-arm superiority design and non-inferiority designs as special cases. For example, for a one-arm design, $c_1 = 1$, and for a two-arm design, $c_1 = -1$ and $c_2 = 1$. Note that a minimal sample size is required when the response and the contrasts have the same shape under a balanced design. If, however, an inappropriate set of contrasts is used, the sample size could be several times larger than the optimal design.

When the shape of the c_i is similar to the shape of u_{ik}, the test statistic is a most powerful test. However, because u_i is usually unknown. In this case, we may consider the adaptive contrasts $c_{ik} = \hat{u}_{ik-1}$ at the kth stage, where $\hat{u}_{ik-1}$ is the observed response at the previous stage, i.e., the $(k-1)^{th}$ stage. Thus, we have

$$Z_k = \sum_{i=1}^{m} (\hat{u}_{ik-1} - \bar{u}_{k-1}) \hat{u}_{ik}, \tag{7.13}$$

which are conditionally, given data at the $(k-1)^{th}$ stage, normally distributed. It can be shown that the correlation between z_{k-1} and z_k is zero since p_k $(=\alpha)$ is independent of $c_m = u_m$, $m = 1, ..., M$ and p_k is independent of Z_{k-1} or p_{k-1}. It follows that Z_1 and Z_2 are independent.

7.4 Comparisons of Seamless Design

There are many possible seamless adaptive designs. It is helpful to classify these designs into the following four categories according to the design features and adaptations: (i) fixed number of regimens, which includes stopping early for futility, biomarker-informed stopping early for futility, and stopping early for futility/efficacy with sample size re-estimation, (ii) flexible number of regimens, which includes a flexible number of regimens, adaptive hypotheses, and response-adaptive randomization, (iii) population adaptation, where the number of patient groups can be changed from the learning phase to the confirmatory phase, and (iv) combinations of (ii) and (iii). For seamless adaptive designs in category (iii), patient groups are often correlated, such as the entire patient population and subpopulation with certain genomic markers. When all patient groups are mutually independent, categories (iii) and (iv) are statistically equivalent. Chang (2005a,b,c) discussed various designs in category (i) and proposed the use of a Bayesian biomarker-adaptive design in a phase II/III clinical program.

In this section, we will focus on seamless adaptive designs with a flexible number of regimens. We will compare four different seamless adaptive designs with normal endpoints. Each design has five treatment groups including a control group in the learning phase. Since there are multiple arms, contract tests are considered for detecting treatment difference under the null hypothesis of

$$H_0 : \Sigma_{i=1}^{5} c_i u_i > 0,$$

where c_i is the contrast for the ith group that has an expected response of u_i. The test statistic is $T = \Sigma_{i=1}^{5} c_i \hat{u}_i$. The four seamless designs considered here include (i) a five-arm group sequential design, (ii) an adaptive hypotheses design, where contracts c_i change dynamically according to the shape of the response (u_i) for achieving the most power, (iii) a drop-the-losers design, where inferior groups (losers) will be dropped, but two groups and the control will be kept in the confirmatory phase, and (iv) a keep-the-winner design, where we keep the best group and the control at the confirmatory phase. Since the maximum power is achieved for a balanced design when the shape of the contrasts is consistent with the shape of the response (Stewart and Ruberg, 2000; Chang and Chow, 2006; Chang, Chow, and Pong, 2006), in the adaptive hypotheses approach, the contrasts in the confirmatory phase are reshaped based on the observed responses in the learning phase. Three different response and contrast shapes are presented (see Table 7.4.1). The powers of the adaptive designs are summarized in Table 7.4.2, where the generalized Fisher combination method (Chang 2005c) with efficacy and futility stopping boundaries of $\alpha_1 = 0.01, \beta_1 = 1, \alpha_2 = 0.0033$ are used. It can be seen that the keep-the-winner design is very robust for different response and contrast shapes.

Table 7.4.1: Response and Contrast Shapes

Shape	u_1	u_2	u_3	u_4	u_5	c_1	c_2	c_3	c_4	c_5
Monotonic	1.0	2.0	3.5	4.0	4.5	-1.9	-0.9	0.1	1.1	1.6
Convex	1.0	1.0	4.0	1.0	3.0	-1.0	-1.0	2.0	-1.0	1.0
Step	1.0	3.4	3.4	3.4	3.4	-1.92	0.48	0.48	0.48	0.48

Table 7.4.2: Power (%) of Contrast Test

		Contrast		
Response	Design	Monotonic	Wave	Step
	Sequential	96.5	27.1	71.0
Monotonic	Adaptive	83.4	50.0	70.0
	Drop-losers	71.2	71.2	71.2
	Keep-winner	84.8	84.8	84.8
	Sequential	26.5	95.8	23.3
Wave	Adaptive	49.5	82.1	48.0
	Drop-losers	47.8	47.8	47.8
	Keep-winner	60.7	60.7	60.7
	Sequential	42.6	14.6	72.4
Step	Adaptive	41.0	26.4	54.6
	Drop-losers	72.7	72.7	72.7
	Keep-winner	83.3	83.3	83.3

Note: $\sigma = 10$, one-sided $\alpha = 0.025$, interim n = 64/group.

Expected total n = 640 under the alternative hypothesis for all the designs.

For simplicity, assume the best arm is correctly predetermined at interim analysis for the drop-losers and keep-winner designs.

It can be seen from Table 7.4.1 and Table 7.4.2, when the contrast shape is consistent with the response shape, it gives the most powerful regardless of the type of design. In addition, given the expected sample size, when the response shape is known, the group sequential design has the most power. This is because that it allows for early stopping for more efficient design. When the response shape is unknown, adaptive design (may be drop–the-losers) is the most powerful design except for the case when the response shape is "step." In such a case, all active dose levels have the same response rates and the contrasts do not really matter. Hence, adaptive design is not helpful. Note that the examples provided here controlled the type I error under the global null hypothesis.

7.5   Drop-the-Loser Adaptive Design

In pharmaceutical research and development, it is desirable to shorten the time of the conduct of clinical trials, data analysis, submission, and regulatory review and approval process in order to bring the drug product to the marketplace as early as possible. Thus, any designs which can help to achieve the goals are very attractive. As a result, various strategies are proposed. For example, Gould (1992) and Zucker et al. (1999) considered using blinded data from the pilot phase to design a clinical trial and then combine the data for final analysis. Proschan and Hunsberger (1995) proposed a strategy which allows re-adjustment of the sample size based upon unblinded data so that a clinical trial is properly powered. Other designs have been proposed to combine studies conducted at different phases of traditional clinical development into a single study. For example, Bauer and Kieser (1999) proposed a two-stage design which enables investigators to terminate the trial entirely or drop a subset of the regimens for lack of efficacy at the end of the first stage. Their procedure is highly flexible and the distributional assumptions are kept to a minimum. Bauer and Kieser's method has the advantage of allowing hypothesis testing at the end of the confirmation stage. However, it is difficult to construct confidence intervals. Brannath, Koening, and Bauer (2003) examined adjusted and repeated confidence intervals in group sequential designs, where the responses are normally distributed. Such confidence intervals are important for interpreting the clinical significance of the results.

In practice, drop-the-losers adaptive designs are useful in combining phase II and phase III clinical trials into a single trial. In this section, we will introduce the application of the drop-the-losers adaptive designs under the assumption of normal distributions. The concept, however, can be similarly applied to other distributions. The drop-the-losers adaptive design consists of two stages with a simple data-based decision made at the interim. In the early phase of the trial, the investigators may administer K experimental treatments (say $\tau_1,...,$ τ_K) to n subjects per treatment. A control treatment, τ_0, is also administered during this phase. Unblinded data on patient responses are collected at end of the first stage. The best treatment group (based on observed mean) and and the control group are retained and other treatment groups are dropped at the second stage.

Cohen and Sackrowitz (1989) provided an unbiased estimate using data from both stages. Cohen and Sackrowitz considered using a conditional distribution on a specific event to construct conditionally unbiased estimators. Following a similar idea, tests and confidence intervals can be derived. The specific conditional distribution used in the final analysis depends on the outcomes from the first stage. Provided the set of possible events from the first stage on which one condition is a partition of the sample space, the *conditional corrections* also hold *unconditionally*. In our setting, conditional level α tests are unconditional level α tests. In other words, if all of the null hypotheses are true for all of the treatments, the probability of rejecting a null hypothesis is never greater than α, regardless of which treatment is selected.

For simplicity, we assume the following ordered outcome after the first stage,

$$Q = \{X : \bar{X}_1 > \bar{X}_2 > ... > \bar{X}_k\}$$

so that τ_1 continues into the second stage (other outcomes would be equivalently handled by relabeling). Typically, at the end of the trial, we want to make inferences on the mean μ_1 of treatment τ_1, and compare them with the control (e.g., test $H_0 : \mu_1 - \mu_0 \leq \Delta_{10}$ or construct a confidence interval about $\mu_1 - \mu_0$). Therefore, we can construct uniformly most powerful (UMP) unbiased tests for hypotheses concerning Δ_1 based upon the conditional distribution of W given $(X*, T)$. To see this, note that the test is based on the conditional event Q. Lehmann (1983) gives a general proof for this family, which shows that conditioning on sufficient statistics associated with nuisance parameters causes them to drop from the distribution. In addition, the theorem states that the use of this conditional distribution to draw inferences about a parameter of interest yields hypothesis testing procedures which are uniformly most powerful unbiased unconditionally (i.e., UMPU before conditioning on the sufficient statistics). The test statistic is

$$W = \frac{n_0 (n_A + n_B)}{(n_0 + n_A + n_B) \sigma^2} (\bar{Z} - \bar{Y}_0),$$

which has the distribution of

$$W \sim f_Q (W | \Delta_1, X^*, T) = C_N \exp \left\{ -\frac{1}{2G} (W - G\Delta_1)^2 \right\} D,$$

where

$$\bar{Z} = \frac{(n_A \bar{X}_M + n_B \bar{Y})}{n_A + n_B},$$

$\bar{X}_M = \max (\bar{X}_1, ..., \bar{X}_k) = $ maximum mean observed mean at first stage,

$$G = \frac{n_0 (n_A + n_B)}{(n_0 + n_A + n_B) \sigma^2},$$

$$T = \frac{n_0 \bar{Y}_0 + (n_A + n_B) \bar{Z}}{n_0 + n_A + n_B},$$

$$D = \Phi \left[\frac{\sqrt{n_A (n_A - n_B)} \left(\sigma^2 W + (n_A + n_B) \left(T - \bar{X}_2 \right) \right)}{\sqrt{n_A (n_A + n_B)} \sigma} \right],$$

and C_N is the normalization constant, which involves integrating W over real line.

In order to test

$$H_0 : \mu_1 - \mu_0 \leq \Delta_{10} \quad vs. \quad H_a : \mu_1 - \mu_0 > \Delta_{10},$$

we consider the following function

$$F_Q (W | \Delta_{10}, X^*, T) = \int_{-\infty}^{W} f_Q (t | \Delta_{10}, X^*, T) \, dt.$$

We can use the function to obtain a critical value, W_u, through $F_Q (W_u | \Delta_{10}, X^*, T) = 1 - \alpha$. Note that $100(1 - \alpha)\%$ confidence intervals, $[\Delta_L, \Delta_U]$, can be constructed from

$$F_Q (W_{obs} | \Delta_L, X^*, T) = 1 - \alpha/2,$$

and

$$F_Q (W | \Delta_{10}, X^*, T) = \alpha/2$$

because $W | X^*, T$ is monotonic likelihood ratio in T. Computer programs are available at

$$\text{http} : //\text{www.gog.org/sdcstaff/mikesily}$$

or

$$\text{http} : //\text{sphhp.buffalo.edoibiostat/}.$$

To illustrate the calculation, Sampson and Sill (2005) simulated a data set from a design, where $k = 7$, $\mu_1 = \ldots = \mu_7 = 0$, $n_A = n_B1 = 100, n_0 = 200$, and $\sigma = 10$. The experimental data have been relabeled in decreasing order. Suppose we want to test

$$H_0 : \mu_1 - \mu_0 \leq 0 \quad vs. \quad H_1 : \mu_1 - \mu_0 > 0.$$

The simulated data are given as follows:

$$\bar{X}_1 = 1.8881,$$
$$\bar{X}_2 = 0.9216,$$
$$\bar{X}_3 = 0.0691,$$
$$\bar{X}_4 = -0.3793,$$
$$\bar{X}_5 = -0.3918,$$
$$\bar{X}_6 = -0.8945,$$
$$\bar{X}_7 = -0.9276,$$
$$\bar{Y} = 0.7888,$$
$$\bar{Y}_0 = -0.4956.$$

Based on these data, $W_{obs} = 1.83$. Thus, the rejection region is given by $(2.13, \infty)$. Hence, we fail to reject H_0. The 95% confidence interval is given by $(-0.742, 3.611)$.

7.6   Summary

The motivation behind the use of an seamless adaptive design is probably the possibility of shortening the time to develop a new medication. As indicated earlier, a seamless phase II/III adaptive design is not only flexible but also efficient as compared to separate phase II and phase III studies. However, benefits and drawbacks for implementing an adaptive seamless phase II/III design must be carefully weighed against each other. In practice, not all clinical developments may be candidates for such a design. Maca et al. (2006) proposed a list of criteria for determining the feasibility of the use of an seamless adaptive design in clinical development plan. These criteria include endpoints and enrollment, clinical development time, and logistical considerations, which are briefly outlined below.

One of the most important feasibility considerations for an adaptive seamless design is the amount of time that a patient needs in order to reach the endpoint, which will be used for dose escalation. If the endpoint duration is too long, the design could result in unacceptable inefficiencies. In this case, a surrogate marker with much shorter duration might be used. Thus, Maca et al. (2006) suggested that well established and understood endpoints (or surrogate markers) be considered when implementing a seamless adaptive design in clinical development. It, however, should be noted that if the goal of a phase II program is to learn about the primary endpoint to be carried forward into phase III, a seamless adaptive design would not be feasible. As the use of a seamless adaptive design is to shorten the time of development, whether the seamless adaptive design would achieve the study objectives within a reduced time frame would be another important factor for feasibility consideration, especially when the adaptive seamless trial is the only pivotal trial required for regulatory submission. In the case where there are two pivotal trials, whether or not the second seamless trial can shorten the overall development time should be taken into feasibility consideration as well. Logistical considerations are referred to drug supply and drug packaging. It is suggested that development programs which do not have costly or complicated drug regimens would be better suited to adaptive seamless designs.

Although seamless phase II/III adaptive designs are efficient and flexible as compared to the traditional separate phase II and phase III studies, potential impact on statistical inference and p-value after adaptations are made should be carefully evaluated. It should be noted that although more adaptations allow higher flexibility, it could result in a much more complicated statistical analysis at the end of trial.

Chapter 8

Adaptive Sample Size Adjustment

In clinical trials, it is desirable to have a sufficient number of subjects in order to achieve a desired power for correctly detecting a clinically meaningful difference, if such a difference truly exists. For this purpose, a pre-study power analysis is often conducted for sample size estimation under certain assumptions such as the variability associated with the observed response of the primary study endpoint (Chow, Shao, and Wang, 2003). If the true variability is much less than the initial guess of the variability, the study may be over-powered. On the other hand, if the variability is much larger than the initial guess of the variability, the study may not achieve the desired power. In other words, the results observed from the study may be due to chance alone and cannot be reproducible. Thus, it is of interest to adjust sample sizes adaptively based on accrued data at interim.

Adaptive sample size adjustment includes planned and unplanned (unexpected) sample size adjustment. Planned sample size adjustment is referred to as sample size re-estimation at interim analyses in a group sequential clinical trial design or an N-adjusted clinical trial design. Most unplanned sample size adjustments are due to changes made to on-going study protocols and/or unexpected administrative looks based on accrued data at interim. Chapter 2 provides an adjustment factor for sample size as the result of protocol amendments. In this chapter, we will focus on the case of planned sample size adjustment in a group sequential design.

In the next section, statistical procedures for sample size re-estimation without unblinding the treatment codes are introduced. Statistical methods such as Cui-Hung-Wang's idea, Proschan-Hunsberger's method, and Bauer and Köhne's approach for sample size re-estimation with unblinding data in group sequential trial designs are given in Sections 8.2, 8.3, and 8.4, respectively. Other methods such as the inverse-normal method and Müller-Schafer's method are discussed in Section 8.5. Some concluding remarks are given in the last section of this chapter.

8.1 Sample Size Re-Estimation without Unblinding Data

In clinical trials, the sample size is determined by a clinically meaningful difference and information on the variability of the primary endpoint. Since the natural history of the distribution is usually not known or the test treatment under investigation is a new class of drug, the estimate of variability for the primary endpoint for sample size estimation may not be adequate during the planning stage of the study. As a result, the planned sample size may need to be adjusted during the conduct of the trial if the observed variability of the accumulated response on the primary endpoint is very different from that used at the planning stage. To maintain the integrity of the trial, it is suggested that sample size re-estimation be performed without unblinding of the treatment codes if the study is to be conducted in a double-blind fashion. Procedures have been proposed for adjusting the sample size during the course of the trial without unblinding and altering the significance level (Gould, 1992, 1995; Gould and Shih, 1992). For simplicity, let us consider a randomized trial with two parallel groups comparing a test treatment and a placebo. Suppose that the distribution of the response of the primary endpoint is normally distributed. Then, the total sample size required for achieving a desired power of $1 - \beta$ for a two-sided alternative hypothesis can be obtained using the following formula (see, e.g., Chow, Shao and Wang, 2003)

$$N = \frac{4\sigma^2(z_{\alpha/2} + z_\beta)}{\Delta^2},$$

where Δ is the difference of clinically importance. In general, σ^2 (the within-group variance) is unknown and need to be estimated based on previous studies. Let σ^{*2} be the within-group variance specified for sample size determination at the planning stage of the trial. At the initiation of the trial, we expect the observed variability to be similar to σ^{*2} so that the trial will have sufficient power to detect the difference of clinically importance. However, if the variance turns out to be much larger than σ^{*2}, we will need to re-estimate the sample size without breaking the randomization codes. If the true within-group variance is in fact σ'^2, then the sample size to be adjusted to achieve the desired power of $1 - \beta$ at the α level of significance for a two-sided alternative is given by

$$N' = N\frac{\sigma'^2}{\sigma^{*2}},$$

where N is the planned sample size calculated based on σ^{*2}. However, σ'^2 is usually unknown and must be estimated from the accumulated data available from a total n of N patients. One simple approach to estimating σ'^2 is based on the sample variance calculated from the n responses, which is given by

$$s^2 = \frac{1}{n-1}\sum\sum(y_{ij} - \bar{y})^2,$$

where y_{ij} is the jth observation in group i and $\bar{y}$ is the overall sample mean, $j = 1, ..., n_i$, $i = 1$ (treatment), 2 (placebo), and $n = n_1 + n_2$. If n is large enough for the mean difference between groups to provide a reasonable approximation to Δ, then it follows that σ'^2 can be estimated by (Gould, 1995)

$$\sigma'^2 = \frac{n-1}{n-2}(s^2 - \frac{\Delta^2}{4}).$$

Note that the estimation of within-group variance σ'^2 does not require the knowledge of the treatment assignment and hence the blindness of the treatment codes is maintained. However, one of the disadvantages of this approach is that it does depend upon the mean difference, which is not calculated and is unknown.

Alternatively, Gould and Shih (1992) and Gould (1995) proposed a procedure based on the concept of EM algorithm for estimating σ'^2 without a value for Δ. This procedure is briefly outline below. Suppose that n observations, say, y_i, $i = 1, ..., n$ on a primary endpoint have been obtained from n patients. The treatment assignments for these patients are unknown. Gould and Shih (1992) and Gould (1995) considered randomly allocate these n observations to either of the two groups assuming that the treatment assignments are missing at random by defining the following π_i as the treatment indicator

$$\pi_i = \begin{cases} 1 & \text{if the treatment is the test drug} \\ 0 & \text{if the treatment is placebo.} \end{cases}$$

The E step is to obtain the provisional values of the expectation of π_i (i.e., the conditional probability that patient i is assigned to the test drug given y_i), which·is given by

$$P(\pi_i = 1|y_i) = \left(1 + \exp\{(\mu_1 - \mu_2)(\mu_1 + \mu_2 - 2y_i)/2\sigma^2]\right)^{-1},$$

where μ_1 and μ_2 are the population mean of the test drug and the placebo, respectively. The M step involves the maximum likelihood estimates of μ_1, μ_2 and σ after updating π_i by their provisional values obtained from the E step in the log-likelihood function of the interim observations, which is given by

$$1 = n\log\sigma + \frac{\sum[\pi_i(y_i - \mu_1)^2 + (1 - \pi_i)(y_i - \mu_2)^2]}{2\sigma^2}.$$

The E and M steps are iterated until the values converge. Gould and Shih (1992) and Gould (1995) indicated that this procedure can estimate within-group variance quite satisfactorily, but failed to provide a reliable estimate of

$\mu_1 - \mu_2$. As a result, the sample size can be adjusted without knowledge of treatment codes. For sample size re-estimation procedure without unblinding treatment codes with respect to binary clinical endpoints, see Gould (1992, 1995). A review of the methods for sample size re-estimation can be found in Shih (2001).

8.2   Cui-Hung-Wang's Method

For a given group sequential trial, let N_k and T_k be the planned sample size and test statistic at stage k. Thus, we have,

$$T_k = \frac{\sqrt{N_k}}{\sqrt{2}\sigma}\left(\frac{1}{N_k}\sum_{i=1}^{N_k} x_i - \frac{1}{N_k}\sum_{i=1}^{N_k} y_i\right).$$

Denote N_L and T_L by the planned cumulative sample size from stage 1 to stage L and the weighted test statistic from stage 1 to stage L. Thus, for a group sequential trial without sample size adjustment, the test statistic for mean difference between two groups at stage k can be expressed as weighted test statistics of the sub-samples from the previous stages as follows (see, e.g., Cui, Hung, and Wang, 1999)

$$T_{L+j} = T_L\left(\frac{N_L}{N_{L+j}}\right)^{1/2} + w_{L+j}\left[\frac{N_{L+j} - N_L}{N_{L+j}}\right]^{1/2}, \qquad (8.1)$$

where

$$w_{L+j} = \frac{\sum_{i=N_L+1}^{N_{L+j}}(x_i - y_i)}{\sqrt{2(N_{L+j} - N_L)}}, \qquad (8.2)$$

in which x_i and y_i are from treatment group 1 and 2, respectively, and M_L is the adjusted cumulative sample from stage 1 to stage L.

For group sequential trials with sample size adjustments, let M be the total sample size after adjustment and N be the original planned sample size. We may consider adjusting sample size with effect size as follows

$$M = \left(\frac{\delta}{\Delta_L}\right)^2 N, \qquad (8.3)$$

where δ is the expected difference (effect size) given by

$$\frac{(\mu_2 - \mu_1)}{\sigma},$$

and Δ_L is observed mean difference $\frac{\Delta\mu_L}{\sigma}$ at stage L. Based on the adjusted sample sizes, test statistic T_{L+j} becomes

$$U_{L+j} = T_L \left(\frac{N_L}{N_{L+j}} \right)^{1/2} + w_{L+j}^* \left[\frac{N_{L+j} - N_L}{N_{L+j}} \right]^{1/2}, \tag{8.4}$$

where

$$w_{L+j}^* = \frac{\sum_{i=N_L+1}^{M_{L+j}} (x_i - y_i)}{\sqrt{2(M_{L+j} - N_L)}}. \tag{8.5}$$

Cui, Hung, and Wang (1999) showed that using U_{L+j} and original boundary from the group sequential trial will not inflate the type I error rate, both mathematically and by means of computer simulation.

Table 8.2.1: Effects of Sample Adjustment Using Original Test Statistic and Stopping Boundaries

Time to N change, t_L	0.20	0.4	0.6	0.8	∞
Type I error rate, α	0.038	0.035	0.037	0.033	0.025
Power	0.84	0.91	0.94	0.96	0.61

Note: $\delta = 0.03$, $\alpha = 0.025$, and power $= 0.9 \Rightarrow N = 250/\text{group}$.
True $\Delta = 0.21$. Sample size adjustment is based on equation 8.3.
Source: Cui, Hung, and Wang (1999).

Table 8.2.2: Effects of Sample Adjustment Using New Test Statistic and Original Stopping Boundaries

Time to N change, t_L	0.20	0.4	0.6	0.8	∞
Type I error rate, α	0.025	0.025	0.025	0.025	0.025
Power	0.86	0.90	0.92	0.91	0.61

Note: $N = 250/\text{group}$, true , $\alpha = 0.025$. True $\Delta = 0.21$;
sample size adjustment is based on equation 8.3.
Source: Cui, Hung, and Wang (1999).

Example 8.2.1

Cui, Hung, and Wang (1999) gave following example: A phase III two-arm trial for evaluating the effect of a new drug for prevention of myocardial infection in patients undergoing coronary artery bypass graft surgery a sample size of 600 [300] patients per group to detect a 50% reduction in incidence from 22% to 11% with 95% power. However, at interim analysis based on data from 600 [300] patients, the test group has 16.5% incidence rate. If this incidence rate is the true rate, the power is about 40%. If using the Cui-Hung-Wang method to increase sample size to 1,400 per group [unrealistically large], the power is 93% based their simulation with 20,000 replications (The calculations seam to be incorrect! All the sample sizes are twice as large as they should be.).

Remarks

Cui-Hung-Wang's method has the following advantages. First, the adjustment of sample size is easy. Second, using the same stopping boundaries from the traditional group sequential trial is straightforward. The disadvantages include that (i) their sample size adjustment is somewhat ad hoc, which does not aim a target power, and (ii) weighting outcomes differently for patients from different stages is difficult to explain clinically.

8.3   Proschan-Hunsberger's Method

For a given two-stage design, Proschan and Hunsberger (1995) and Proschan (2005) considered adjusting the sample size at the second stage based on the evaluation of conditional power given the data observed at the first stage. We will refer to their method as Proschan-Hunsberger's method. Let $P_c(n_2, z_\alpha | z_1, \delta)$ be the conditional probability that Z exceeds z_α, given that $Z_1 = z_1$ and $\delta = (\mu_x - \mu_y)/\sigma$ based on $n = n_1 + n_2$ observations. That is,

$$
\begin{aligned}
&P_c(n_2, z_\alpha | z_1, \delta) \\
&= \Pr\left(Z > z_\alpha | Z_1 = z_1, \delta\right) \\
&= \Pr\left[\frac{n_1\left(\bar{Y}_1 - \bar{X}_1\right) + n_2\left(\bar{Y}_2 - \bar{X}_2\right)}{\sqrt{2\hat{\sigma}^2 n}} > z_\alpha | Z_1 = z_1, \delta\right] \\
&= \Pr\left[\frac{n_2\left(\bar{Y}_2 - \bar{X}_2\right) - n_2\delta\sigma}{\sqrt{2n_2\hat{\sigma}^2}} > \frac{z_\alpha\sqrt{2\hat{\sigma}^2 n} - z_1\sqrt{2n_1\hat{\sigma}^2} - n_2\delta\sigma}{\sqrt{2n\hat{\sigma}^2}} | \delta\right].
\end{aligned}
$$

If we treat $\hat{\sigma}$ as the true σ, we have

$$
P_c(n_2, z_\alpha | z_1, \delta) = 1 - \Phi\left[\frac{z_\alpha\sqrt{2n} - z_1\sqrt{2n_1} - n_2\delta}{\sqrt{2n_2}}\right]. \tag{8.6}
$$

Since Z_1 is normally distributed, the type I error rate of this two-stage process without early stopping is given by

$$
\int_{-\infty}^{\infty} P_c(n_2, z_\alpha | z_1, 0)\phi(z_1)dz_1 = \int_{-\infty}^{\infty}\left\{1 - \Phi\left[\frac{z_\alpha\sqrt{2n} - z_1\sqrt{2n_1}}{\sqrt{2n_2}}\right]\right\}\phi(z_1)dz_1.
$$

Proschan and Hunsberger (1995) showed that without adjustment of reject regions, the type I error rate caused by sample size adjustment could be as high as

$$
\alpha_{\max} = \alpha + 0.25e^{-z_\alpha^2/2}.
$$

In the interest of controlling the type I error rate at the nominal level, we may consider modifying the rejection region from z_α to z_c such that

$$\int_{-\infty}^{\infty} P_c(n_2, z_c | z_1, 0)\phi(z_1)dz_1 = \alpha, \qquad (8.7)$$

where z_c is a function of z_1, n_1, and n_2. Since the integration is a constant α, we wish to find z_c such that $P_c(n_2, z_c | z_1, 0)$ depends only upon a function of z_1, say $A(z_1)$, i.e.,

$$P_c(n_2, z_c | z_1, 0) = A(z_1). \qquad (8.8)$$

From (8.7) and (8.8), we can solve for z_c as follows

$$z_c = \frac{\sqrt{n_1}\, z_1 + \sqrt{n_2}\, z_A}{\sqrt{n_1 + n_2}}, \qquad (8.9)$$

where $z_A = \Phi^{-1}(1 - A(z_1))$ and $A(z_1)$ is any increasing function with the range of $[0, 1]$ satisfying

$$\int_{-\infty}^{\infty} A(z_1)\phi(z_1)dz_1 = \alpha. \qquad (8.10)$$

To find the function of $A(z_1)$, It may be convenient to write $A(z_1)$ in the form of $A(z_1) = f(z_1)/\phi(z_1)$.(8.10) provides the critical value for rejecting the null hypothesis while protecting the overall α. The next step is to choose the additional sample size n_2 at stage 2. At stage 1 we have the empirical estimate $\hat{\delta} = (\bar{y}_1 - \bar{x}_1)/\hat{\sigma}$ of the standard treatment difference. We may wish to power the trial to detect a value somewhere between the originally hypothesized difference and the empirical estimate. Whichever target difference δ we use, if we plug z_c from (8.9) into (8.6), we obtain the conditional power

$$P_c(n_2, z_c | z_1, \delta) = 1 - \Phi\left(z_A - \sqrt{n_2/2}\,\delta\right). \qquad (8.11)$$

Suppose that the desired power is $1 - \beta_2$, we can immediately obtain the required sample size as follows

$$n_2 = \frac{2(z_A + z_{\beta_2})^2}{\delta^2}. \qquad (8.12)$$

Plugging this into (8.9), we have

$$z_c = \frac{\delta\sqrt{\frac{n_1}{2}}\, z_1 + (z_A + z_{\beta_2})\, z_A}{\sqrt{\frac{n_1}{2}\delta^2 + (z_A + z_{\beta_2})^2}}. \qquad (8.13)$$

Note that z_c is the reject region in n terms of $(\sqrt{n_1}z_1 + \sqrt{n_2}z_2)/\sqrt{n}$, usual z score on all $2n$ observations. If we use the empirical estimate $\hat{\delta}$, (8.12) and (8.13) become

$$n_2 = \frac{n_1(z_A + z_{\beta_2})^2}{z_1^2}, \qquad (8.14)$$

and

$$z_c = \frac{z_1^2 + (z_A + z_{\beta_2}) z_A}{\sqrt{z_1^2 + (z_A + z_{\beta_2})^2}}. \tag{8.15}$$

The fact that the value of β_2 can be changed after observing $Z_1 = z_1$ underscores the flexibility of the procedure. Note that (8.14) is the sample size formula to achieve power $1 - \beta$ in the fixed sample test at level $A(z_1)$. This interpretation allows us to see the benefit of extending our study relative to starting a new one. If $A(z_1) < \alpha$, we would be better off starting a new study than extending the old. We can extend the test procedure for two stages with negative or positive early stopping with stopping rules in the first stage being

$$\begin{cases} \text{Stop not to reject } H_o, & z_1 < z_{cl}; \\ \text{Continue to stage 2,} & z_{cl} \le z_1 \le z_{cu}; \\ \text{Stop to reject } H_o, & z_1 > z_{cu}. \end{cases} \tag{8.16}$$

then (8.7) should be modified as follows:

$$\alpha_1 + \int_{z_{cl}}^{z_{cu}} P_c(n_2, z_c|z_1, 0)\phi(z_1)dz_1 = \alpha \tag{8.17}$$

where $\phi(z_1)$ is the standard normal density function $\alpha_1 = \int_{z_{cu}}^{+\infty} \phi(z_1)dz_1$.
    Define

$$\tilde{P}_c(z_1; z_{c1}; \delta) = \begin{cases} 0 & z_1 < z_{cl}; \\ P_c(n_2, z_c|z_1, \delta) & z_{cl} \le z_1 \le z_{cu}; \\ 1 & z_1 > z_{cu}. \end{cases} \tag{8.18}$$

Note that

$$\alpha_1 = \int_{z_{cl}}^{z_{cu}} P_c(n_2, z_c|z_1, 0)\phi(z_1)dz_1.$$

Then (8.17) can be written

$$\alpha = \int_{-\infty}^{\infty} \tilde{P}_c(n_2, z_c|z_1, 0)\phi(z_1)dz_1, \tag{8.19}$$

which in the same format as (8.7). Let $\tilde{P}_c(z_1; z_{c1}; \delta) = A(z_1)$, i.e.,

$$A(z_1) = \begin{cases} 0 & z_1 < z_{cl}; \\ P_c(n_2, z_c|z_1, \delta) & z_{cl} \le z_1 \le z_{cu}; \\ 1 & z_1 > z_{cu}. \end{cases} \tag{8.20}$$

(8.10)-(8.18) are still valid and $A(z_1)$ is any increasing function with range [0, 1] satisfying takes the form of

$$A(z_1) = \begin{cases} 0 & z_1 < z_{cl}; \\ f(z_1)/\phi(z_1) & z_{cl} \le z_1 \le z_{cu}; \\ 1 & z_1 > z_{cu}. \end{cases} \qquad (8.21)$$

Proschan (1995) and Hunsberger (2004) gave the following linear-error function:

$$A(z_1) = 1 - \Phi(\sqrt{2}z_\alpha - z_1).$$

Given observed treatment difference δ, we can use (8.12) or (8.14) re-estimate sample size and substitute (8.21) into (8.13) or (8.15) to determine reject region z_c. Note that this is a design without early stopping.

Example 8.3.1 Consider the following circular-function:

$$A(z_1) = \begin{cases} 0 & z_1 < z_{cl}; \\ 1-\Phi(\sqrt{z_{cu}^2 - z_1^2}) & z_{cl} \le z_1 \le z_{cu}; \\ 1 & z_1 > z_{cu}. \end{cases} \qquad (8.22)$$

For each z_{cl}, the corresponding z_{cu} can be calculated by substituting (8.21) into (8.11). and then calculating z_c from (8.12) or (8.14) with $A(z_1)$ of (8.21). For convenience's sake, we tabulate z_{cl}, z_{cu} and z_c in Table 8.3.1 for overall one-sided $\alpha = 0.025$ and 0.5.

Table 8.3.1: Corresponding Values z_{cu} for Different z_{cl}

α	$\alpha_0 = \Phi(1 - z_{cl})$								
	.10	.15	.20	.25	.30	.35	.40	.45	.50
0.025	2.13	2.17	2.19	2.21	2.22	2.23	2.25	2.26	2.27
0.050	1.77	1.82	1.85	1.88	1.89	1.91	1.93	1.94	1.95

Source: Proschan and Hunsberger (1995).

8.4 Müller-Schafer Method

Müller and Schafer (2001) showed how one can make any data dependent change in an on-going adaptive trial and still preserve the overall type-1 error. To achieve that, all one needs to do is preserve the conditional type-1 error of the remaining portion of the trial. Therefore, Müller-Schafer method is special conditional error approach.

8.5   Bauer-Köhne Method

Two-stage Design

Bauer-Köhne's method is based on the fact that under H_0 the p-value for the test of a particular null hypothesis, H_{0k}, in a stochastically independent sample, which is generally uniformly distributed on [0,1], where continuous test statistics are assumed (Bauer and Köhne, 1994, 1996). Usually, however, one obtains conservative combination tests when under H_0 the distribution of the p-values is stochastically larger than the uniform distribution.

Moreover, under H_0 the distribution of the resultant p-value is stochastically independent of previously measured random variables. Hence, provided H_0 is true, data-dependent planning (e.g., sample size change) does not change the convenient property of independently and uniformly distributed p-values, but some care is needed (Liu, Proschan, and Pledger, 2002). The modification considered here would imply that data are not allowed to be pooled over the whole trial. Data from the stages before and after that adaptive interim analysis have to be looked at separately. In the analysis, p-values from the partitioned sample have to be used. These are general measures of "deviation" from the respective null hypotheses. There are many ways to test the intersection H_o of two or more individual null hypotheses based on independently and uniformly distributed p-values for the individual test (Hedges and Olkin, 1985; Sonnesmann, 1991). Fisher's criterion using the product of the p-values has good properties. One obvious questions is whether combination tests could be used that explicitly include a weighting of the p-values by the sample size. If the sample size itself is open to adaptation, then clearly the answer is no. To derive critical regions for test statistics explicitly containing random sample sizes, one would need to know or pre-specify the distribution. This, however, contradicts the intended flexibility of general approach.

Let P_1 and P_2 be the p-values for the sub-samples obtained from the first stage and second stage, respectively. Fisher's criterion leads to rejection of H_0 at the end of trial if

$$P_1 P_2 \le c_\alpha = e^{-\frac{1}{2}\chi^2_{4,1-\alpha}}, \qquad (8.24)$$

where $\chi^2_{4,1-\alpha}$ is the $(1-\alpha)$-quantile of the central χ^2 distribution with 4 degrees of freedom. Decision rules at the first stage:

$$\begin{cases} P_1 \le \alpha_1, & \text{Stop trial and reject } H_0 \\ P_1 > \alpha_0, & \text{Stop trial and accept } H_0 \\ \alpha_1 < P_1 \le \alpha_0, & \text{Continue to the second stage.} \end{cases} \qquad (8.25)$$

For determination of α_1 and α_0, the overall type I error rate is given by

$$\alpha_1 + \int_{\alpha_1}^{\alpha_0} \int_0^{\frac{c_\alpha}{P_1}} dP_2 dP_1 = \alpha_1 + c_\alpha \ln \frac{\alpha_0}{\alpha_1}. \qquad (8.26)$$

Letting this error rate equal to α, and using the relationship

$$c_\alpha = e^{-\frac{1}{2}\chi^2_{4,1-\alpha}},$$

we have

$$\alpha_1 + \ln \frac{\alpha_0}{\alpha_1} e^{-\frac{1}{2}\chi^2_{4,1-\alpha}} = \alpha. \tag{8.27}$$

Table 8.5.1: Stopping Boundaries α_0, α_1, and C_α

α	C_α		α_0 0.3	0.4	0.5	0.6	0.7	1.0
0.1	0.02045		0.0703	0.0618	0.0548	0.0486	0.0429	0.02045
0.05	0.00870	α_1	0.0299	0.0263	0.0233	0.0207	0.0183	0.00870
0.025	0.00380		0.0131	0.0115	0.0102	0.0090	0.0080	0.00380

Source: Table 1 of Bauer (1994).

Decision rules at final stage are given by

$$\begin{cases} P_1 P_2 \le e^{-\frac{1}{2}\chi^2_{4,1-\alpha}}, & \text{Reject } H_0 \\ \text{Otherwise}, & \text{Accept } H_0. \end{cases}$$

Assuming that z_i and n_i are the standardized mean and sample size for the sub-sample at stage i, under the condition that $n_1 = n_2$, the uniformly most powerful test is given by

$$\frac{z_1 + z_2}{\sqrt{2}} \ge z_{1-\alpha}.$$

Equivalently,

$$\Phi_o^{-1}(1 - P_1) + \Phi_o^{-1}(1 - P_2) \ge \sqrt{2}\Phi_o^{-1}(1 - \alpha).$$

Three-Stage Design

Let p_i (i=1,2,3) be the p-values for the hypothesis tests based on sub-sample obtained at stage 1, 2, and 3, respectively.

Decision rules:

Stage 1:
$$\begin{cases} \text{Stop with rejection of } H_0 \text{ if } p_1 \le \alpha_1, \\ \text{Stop without rejection of } H_0 \text{ if } p_1 > \alpha_0, \\ \text{Otherwise continue to stage 2.} \end{cases}$$

Stage 2:
$$\begin{cases} \text{Stop with rejection of } H_0 \text{ if } p_1 p_2 \le c_{a_2} = e^{-\frac{1}{2}\chi_4^2(1-\alpha_2)}, \\ \text{Stop without rejection of } H_0 \text{ if } p_2 > \alpha_0, \\ \text{Otherwise continue.} \end{cases}$$

Stage 3:
$$\begin{cases} \text{Stop with rejection of } H_0 \text{ if } p_1 p_2 p_3 \le d_\alpha = e^{-\frac{1}{2}\chi_6^2(1-\alpha)}, \\ \text{Otherwise stop without rejection of } H_0. \end{cases}$$

To avoid qualitative interaction between stages and treatments, choose

$$c_{a_2} = d_\alpha / \alpha_0.$$

Then, no values of $p_3 \ge \alpha_0$ can lead to the rejection of H_0 because the procedure would have stopped beforehand. On the other hand, if

$$\alpha_1 \ge c_{a_2} / \alpha_0,$$

then no $p_2 \ge \alpha_0$ can lead to the rejection of H_0. Note that

$$\alpha_1 + \int_{\alpha_1}^{\alpha_0} \int_0^{d_\alpha/(\alpha_0 p_1)} dp_1 dp_2 + \int_{\alpha_1}^{\alpha_0} \int_{d_\alpha/(\alpha_0 p_1)}^{\alpha_0} \int_0^{d_\alpha/(p_1 p_2)} dp_1 dp_2 dp_3$$

$$= a_1 + \frac{d_\alpha}{\alpha_0}(\ln \alpha_0 - \ln \alpha_1) + d_a(2 \ln \alpha_0 - \ln d_\alpha)(\ln \alpha_0 - \ln \alpha_1)$$

$$+ \frac{d_\alpha}{2}(\ln^2 \alpha_0 - \ln^2 \alpha_1).$$

Now, let it be equal to α. We can then solve for α_1 given α and α_0. For $\alpha_0 = 0.025$, $d_\alpha = 0.000728$.

Table 8.5.2: Stopping Boundaries

α_0	α_1	α_2
.4	.0265	.0294
.6	.0205	.0209
.8	.0137	.0163

Source: Bauer and Köhne (1995).

8.6 Generalization of Independent P-value Approaches

General Approach

Consider a clinical trial with K stages and at each stage a hypothesis test is performed, followed by some actions that are dependent on the analysis results. Such actions could be an early futility or efficacy stopping, sample size re-estimation, modification of randomization, or other adaptations. The objective of the trial (e.g., testing the efficacy of the experimental drug) can be formulated using a global hypothesis test, which is the intersection of the individual hypothesis tests from the interim analyses.

$$H_0 : H_{01} \cap ... \cap H_{0K}, \tag{8.29}$$

where H_{0k} $(k = 1, ..., K)$ is the null hypothesis test at the kth interim analysis. Note that the H_{0k} have some restrictions, that is, rejection of any H_{0k} $(k = 1, ..., K)$ will lead to the same clinical implication (e.g., drug is efficacious). Otherwise the global hypothesis can not be interpreted. In the rest of the paper, H_{0k} will be based on sub-sample from each stage with the corresponding test statistic denoted by T_k and p-value denoted by p_k. The stopping rules are given by

$$\begin{cases} \text{Stop for efficacy} & \text{if } T_k \le \alpha_k, \\ \text{Stop for futility} & \text{if } T_k > \beta_k, \\ \text{Continue with adaptations if } \alpha_k < T_k \le \beta_k, \end{cases} \tag{8.30}$$

where $\alpha_k < \beta_k$ $(k = 1, ..., K - 1)$, and $\alpha_K = \beta_K$. For convenience, α_k and β_k are called the efficacy and futility boundaries, respectively.

To reach the kth stage, a trial has to pass the 1st to $(k - 1)$th stages, therefore the cumulative distribution function (CDF) of T_k is given by

$$\begin{aligned} \varphi_k(t) &= \Pr(T_k < t, \alpha_1 < t_1 \le \beta_1, ..., \alpha_{k-1} < t_{k-1} \le \beta_{k-1}) \\ &= \int_{\alpha_1}^{\beta_1} ... \int_{\alpha_{k-1}}^{\beta_{k-1}} \int_0^t f_{T_1...T_k} \, dt_k \, dt_{k-1}...dt_1, \end{aligned} \tag{8.31}$$

where $f_{T_1...T_k}$ is the joint PDF of $T_1, ...,$ and T_k. The error rate (α spent) at the kth stage is given by $\Pr(T_k < \alpha_k)$, that is,

$$\pi_k = \varphi_k(\alpha_k). \tag{8.32}$$

When the efficacy is claimed at a certain stage, the trial is stopped. Therefore, the type I errors at different stages are mutually exclusive. Hence the experiment-wise type I error rate can be written as

$$\alpha = \sum_{k=1}^{K} \pi_k. \tag{8.33}$$

(8.33) is the key to determining the stopping boundaries as illustrated in the next four sections with two-stage adaptive designs.

There are different p-values that can be calculated: unadjusted p-value and adjusted p-value. Both are measures of the statistical strength for treatment effect. The unadjusted p-value (p_u) associates with π_k when the trial stops at the kth stage, while the adjusted p-value associates with the overall α. The unadjusted p-value corresponding with an observed t when the trial stops at the kth stage is given by

$$p_u(t; k) = \varphi_k(t), \tag{8.34}$$

where $\varphi_k(t)$ is obtained from (8.31). The adjusted p-value corresponding an observed test statistic $T_k = t$ at the kth stage is given by

$$p(t; k) = \sum_{i=1}^{k-1} \pi_i + p_u(t; k), \quad k = 1, ...K. \tag{8.35}$$

Note that the adjusted p-value is a measure of over statistical strength for rejecting H_0. The later the H_0 is rejected, the larger the adjusted p-value is and the weaker the statistical evidence is.

Selection of Test Statistic

Without losing generality, assume H_{0k} is a test for the efficacy of the experimental drug, which can be written as

$$H_{0k} : \eta_{k1} \geq \eta_{k2} \quad \text{vs.} \quad H_{ak} : \eta_{k1} < \eta_{k2} \tag{8.36}$$

where η_{k1} and η_{k2} are the treatment response (mean, proportion or survival) in the two comparison groups at the kth stage. The joint probability density function (PDF) $f_{T_1...T_k}$ in (8.31) can be any density function, however, it is desirable to chose T_k such that $f_{T_1...T_k}$ has a simple form. Note that when $\eta_{k1} = \eta_{k2}$, the p-value p_k from the sub-sample at the kth stage is uniformly distributed on [0,1] under H_0. This desirable property can be used to construct test statistics for adaptive designs.

In what follows, two different combinations of the p-values will be studied: (i) linear combination of p-values (Chang, 2005c), and (ii) product of p-values. The linear combination is given by

$$T_k = \Sigma_{i=1}^{k} w_{ki} p_i, \quad k = 1, ..., K, \tag{8.37}$$

where $w_{ki} > 0$, and K is the number of analyses planed in the trial. There are two interesting cases of (8.37) that will be studied. They are the tests based on the individual p-value for the sub-sample obtained at each stage and the test based on the sum of the p-values from the sub-samples.

The test statistic using the product of p-values is given by

$$T_k = \Pi_{i=1}^k p_i, \ k = 1, ..., K. \tag{8.38}$$

This form has been proposed by Bauer and Köhne (1994) using Fisher's criterion. Here, it will be generalized without using Fisher's criterion so that the selection of stopping boundaries is more flexible. Note that p_k in (8.37) and (8.38) is the p-value from the sub-sample at the kth stage, while $p_u(t; k)$ and $p(t; k)$ in the previous section are unadjusted and adjusted p-values, respectively, calculated from the test statistic, which are based on the cumulative sample up to the kth stage where the trial stops.

Test Based on Individual P-values

The test statistic in this method is based on individual p-values from different stages. The method is referred to as method of individual p-values (MIP). By defining the weighting function as $w_{ki} = 1$ if $i = k$, and $w_{ki} = 0$ otherwise, (8.37) becomes

$$T_k = p_k \tag{8.39}$$

due to the independence of p_k, $f_{T_1...T_k} = 1$ under H_0 and

$$\varphi_k(t) = t \prod_{i=1}^{k-1} L_i. \tag{8.40}$$

where $L_i = (\beta_i - \alpha_i)$ and for convenience, when the upper bound exceeds the lower bound, define $\prod_{i=1}^0 (\cdot) = 1$. The family experiment-wise type I error rate is given by,

$$\alpha = \sum_{k=1}^K \alpha_k \prod_{i=1}^{k-1} L_i. \tag{8.41}$$

(8.41) is the necessary and sufficient condition for determining the stopping boundaries, (α_i, β_i).

For a two-stage design, (8.41) becomes

$$\alpha = \alpha_1 + \alpha_2(\beta_1 - \alpha_1) \tag{8.42}$$

For convenience, a table of stopping boundaries has been constructed using (8.42) (Table 8.6.1). The adjusted p-value is given by

$$p(t, k) = \begin{cases} t & \text{if } k - 1, \\ \alpha_1 + (\beta_1 - \alpha_1)t & \text{if } k = 2. \end{cases} \quad (8.43)$$

Table 8.6.1: Stopping Boundaries with MIP

α_1	0.000	0.005	0.010	0.015	0.020
β_1					
0.15	0.1667	0.1379	0.1071	0.0741	0.0385
0.20	0.1250	0.1026	0.0789	0.0541	0.0278
0.25	0.1000	0.0816	0.0625	0.0426	0.0217
0.30	0.0833	0.0678	0.0517	0.0351	0.0179
0.35 α_2	0.0714	0.0580	0.0441	0.0299	0.0152
0.40	0.0625	0.0506	0.0385	0.026	0.0132
0.50	0.0500	0.0404	0.0306	0.0206	0.0104
0.80	0.0312	0.0252	0.0190	0.0127	0.0064
1.00	0.0250	0.0201	0.0152	0.0102	0.0051

Note: One-sided $\alpha = 0.025$.

Test Based on Sum of P-values

This method is referred to as the method of sum of p-values (MSP). The test statistic in this method is based on the sum of the p-values from the subsamples. Defining the weights as $w_{ki} = 1$, (8.37) becomes

$$T_k = \Sigma_{i=1}^k p_i, \quad k = 1, ..., K. \quad (8.44)$$

For two-stage designs, the α spent at stage 1 and stage 2 are given by.

$$\Pr(T_1 < \alpha_1) = \int_0^{\alpha_1} dt_1 = \alpha_1, \quad (8.45)$$

and

$$\Pr(T_2 < \alpha_2, \alpha_1 < T_1 \le \beta_1) = \begin{cases} \int_{\alpha_1}^{\beta_1} \int_{t_1}^{\alpha_2} dt_2 dt_1, & \text{for } \beta_1 \le \alpha_2, \\ \int_{\alpha_1}^{\alpha_2} \int_{t_1}^{\alpha_2} dt_2 dt_1, & \text{for } \beta_1 > \alpha_2, \end{cases} \quad (8.46)$$

respectively. Carrying out the integrations in (8.46) and substituting the results into (8.33), it is immediately obtained that

$$\alpha = \begin{cases} \alpha_1 + \alpha_2(\beta_1 - \alpha_1) - \frac{1}{2}(\beta_1^2 - \alpha_1^2), & \text{for } \beta_1 < \alpha_2, \\ \alpha_1 + \frac{1}{2}(\alpha_2 - \alpha_1)^2, & \text{for } \beta_1 \ge \alpha_2. \end{cases} \quad (8.47)$$

Various stopping boundaries can be chosen from (8.47). See Table 8.6.2 for examples of the stopping boundaries.

Table 8.6.2: Stopping Boundaries with MSP

α_1		0.000	0.005	0.010	0.015	0.020
β_1						
0.05		0.5250	0.4719	0.4050	0.3182	0.2017
0.10		0.3000	0.2630	0.2217	0.1751	0.1225
0.15	α_2	0.2417	0.2154	0.1871	0.1566	0.1200
0.20		0.2250	0.2051	0.1832	0.1564	0.1200
>0.25		0.2236	0.2050	0.1832	0.1564	0.1200

Note: One-sided $\alpha = 0.025$.

The adjusted p-value can be obtained by replacing α_1 with t in (8.45) if the trial stops at stage 1 and by replacing α_2 with t in (8.47) if the trial stops at stage 2.

$$p(t; k) = \begin{cases} t, & k = 1, \\ \alpha_1 + t(\beta_1 - \alpha_1) - \frac{1}{2}(\beta_1^2 - \alpha_1^2), & k = 2 \text{ and } t \leq \alpha_2, \\ \alpha_1 + \frac{1}{2}(t - \alpha_1)^2, & k = 2 \text{ and } t > \alpha_2, \end{cases} \qquad (8.48)$$

where $t = p_1$ if the trial stops at stage 1 $(k = 1)$ and $t = p_1 + p_2$ if the trial stops at stage 2 $(k = 2)$.

Test Based on Product of P-values

This method is known as the method of products of p-values (MPP). The test statistic in this method is based on the product of the p-values from the sub-samples. For two-stage designs, (8.37) becomes

$$T_k = \Pi_{i=1}^k p_i, \quad k = 1, 2. \qquad (8.49)$$

The α spent in the two stages are given by

$$\Pr(T_1 < \alpha_1) = \int_0^{\alpha_1} dt_1 = \alpha_1 \qquad (8.50)$$

and

$$\Pr(T_2 < \alpha_2, \alpha_1 < T_1 \leq \beta_1) = \int_{\alpha_1}^{\beta_1} \int_0^{\min(\alpha_2, t_1)} \frac{1}{t_1} dt_2 dt_1. \qquad (8.51)$$

(8.51) can also be written as

$$\Pr(T_2 < \alpha_2, \alpha_1 < T_1 \leq \beta_1)$$
$$= \begin{cases} \int_{\alpha_1}^{\beta_1} \int_0^{\alpha_2} \frac{1}{t_1} dt_2 dt_1, & \text{for } \beta_1 \leq \alpha_2; \\ \int_{\alpha_1}^{\alpha_2} \int_0^{\alpha_2} \frac{1}{t_1} dt_2 dt_1 + \int_{\alpha_2}^{\beta_1} \int_0^{t_1} \frac{1}{t_1} dt_2 dt_1, & \text{for } \beta_1 > \alpha_2. \end{cases} \qquad (8.52)$$

Carrying out the integrations in (8.52) and substituting the results into (8.33), it is immediately obtained that

$$\alpha = \begin{cases} \alpha_1 + \alpha_2 \ln \frac{\beta_1}{\alpha_1}, & \text{for } \beta_1 \leq \alpha_2, \\ \alpha_1 + \alpha_2 \ln \frac{\beta_1}{\alpha_1} + (\beta_1 - \alpha_2), & \text{for } \beta_1 > \alpha_2. \end{cases} \tag{8.53}$$

Note that the stopping boundaries based on Fisher's criterion are special cases of (8.53), where

$$\beta_1 < \alpha_2$$

and

$$\alpha_2 = \exp\left[-\frac{1}{2}\chi_4^2(1-\alpha)\right], \tag{8.54}$$

that is, $\alpha_2 = 0.0380$ for $\alpha = 0.025$. Examples of the stopping boundaries using (8.49) are provided in Table 8.6.3.

Table 8.6.3: Stopping Boundaries with MPP

α_1	0.005	0.010	0.015	0.020
β_1				
0.15	0.0059	0.0055	0.0043	0.0025
0.20	0.0054	0.0050	0.0039	0.0022
0.25	0.0051	0.0047	0.0036	0.0020
0.30	0.0049	0.0044	0.0033	0.0018
0.35 α_2	0.0047	0.0042	0.0032	0.0017
0.40	0.0046	0.0041	0.0030	0.0017
0.50	0.0043	0.0038	0.0029	0.0016
0.80	0.0039	0.0034	0.0025	0.0014
1.00	0.0038	0.0033	0.0024	0.0013

Note: One-sided $\alpha = 0.025$.

The adjusted p-value can be obtained by replacing α_1 with t in (8.50) if the trial stops at stage 1 and replacing α_2 with t in (8.53) if the trial stops at stage 2.

$$p(t;k) = \begin{cases} t, & k = 1, \\ \alpha_1 + t \ln \frac{\beta_1}{\alpha_1}, & k = 2 \text{ and } t \leq \alpha_2, \\ \alpha_1 + t \ln \frac{\beta_1}{\alpha_1} + (\beta_1 - t), & k = 2 \text{ and } t > \alpha_2, \end{cases} \tag{8.55}$$

where $t = p_1$ if the trial stops at stage 1 ($k = 1$) and $t = p_1 + p_2$ if the trial stops at stage 2 ($k = 2$).

Rules for Sample Size Adjustment The primary rule for adjustment is based on the ratio of the initial estimate of effect size (E_0) to the observed effect size (E), specifically,

$$N = \left| \frac{E_0}{E} \right|^a N_0, \tag{8.56}$$

where N is the newly estimated sample size, N_0 is the initial sample size which can be estimated from a classic design, and a is a constant,

$$E = \frac{\hat{\eta}_{i2} - \hat{\eta}_{i1}}{\hat{\sigma}_i}. \tag{8.57}$$

With large sample size assumption, the common variance for the two treatment groups is given by

$$\hat{\sigma}_i^2 = \begin{cases} \hat{\sigma}_i^2, & \text{for normal endpoint,} \\ \bar{\eta}_i(1 - \bar{\eta}_i), & \text{for binary endpoint,} \\ \bar{\eta}_i^2 \left[1 - \frac{e^{\bar{\eta}_i T_0} - 1}{T_0 \bar{\eta}_i e^{\bar{\eta}_i T_s}} \right]^{-1}, & \text{for survival endpoint,} \end{cases} \tag{8.58}$$

where

$$\bar{\eta}_i = \frac{\hat{\eta}_{i1} + \hat{\eta}_{i1}}{2}.$$

$\bar{\eta}_i = \frac{\hat{\eta}_{i1} + \hat{\eta}_{i2}}{2}$ and the logrank test is assumed to be used for the survival analysis. Note that the standard deviations for proportion and survival have several versions. There are usually slight differences in sample size or power among the different versions.

The sample size adjustment in (8.56) should have the following additional constraints: (i) It should be smaller than $N_{\max}$ (due to financial and or other constraints) and greater than or equal to $N_{\min}$ (the sample size for the interim analysis), and (ii) If E and E_0 have different signs, no adjustment will be made.

Operating Characteristics

The operating characteristics are studied using the following example, which is modified slightly from an oncology trial.

Example 8.6.1 In a two-arm comparative oncology trial, the primary efficacy endpoint is time to progression (TTP). The median TTP is estimated to be 8 months (hazard rate = 0.08664) for the control group, and 10.5 months (hazard rate = 0.06601) for the test group. Assume a uniform enrollment with an accrual period of 9 months and a total study duration of 24 months. The logrank test will be used for the analysis. An exponential survival distribution is assumed for the purpose of sample size calculation.

When there is a 10.5 month median time for the test group, the classic design requires a sample size of 290 per group with 80% power at a level of significance (one-sided) α of 0.025. To increase efficiency, an adaptive design with an interim sample size of 175 patients per group is used. The interim analysis allowing for early efficacy stopping with stopping boundaries (from Tables 8.6.1, 8.6.2, and 8.6.3) $\alpha_1 = 0.01$, $b_1 = 0.25$ and $\alpha_2 = 0.0625$ (MIP), 0.1832 (MSP), 0.00466 (MPP). The sample size adjustment is based on the rules described in the appendix where $a = 2$. The maximum sample size allowed for adjustment is $N_{max} = 350$. The simulation results are presented in Table 8.6.4, where the abbreviations EESP and EFSP stand for early efficacy stopping probability and early futility stopping probability, respectively.

Table 8.6.4: Operating Characteristics of Adaptive Methods

| Median time | | EESP | EFSP | Expected | Power (%) |
Test	Control			N	MIP/MSP/MPP
0	0	0.010	0.750	216	2.5/2.5/2.5
9.5	8	0.174	0.238	273	42.5/44.3/45.7
10.5	8	0.440	0.067	254	78.6/80.5/82.7
11.5	8	0.703	0.015	219	94.6/95.5/96.7

Note: 1,000,000 simulation runs.

Note that power is the probability of rejecting the null hypothesis. Therefore when the null hypothesis is true, the power is the type I error rate α. From Table 8.6.4, it can be seen that the one-sided α is controlled at a 0.025 level as expected for all three methods. The expected sample sizes under all four scenarios are smaller than the sample size for the classic design (290/group). In terms of power, MPP has 1% more power than MSP, and MSP has about 1% more power than MIP. If the stopping boundaries are changed to $\alpha_1 = 0.005$ and $\beta_1 = 0.2$, then the power (median TTP =10.5 months for the test group) will be 76, 79, and 82 for MIP, MSP and MPP, respectively. The detailed results are not presented.

To demonstrate how to calculate the adjusted p-value (e.g. using MSP), assume that naive p-values from logrank test (or other test) are $p_1 = 0.1$, $p_2 = 0.07$, and the trial stops at stage 2. Therefore, $t = p_1 + p_2 = 0.17 < \alpha_2$, and the null hypothesis of no treatment difference is rejected. In fact, the adjusted p-value is 0.0228 (< 0.025) which is obtained from Eq.5-5 using $t = 0.17$ and $\alpha_1 = 0.01$.

Remarks

With respect to the accuracy of proposed methods, a larger portion of the stopping boundaries in Tables 8.6.1 through 8.6.3 is validated using computer simulations with 1,000,000 runs for each set of boundaries $(\alpha_1, \beta_1, \alpha_2)$. To conduct an adaptive design using the methods proposed, follow the steps below:

Step 1: If MIP is used for the design, use (8.42) or Table 8.6.1 to determine the stopping boundaries $(\alpha_1, \beta_1, \alpha_2)$, and use (8.43) to calculate the adjusted p-value when the trial is finished.

Step 2: If MSP is used for the design, use (8.45) or Table 8.6.2 to determine the stopping boundaries, and use (8.48) to calculate the adjusted p-value.

Step 3: If MPP is used for the design, use (8.53) or Table 8.6.3 to determine the stopping boundaries, and (8.54) to calculate the adjusted p-value.

To study the operating characteristics before selecting an optimal design, simulations must be conducted with various scenarios. A SAS program for the simulations can be obtained from the author. The program has fewer than 50 lines of executable code and is very user-friendly.

8.7 Inverse-Normal Method

Lehmacher and Wassmer (1999) proposed normal-inverse method. The test statistic that results from the inverse normal method of combining independent p values (Hedges and Olkin, 1985) is given by

$$\frac{1}{\sqrt{k}} \sum_{i=1}^{k} \Phi^{-1}(1 - p_i) \tag{8.59}$$

where $\Phi^{-1}(\cdot)$ denotes the inverse cumulative standard normal distribution function. Then proposed approach involves using the classical group sequential boundaries for the statistics (8.59). Since the

$$\Phi^{-1}(1 - p_i)'s, k = 1, 2, ..., K,$$

are independent and standard normally distributed, the proposed approach maintains α exactly for any (adaptive) choice of sample size.

Example 8.7.1

Lahmacher and Wassmer gave the following example to demonstrate their method. In a randomized, placebo-controlled, double-blind study involving patients with acne papulopustulosa, Plewig's grade Il-Ill, the effect of treatment under a combination of 1% chloramphenicol (CAS 56-75-7) and 0.5% pale sulfonated shale oil vs. the alcoholic vehicle (placebo) was investigated (Fluhr et al., 1998). After 6 weeks of treatment, reduction of bacteria from baseline, examined on agar plates (log CFU/cm^2; CFU, colony forming units), of the active group as compared to the placebo group were assessed. The available data were from 24 and 26 patients in the combination drug and the placebo groups, respectively. The combination therapy resulted in a highly significant reduction in bacteria as compared to placebo using a two-sided t-test for the changes (p = 0.0008).

They further illustrated the method. Suppose that it was intended to perform a three-stage adaptive Pocock's design with $\alpha = 0.01$ and after 2 x 12 patients the first interim analysis was planned. The two-sided critical bounds for this method are $\alpha_1 = \alpha_2 = \alpha_3 = 2.873$ (Pocock, 1977). After ni = 12 patients per group, the test statistic of the t-test is 2.672 with one-sided p-value $p_1 = 0.0070$, resulting from an observed effect size $\bar{x}_{ii} - \bar{x}_{21} = 1.549$ and an observed standard deviation $s_i = 1.316$. The study should be continued since

$$\Phi^{-1}(i - P_1) = 2.460 < \alpha_1.$$

The observed effect is fairly near to significance. We therefore plan the second interim analysis to be conducted after observing the next 2 x 6 patients, i.e., the second interim analysis will be performed after fewer patients than the first. The t-test statistic of the second stage is equal to 1.853 with one-sided p value $P_2 = 0.0468$ ($\bar{x}_{12} - \bar{x}_{22} = 1.580$, standard deviation of the second stage $s_2 = 1.472$). The test statistic becomes

$$\sqrt{2}(\Phi^{-1}(1 - p_1) + \Phi^{-1}(1 - p_2)) = 2.925,$$

yielding a significant result after the second stage of the trial. Corresponding approximate 99% RCIs are (0.12, 3.21) and (0.21, 2.92) for the first and the second stages, respectively.

8.8   Concluding Remarks

One of the purposes for adaptive sample size adjustment based on accrued data at interim in clinical trials is not only to achieve statistical significance with a desired power for detecting a clinically significant difference, but also to have option for stopping the trial early for safety or futility/benefits. To maintain the integrity of the trial, it is strongly recommended that an independent data monitoring committee (DMC) should be established to perform (safety) data monitoring and interim analyses for efficacy/benefits regardless the review or analysis is blinded or unblinded. Based on sample size re-assessment, the DMC can then recommend one of the following that (i) continue the trial with no changes, (ii) decrease/increase the sample size for achieving statistical significance with a desired power, (iii) stop the trial early for safety, futility or benefits, and (iv) make modifications to the study protocol. In a recent review article by Montori et al. (2005), it is indicated that there is a significant increasing trend that the percentage of randomized clinical trials are stopped early for benefits in the past decade. Pocock (2005), however, criticized that the majority of the trails that stop early for benefits do not have the correct infrastructure/system in place, and hence the decisions/recommendations for stopping early may not be appropriate. Chow (2005) suggested that so-called reproducibility probability be carefully evaluated if a trial is to be stopped early for benefits in addition to an observed small p-value.

It should be noted that current methods for adaptive sample size adjustment are mostly developed in the interest of controlling an overall type I error rate at the nominal level. These methods, however, are conditional and may not be feasible to reflect current best medical practice. As indicated in Chapter 2, the use of adaptive design methods in clinical trials could result in a moving target patient population after protocol amendments. As a result, the sample size required in order to have an accurate and reliable statistical inference on the moving target patient population is necessarily adjusted unconditionally. In practice, it is then suggested that current statistical methods for group sequential designs should be modified to incorporate the randomness of the target patient population over time. In other words, sample sizes should be adjusted adaptively to account for random boundaries at different stages.

Chapter 9

Two-Stage Adaptive Design

9.1 Introduction

As indicated in Chapter 7, a seamless trial design is referred to as a program that addresses study objectives within a single trial that are normally achieved through separate trials in clinical development. A two-stage (seamless) adaptive design is a seamless trial design that would use data from patients enrolled before and after the adaptation in the final analysis. Thus, a two-stage seamless adaptive design consists of two phases (stages), namely a learning (or exploratory) phase (stage 1) and a confirmatory phase (stage 2). The learning phase provides an opportunity for adaptations such as stopping the trial early due to safety and/or futility/efficacy based on accrued data at the end of the learning phase. A two-stage seamless adaptive trial design reduces lead time between the learning (i.e., the first study for the traditional approach) and confirmatory (i.e., the second study for the traditional approach) phases. Most importantly, data collected at the learning phase can be combined with those data obtained at the confirmatory phase for final analysis.

Chow and Tu (2008) classified two-stage (seamless) adaptive trial designs into four categories, namely SS, SD, DS, and DD designs depending upon whether the study objectives and study endpoints are the same at different stages, where SD designs are the two-stage designs with same study objectives but different study endpoints that are used at different stages (see also Pong and Chow, 2010). In practice, the SS two-stage designs are similar to group sequential designs with one planned interim analysis (at the end of the first stage). As a result, the SS designs are considered well-understood designs as described in the FDA draft guidance. Other two-stage adaptive designs (i.e., SD, DS, and DD designs) are considered less well-understood designs. Consequently, the following issues/concerns exist (i) strategies for preventing possible operational biases that may be introduced by the adaptations applied, (ii) the control of the overall type I error rate, (iii) the use of data collected from both stages for a valid final analysis, (iv) the feasibility of O'Brien-Fleming type of boundaries, and (v) sample size calculation and allocation. It is then suggested that the above issues/concerns be addressed before the SD, DS, and DD designs can be used in clinical trials (i.e., the less well-understood designs have become well-understood designs).

In the next section, some practical issues regarding the flexibility, efficiency, validity, and integrity of clinical trials utilizing two-stage adaptive trial designs are discussed. Also included in the section are regulatory perspectives/concerns of the use of less well-understood two-stage adaptive designs in clinical trials. Types of two-stage (seamless) adaptive trial designs depending upon whether the study objectives and/or the study endpoints at different stages are the same are described in Section 9.3. Sections 9.4-9.6 summarize statistical methods for analysis of various types of two-stage designs depending upon study objectives and the study endpoints used at different stages. Some concluding remarks are provided in the last section of this chapter.

9.2   Practical Issues

The use of adaptive design methods for modifying the trial and/or statistical procedures of on-going clinical trials based on accrued data has been in practice for years in clinical research. Adaptive design methods in clinical research are very attractive to clinical scientists due to the following reasons. First, it reflects medical practice in real world. Second, it is ethical with respect to both efficacy and safety (toxicity) of the test treatment under investigation. Third, it is not only flexible, but also efficient in the early phase of clinical development. However, some concerns regarding the validity and integrity of the clinical trials utilizing adaptive trial designs have been raised and discussed tremendously within the pharmaceutical industry and the regulatory agencies (Chang, Chow and Pong, 2006; Chow and Chang, 2008; Chow, 2011). In what follows, controversial issues regarding the flexibility, efficiency, validity, and integrity of a clinical trial utilizing adaptive trial design are briefly described.

9.2.1   Flexibility and efficiency

As discussed in Chapter 7, a two-stage seamless adaptive design is considered a more efficient and flexible study design as compared to the traditional approach of having separate studies (e.g., a phase II study and a phase III study) in terms of controlling the type I error rate and power. The type I error rate for a two-stage seamless phase II/III adaptive design is $1/\alpha_{II}$ times larger than the traditional approach for having two separate phase II and phase III studies, while the corresponding power is $1/Power_{II}$ times larger than the traditional approach for having two separate phase II and phase III studies, where α_{II} and $Power_{II}$ are the type I error rate and power for a phase II study, respectively.

In addition, a two-stage seamless adaptive trial design that combines two separate (independent) studies can help in reducing lead time between studies. In practice, the lead time between studies is estimated about six months to a year. As a common clinical practice, the phase III study will not be initiated until the final report of the phase II trial is reviewed and issued. After the completion of a phase II study, on average, it will usually take about four months to lock database (including data entry/verification and data query/validation), programming and data analysis, and final integrated statistical/clinical report. During the preparation of the phase III trial, the development of study protocol and IRB (Institutional Review Board) review/approval will also take some time. As a result, the application of a two-stage phase II/III seamless adaptive trial design will not only reduce the lead time between studies, but also allow the sponsor (investigator) to make a go/no-go decision at the end of the first stage (phase II study) early. In some cases, a two-stage phase II/III seamless adaptive trial design may require a smaller sample size as compared to the traditional approach of two separate studies for phase II and phase III since data collected from both stages would be combined for a final assessment of the test treatment effect under investigation.

9.2.2 Validity and integrity

In practice, before an adaptive design can be implemented, some practical issues such as the feasibility, validity, and robustness are necessarily addressed. For feasibility, several questions arise. For example, does the adaptive design require extra efforts in implementation? Do the level of difficulty and the associated cost justify the gain from implementing the adaptive design? Does the implementation of adaptive design delay patient recruitment and prolong study duration? How often are the unblinded analyses practical and to whom should the data should be unblinded? How should the impact of the DMC's decision regarding the trial (e.g., recommending an early stopping or other adaptations due to safety concern) be considered at the design stage?

For the issue of validity, it is reasonable to ask the following questions. Does the unblinding cause potential bias in treatment assessment? Does the implementation of an adaptive design destroy the randomness? For example, response-adaptive randomization is used to assign more patients to the superior treatment groups by changing the randomization schedule. However, for ethical reasons, the patients should be informed that the later they come into the study, the greater the chance of being assigned to the superior groups. For this reason, patients may prefer to wait for late entry into the study. This could cause bias because sicker patients might enroll earlier just because they cannot wait. When this happens, the treatment effect is confounded by the patients disease background. The bias could occur for a drop-losers design and other adaptive designs.

Regarding the issue of robustness, virtually without any exception, a trial can-not be conducted exactly as specified in the protocol. Would protocol deviations invalidate the adaptive method? For example, if an actual interim analysis was performed at a different (information) time than the scheduled one, how does it impact the type I error of the adaptive design? How does an unexpected

DMC action affect the power and validity of the design? Would a protocol amendment such as endpoint change or inclusion/exclusion change invalidate the design and analysis? Would delayed responses diminish the advantage of implementing an adaptive design such as CRM in an adaptive dose-escalation design and trials with a survival endpoint?

Adaptive designs usually involve multiple comparisons and often invoke a dependent sampling procedure or an adaptive combination of subsamples from different stages. Therefore, studies with adaptive designs are much more complicated than those with classic designs. The theoretical challenges that arise from a typical adaptive design include (i) alpha adjustment to control overall type I error rates for multiple comparisons, (ii) the p-value adjustment due to the dependent sampling procedure, (iii) finding a robust unbiased point estimate, and (iv) finding a reliable confidence interval. In practice, it is not always easy to derive an analytical form for correctly adjusted alpha and p-values due to the flexibility of adaptations. However, they can be addressed through computer simulations regardless of the complexity of the adaptive designs. To do this, it is necessary to define an appropriate test statistic that can be applied before and after adaptations. A simulation can then be conducted under the null hypothesis for obtaining the sampling distribution of the test statistic. Based on the simulated distribution, the rejection region, adjusted alpha, and adjusted p-values can be obtained. The simulations can be done during protocol design to provide justification for choosing an appropriate design. More details regarding the use of clinical trial simulation in adaptive trial designs can be found in Chapter 15.

9.2.3　Regulatory perspectives/concerns

As it is recognized by the regulatory agencies, there are some possible benefits when utilizing adaptive design methods in clinical trials. For example, the use of adaptive design methods in clinical trials allows the investigator to correct wrong assumptions and select the most promising option early. In addition, adaptive designs make use of cumulative information of the on-going trial and emerging external information to the trial, which allows the investigator to react earlier to *surprises* regardless of positive or negative results. As a result, the use of adaptive design methods may speed up the development process.

Although the investigator may have a second chance to re-design the trial after seeing data from the trial itself at interim (or externally), it is flexible but more problematic operationally due to potential bias that may have been introduced to the conduct of the trial. For example, it is a major concern that unblinding during an interim analysis may have introduced potential bias by a change in clinical practice resulting from feedback from the analysis. As a result, we may have compromised scientific integrity of trial conduct due to operational bias. As indicated by the U.S. FDA, operational biases commonly occur when adaptations in trial and/or statistical procedures are applied. Trial procedures are referred to as eligibility criteria, dose/dose regimen and duration, assessment of study endpoints, and/or diagnostic/laboratory testing procedures that are employed during the conduct of the trial. Statistical procedures include (i) selection and/or modification of study design, (ii) formulation and/or modification of statistical hypotheses (according study objectives), (iii) selection and/or modification of study endpoints, (iv) sample size calculation, re-estimation, and/or adjustment, (v) generation of randomization schedules, and (vi) development of statistical analysis plan (SAP). As a result, commonly seen operational biases due to adaptations include (i) sample size re-estimation at interim analysis, (ii) sample size allocation to treatments (e.g., change from 1:1 ratio to an unequal ratio), (iii) delete, add, or change treatment arms after the review of interim analysis results, (iv) shift in patient population after the application of adaptations (e.g., change in inclusion/exclusion criteria and/or subgroups), (v) change in statistical test strategy (e.g., change logrank to other tests), (vi) change study endpoints (e.g., change survival to time-to-disease progression and/or response rate in cancer trials), and (vii) change study objectives (e.g., switch a superiority hypothesis to a non-inferiority hypothesis).

In summary, regulatory agencies do not object to the use of the adaptive design methods in clinical trials due to their flexibility, efficiency and potential benefits as described above. However, the validity and integrity of the clinical trials after the implementation of various adaptations have raised critical concerns to the drug evaluation and approval process. These concerns include, but are not limited to (i) that we may not be able to control (preserve) the overall type I error rate at a pre-specified level of significance, (ii) that the obtained p-values may not be correct, (iii) that the obtained confidence interval may not be reliable, and (iv) that major (significant) adaptations may have resulted in a totally different trial that is unable to address the scientific/medical questions the original study intended to answer.

9.3 Types of Two-Stage Adaptive Designs

In practice, two-stage (seamless) adaptive trial designs can be classified into the following four categories depending upon study objectives and study endpoints at different stage (see, e.g., Chow and Tu, 2008; Pong and Chow, 2010).

Table 9.3.1: Types of Two-stage Seamless Adaptive Designs

Study Objectives	Study Endpoints	
	Same (S)	Different (D)
Same (S)	I = SS	II = SD
Different (D)	III = DS	IV = DD

In other words, we have (i) Category I (SS) - same study objectives and same study endpoints, (i) Category II (SD) - same study objectives but different study endpoints, (iii) Category III (DS) - different study objectives but same study endpoints, and (iv) Category IV (DD) - different study objectives and different study endpoints. Note that different study objectives are usually referred to dose finding (selection) at the first stage and efficacy confirmation at the second stage, while different study endpoints are directed to biomarker vs. clinical endpoint or the same clinical endpoint with different treatment durations. Category I trial design is often viewed as a similar design to a group sequential design with one interim analysis despite the fact that there are differences between a group sequential design and a two-stage seamless design. In this chapter, our emphasis will be placed on Category II designs. The results obtained can be similarly applied to Category III and Category IV designs with some modification for controlling the overall type I error rate at a pre-specified level. In practice, typical examples for a two-stage seamless adaptive design include a two-stage seamless phase I/II adaptive design and a two-stage seamless phase II/III adaptive design. For the two-stage seamless phase I/II adaptive design, the objective at the first stage is for biomarker development, and the study objective for the second stage is to establish early efficacy. For a two-stage seamless phase II/III adaptive design, the study objective is for treatment selection (or dose finding) while the study objective at the second stage is for efficacy confirmation.

Statistical consideration for the first kind of two-stage seamless designs is similar to that of a group sequential design with one planned interim analysis. Sample size calculation and statistical analysis for this kind of study design can be found in Chow and Chang (2006). For other kinds of two-stage seamless trial designs, standard statistical methods for group sequential design are not appropriate and hence should not be applied directly. In this chapter, statistical methods for a two-stage seamless adaptive design with different study endpoints (e.g., a biomarker vs. clinical endpoint or the same clinical endpoint with different treatment durations) but the same study endpoint will be developed. Modification to the derived results is necessary if the study endpoints and study objectives are different at different stages.

One of the questions that is commonly asked when applying a two-stage seamless adaptive design in clinical trials is sample size calculation/allocation. For the first kind of two-stage seamless designs, the methods based on individual p-values as described in Chow and Chang (2006) can be applied. However, these methods are not appropriate for Category IV (DD) trial designs with different study objectives and endpoints at different stages. For Category IV (DD) trial designs, the following issues are challenging to the investigator and the biostatistician. First, how do we control the overall type I error rate at a pre-specified level of significance? Second, is the typical O'Brien-Fleming type of boundaries feasible? Third, how to perform a valid final analysis that combines data collected from different stages? Cheng and Chow (2011) attempt to address these questions by proposing a new multiple-stage transitional seamless adaptive design accompanied by valid statistical tests to incorporate different study endpoints for achieving different study objectives at different stages.

9.4 Analysis for Seamless Design with Same Study Objectives/Endpoints

In practice, since a two-stage seamless design with same study objectives and same study endpoints at different stages is similar to a typical group sequential design with one planned interim analysis, standard statistical methods for group sequential design are often employed. With various adaptations that applied, many interesting methods have been developed in the literature. For example, the following is a list of methods that are commonly employed: (i) Fisher's criterion for combination of independent p-values from subsamples collected between two consecutive adaptations (Bauer and Köhne, 1994; Bauer and Röhmel, 1995; Posch and Bauer, 2000), (ii) weighting the samples differently before and after each adaptation (Cui, Hung, and Wang, 1999), (iii) the conditional error function approach (Proschan and Hunsberger, 1995; Liu and Chi 2001), and (iv) conditional power approaches (Li, Shih, and Wang, 2005). The method using Fisher's combination of p-values provides great flexibility in the selection of statistical methods for individual hypothesis testing based on subsamples. However, as pointed out by Müller and Schafer (2001), the method lacks flexibility in the choice of boundaries. Among other interesting studies, Proschan and Wittes (2000) constructed an unbiased estimate that uses all of the data from the trial. Adaptive designs featuring response-adaptive randomization were studied by Rosenberger and Lachin (2003). The impact of study population changes due to protocol amendments was studied by Chow, Chang, and Pong (2005). An adaptive design with a survival endpoint was studied by Li, Shih, and Wang (2005). Hommel, Lindig, and Faldum (2005) studied a two-stage adaptive design with correlated data. An adaptive approach for a bivariate-endpoint was studied Todd (2003). Tsiatis and Mehta (2003) showed that for any adaptive design with sample size adjustment, there exists a more powerful group sequential design.

In what follows, for illustration purposes, we will introduce the method based on sum of p-values (MSP) by Chow and Chang (2006) and Chang (2007). The MSP following the idea of considering a linear combination of the p-values calculated using sub-samples from the current and previous stages. Because of the simplicity of this method, it has been widely used in clinical trials. The theoretical framework of the MSP is described in the next subsection. Chang (2007) derived the stopping boundaries and p-value formula for three different types of adaptive designs that allow (i) early efficacy stopping, (ii) early stopping for both efficacy and futility; and (iii) early futility stopping. The formulation can be applied to both superiority and non-inferiority trials with or without sample size adjustment.

9.4.1 Early efficacy stopping

Based on the discussion given in Section 8.6, for a two-stage design ($K = 2$) allowing for early efficacy stopping ($\beta_1 = 1$), the type I error rates to spend at

Stage 1 and Stage 2 are

$$\pi_1 = \psi_1(\alpha_1) = \int_0^{\alpha_1} dt_1 = \alpha_1, \tag{9.1}$$

and

$$\pi_2 = \psi_2(\alpha_2) = \int_{\alpha_1}^{\alpha_2} \int_t^{\alpha_1} dt_2 dt_1 = \frac{1}{2}(\alpha_2 - \alpha_1)^2, \tag{9.2}$$

respectively. By (9.1) and (9.2), we have

$$\alpha = \alpha_1 + \frac{1}{2}(\alpha_2 - \alpha_1)^2. \tag{9.3}$$

Solving for α_2, we obtain

$$\alpha_2 = \sqrt{2(\alpha - \alpha_1)} + \alpha_1. \tag{9.4}$$

Note that when the test statistic $t_1 = p_1 > \alpha_2$, it is certain that $t_2 = p_1 + p_2 > \alpha_2$. Therefore, the trial should stop when $p_1 > \alpha_2$ for futility. The clarity of the method in this respect is unique, and the futility stopping boundary is often hidden in other methods. Furthermore, α_1 is the stopping probability (error spent) at the first stage under the null hypothesis condition and $\alpha - \alpha_1$ is the error spent at the second stage. Table 9.4.1 provides some examples of the stopping boundaries from (9.4).

Table 9.4.1: Stopping Boundaries for Two-Stage Efficacy Designs

One-sided α	α_1	0.005	0.010	0.015	0.020	0.025	0.030
0.025	α_2	0.2050	0.1832	0.1564	0.1200	0.0250	—
0.05	α_2	0.3050	0.2928	0.2796	0.2649	0.2486	0.2300

Source: Chang (2007) Statistics in Medicine, 26, 2772-2784.

The adjusted p-value is given by

$$p(t; k) = \begin{cases} t & \text{if } k = 1 \\ \alpha_1 + \frac{1}{2}(t - \alpha_1)^2 & \text{if } k = 2 \end{cases}, \tag{9.5}$$

where $t = p_1$ if the trial stops at Stage 1 and $t = p_1 + p_2$ if the trial stops at Stage 2.

9.4.2   Early efficacy or futility stopping

It is obvious that if $\beta_1 \geq \alpha_2$, the stopping boundary is the same as it is for the design with early efficacy stopping. However, futility boundary β_1 when $\beta_1 \geq \alpha_2$ is expected to affect the power of the hypothesis testing. As discussed in Section 8.6, we have

$$\alpha = \begin{cases} \alpha_1 + \alpha_2(\beta_1 - \alpha_1) - \frac{1}{2}(\beta_1^2 - \alpha_1^2) & \text{for } \beta_1 < \alpha_2 \\ \alpha_1 + \frac{1}{2}(\alpha_2 - \alpha_1)^2 & \text{for } \beta_1 \geq \alpha_2 \end{cases} \tag{9.6}$$

Various stopping boundaries can be chosen from (9.6). A trial featuring early futility stopping is a special case of the previous design, where $\alpha_1 = 0$ in (9.6). Hence, we have

$$\alpha = \begin{cases} \alpha_2\beta_1 - \frac{1}{2}\beta_1^2 \text{ for } \beta_1 < \alpha_2 \\ \frac{1}{2}\alpha_2^2 \text{ for } \beta_1 \geq \alpha_2 \end{cases} \qquad (9.7)$$

Solving for α_2, it can be obtained that

$$\alpha_2 = \begin{cases} \frac{\alpha}{\beta_1} + \frac{1}{2}\beta_1 \text{ for } \beta_1 < \sqrt{2\alpha} \\ \sqrt{2\alpha} \text{ for } \beta_1 \geq \alpha_2. \end{cases} \qquad (9.8)$$

Examples of the stopping boundaries generated using (9.8) are presented in Table 9.4.2. The adjusted p-value can be obtained from (9.6), where $\alpha_1 = 0$, that is,

$$p(t; k) = \begin{cases} t \text{ if } k = 1 \\ \alpha_1 + t\beta_1 - \frac{1}{2}\beta_1^2 \text{ if } k = 2 \text{ and } \beta_1 < \alpha_2 \\ \alpha_1 + \frac{1}{2}t^2 \text{ if } k = 2 \ \beta_1 \geq \alpha_2. \end{cases} \qquad (9.9)$$

Table 9.4.2: Stopping Boundaries for Two-Stage Futility Design

One-sided α	β_1	0.1	0.2	0.3	≥ 0.4
0.025	α_2	0.3000	0.2250	0.2236	0.2236
0.05	α_2	0.5500	0.3500	0.3167	0.3162

Source: Chang (2007) Statistics in Medicine, 26, 2772-2784.

9.4.3 Conditional power

Conditional power is a very useful operating characteristic of adaptive designs. It can be used for interim decision-making and drawing comparisons among different designs and different statistical methods for adaptive designs. Because the stopping boundaries for the most existing methods are either based on z-scale or p-scale, for the purpose of comparison, we will use the transformation $p_k = 1 - \Phi(z_k)$ and inversely, $z_k = \Phi^{-1}(1 - p_k)$, where z_k and p_k are the normal z-score and the naive p-value from the sub-sample at the kth stage, respectively. Note that z_2 has asymptotically normal distribution with $N(\delta/se(\hat{\delta}_2), 1)$ under the alternative hypothesis, where $\hat{\delta}_2$ is the estimation of treatment difference in the second stage and

$$se(\hat{\delta}_2) = \sqrt{2\hat{\sigma}^2/n_2} \approx \sqrt{2\sigma^2/n_2}.$$

To derive the conditional power, we express the criterion for rejecting H_0 as

$$z_2 \geq B(\alpha_2, p_1). \qquad (9.10)$$

From (9.10), we can immediately obtain the conditional probability given the first stage naive p-value, p_1 at the second stage as

$$P_C(p_1, \delta) = 1 - \Phi\left(B(\alpha_2, p_1) - \frac{\delta}{\sigma}\sqrt{\frac{n_2}{2}}\right), \quad \alpha_1 < p_1 \le \beta_1. \quad (9.11)$$

For the method based on the product of stage-wise p-values (MPP), the rejection criterion for the second stage is $p_1 p_2 \le \alpha_2$, i.e., $z_2 \ge \Phi^{-1}(1 - \alpha_2/p_1)$. Therefore, $B(\alpha_2, p_1) = \Phi^{-1}(1 - \alpha_2/p_1)$. Similarly, for the method based on the sum of stage-wise p-values (MSP), the rejection criterion for the second stage is $p_1 + p_2 \le \alpha_2$, i.e., $z_2 = B(\alpha_2, p_1) = \Phi^{-1}(1 - \max(0, \alpha_2 - p_1))$. For the inverse normal method (Lehmacher and Wassmer, 1999), the rejection criterion for the second stage is $w_1 z_1 + w_2 z_2 \ge \Phi^{-1}(1 - \alpha_2)$, i.e., $z_2 \ge (\Phi^{-1}(1 - \alpha_2) - w_1\Phi^{-1}(1 - p_1))/w_2$, where w_1 and w_2 are prefixed weights satisfying the condition of $w_1^2 + w_2^2 = 1$. Note that the group sequential design and CHW method (Cui, Hung, and Wang, 1999) are special cases of the inverse-normal method. For simplicity, we will compare only MPP and MSP analytically because the third method also depends on two additional parameters, w_1 and w_2. To compare the conditional power, the same α_1 should be used for both methods, otherwise the comparison will be much less informative. From (9.11), we can see that the comparison of the conditional power is equivalent to the comparison of function $B(\alpha_2, p_1)$. Equating the two $B(\alpha_2, p_1)$, we have

$$\frac{\hat{\alpha}_2}{p_1} = \tilde{\alpha}_2 - p_1, \quad (9.12)$$

where $\hat{\alpha}_2$ and $\tilde{\alpha}_2$ are the final rejection boundaries for MPP and MSP, respectively. Solving (9.12) for p_1, we obtain the critical point for p_1

$$\eta = \frac{\tilde{\alpha}_2 \mp \sqrt{\tilde{\alpha}_2^2 - 4\tilde{\alpha}_2}}{2} \quad (9.13)$$

such that when $p_1 < \eta_1$ or $p_2 > \eta_2$ MPP has a higher conditional power than MSP. When $\eta_1 < p_1 < \eta_2$, MSP has a higher conditional power than MPP. For example, for overall one-sided $\alpha = 0.025$, if we choose $\alpha_1 = 0.01$ and $\beta_1 = 0.3$, then $\hat{\alpha}_2 = 0.0044$, and $\tilde{\alpha}_2 = 0.2236$, and finally $\eta_1 = 0.0218$, $\eta_2 = 0.2018$ from (9.13). The unconditional power P_w is the expectation of conditional power, i.e.

$$P_w = E_\delta[P_C(p_1, \delta)]. \quad (9.14)$$

Therefore, the difference in unconditional power between MSP and MPP is dependent on the distribution of p_1, and consequently, dependent on the true difference δ, and the stopping boundaries at the first stage (α_1, β_1).

Note that in Bauer and Köhne's (Bauer and Köhne, 1994) method using Fisher's combination, which leads to the equation $\alpha_1 + \ln(\beta_1/\alpha_1)e^{-(1/2)\chi_{4,1-\alpha}^2} = \alpha$, it is obvious that determination of β_1 leads to a unique α_1, consequently α_2. This is a non-flexible approach. However, it can be verified that the method can be generalized to $\alpha_1 + \alpha_2 \ln \beta_1/\alpha_1 = \alpha$, where α_2 does not have to be $e^{-(1/2)\chi^2_{4,1-\alpha}}$.

Note that Tsiatis and Mehta (2003) indicated that there is an optimal (uniformly more powerful) design for any class of sequential design with a specified error spending function. In other words, for any adaptive design, one can always construct a classic group sequential test statistic that, for any parameter value in the space of alternatives, will reject the null hypothesis earlier with equal or higher probability, and, for any parameter value not in the space of alternatives, will accept the null hypothesis earlier with equal or higher probability. However, the efficacy gain by the classic group sequential design comes with a cost—for example, an increased number of interim analyses increases (e.g. from 3 to 10)—which definitely has an associated cost practically. Also, the optimal design is under the condition of a pre-specified error-spending function, but adaptive designs do not require in general a fixed error-spending function.

9.5 Analysis for Seamless Design with Different Endpoints

9.5.1 Continuous endpoint

For illustration purposes, consider a two-stage seamless phase II/III adaptive trial design with different (continuous) study endpoints. Let x_i be the observation of one study endpoint (e.g., a biomarker) from the ith subject in phase II, $i = 1, ..., n$ and y_j be the observation of another study endpoint (the primary clinical endpoint) from the jth subject in phase III, $j = 1, ..., m$. Assume that $x_i's$ are independently and identically distributed with $E(x_i) = \nu$ and $Var(x_i) = \tau^2$; and $y_j's$ are independently and identically distributed with $E(y_j) = \mu$ and $Var(y_j) = \sigma^2$. Chow, Lu and Tse (2007) proposed using the established functional relationship to obtain predicted values of the clinical endpoint based on data collected from the biomarker (or surrogate endpoint). Thus, these predicted values can be combined with the data collected at the confirmatory phase to develop a valid statistical inference for the treatment effect under study. Suppose that x and y can be related in a straight-line relationship

$$y = \beta_0 + \beta_1 x + \varepsilon \qquad (9.15)$$

where ε is an error term with zero mean and variance ς^2. Furthermore, ε is independent of x. In practice, we assume that this relationship is well-explored and the parameters β_0 and are known. Based on (9.15), the observations x_i observed in the learning phase would be translated to $\beta_0 + \beta_1 x_i$ (denoted by $\hat{y}_i$) and are combined with those observations y_i collected in the confirmatory phase. Therefore, $\hat{y}_i$'s and y_i's are combined for the estimation of the treatment mean μ. Consider the following weighted-mean estimator,

$$\hat{\mu} = \omega \bar{\hat{y}} + (1 - \omega)\bar{y} \qquad (9.16)$$

where $\bar{\hat{y}} = \frac{1}{n} \sum\limits_{i=1}^{n} \hat{y}_i$, $\bar{y} = \frac{1}{m} \sum\limits_{j=1}^{m} y_j$ and $0 \le \omega \le 1$. It should be noted that $\hat{\mu}$ is the minimum variance unbiased estimator among all weighted-mean estimators when the weight is given by

$$\omega = \frac{n/(\beta_1^2 \tau^2)}{n/(\beta_1^2 \tau^2) + m/\sigma^2}, \tag{9.17}$$

if β_1, τ^2 and σ^2 are known. In practice, τ^2 and σ^2 are usually unknown and ω is commonly estimated by

$$\hat{\omega} = \frac{n/s_1^2}{n/s_1^2 + m/s_2^2} \tag{9.18}$$

where s_1^2 and s_2^2 are the sample variances of $\hat{y}_i$'s and y_j's, respectively. The corresponding estimator of μ, which is denoted by

$$\hat{\mu}_{GD} = \hat{\omega}\bar{\hat{y}} + (1 - \hat{\omega})\bar{y}, \tag{9.19}$$

is called the Graybill-Deal (GD) estimator of μ. The GD estimator is often called the weighted mean in metrology. Khatri and Shah (1974) gave an exact expression of the variance of this estimator in the form of an infinite series. An approximate unbiased estimator of the variance of the GD estimator, which has bias of order $O(n^{-2} + m^{-2})$, was proposed by Meier (1953). In particular, it is given as

$$\widehat{Var}(\hat{\mu}_{GD}) = \frac{1}{n/S_1^2 + m/S_2^2} \left[1 + 4\hat{\omega}(1 - \hat{\omega}) \left(\frac{1}{n-1} + \frac{1}{m-1} \right) \right].$$

For the comparison of the two treatments, the following hypotheses are considered

$$H_0 : \mu_1 = \mu_2 \ v.s. \ H_1 : \mu_1 \ne \mu_2. \tag{9.20}$$

Let $\hat{y}_{ij}$ be the predicted value $\beta_0 + \beta_1 x_{ij}$, which is used as the prediction of y for the jth subject under the ith treatment in phase II. From (9.19), the Graybill-Deal estimator of μ_i is given as

$$\hat{\mu}_{GDi} = \hat{\omega}_i \bar{\hat{y}}_i + (1 - \hat{\omega}_i)\bar{y}_i, \tag{9.21}$$

where $\bar{\hat{y}}_i = \frac{1}{n_i} \sum\limits_{j=1}^{n_i} \hat{y}_{ij}$, $\bar{y}_i = \frac{1}{m_i} \sum\limits_{j=1}^{m_i} y_{ij}$ and $\hat{\omega}_i = \frac{n_i/S_{1i}^2}{n_i/S_{1i}^2 + m_i/S_{2i}^2}$ with S_{1i}^2 and S_{2i}^2 being the sample variances of $(\hat{y}_{i1}, \cdots, \hat{y}_{in_i})$ and $(y_{i1}, \cdots, y_{im_i})$, respectively. For hypotheses (9.20), consider the following test statistic,

$$\tilde{T}_1 = \frac{\hat{\mu}_{GD1} - \hat{\mu}_{GD2}}{\sqrt{\widehat{Var}(\hat{\mu}_{GD1}) + \widehat{Var}(\hat{\mu}_{GD2})}} \tag{9.22}$$

where

$$\widehat{Var}(\hat{\mu}_{GDi}) = \frac{1}{n_i/S_{1i}^2 + m_i/S_{2i}^2} \left[1 + 4\hat{\omega}_i(1 - \hat{\omega}_i) \left(\frac{1}{n_i - 1} + \frac{1}{m_i - 1} \right) \right]$$

is an estimator of $Var(\hat{\mu}_{GDi})$, $i = 1, 2$. Using arguments similar to those given earlier, it can be verified that $\hat{T}_1$ has a limiting standard normal distribution under the null hypothesis H_0 if $Var(S_{1i}^2)$ and $Var(S_{2i}^2) \to 0$ as n_i and $m_i \to \infty$. Consequently, an approximate $100(1-\alpha)\%$ confidence interval of $\mu_1 - \mu_2$ is given as

$$\left(\hat{\mu}_{GD1} - \hat{\mu}_{GD2} - z_{\alpha/2}\sqrt{V_T}, \ \hat{\mu}_{GD1} - \hat{\mu}_{GD2} + z_{\alpha/2}\sqrt{V_T} \right) \qquad (9.23)$$

where $V_T = \widehat{Var}(\hat{\mu}_{GD1}) + \widehat{Var}(\hat{\mu}_{GD2})$. Therefore, hypothesis H_0 is rejected if the confidence interval (9.23) does not contain 0. Thus, under the local alternative hypothesis that $H_a : \mu_1 - \mu_2 = \delta \neq 0$, the required sample size to achieve a $1 - \beta$ power satisfies

$$-z_{\alpha/2} + |\delta| \Big/ \sqrt{Var(\hat{\mu}_{GD1}) + Var(\hat{\mu}_{GD2})} = z_\beta.$$

Let $m_i = \rho n_i$ and $n_2 = \gamma n_1$. Then, denoted by N_T the total sample size for two treatment groups is $(1 + \rho)(1 + \gamma)n_1$ with n_1 given as

$$n_1 = \frac{1}{2}AB\left(1 + \sqrt{1 + 8(1 + \rho)A^{-1}C}\right) \qquad (9.24)$$

where $A = \frac{(z_{\alpha/2}+z_\beta)^2}{\delta^2}, B = \frac{\sigma_1^2}{\rho+r_1^{-1}} + \frac{\sigma_2^2}{\gamma(\rho+r_2^{-1})}$ and $C = B^{-2}\left[\frac{\sigma_1^2}{r_1(\rho+r_1^{-1})^3} + \frac{\sigma_2^2}{\gamma^2 r_2(\rho+r_2^{-1})^3}\right]$ with $r_i = \beta_1^2\tau_i^2/\sigma_i^2$, $i = 1, 2$.

For the case of testing for superiority, consider the following local alternative hypothesis that $H_a: \mu_1 - \mu_2 = \delta_1 > \delta$.

The required sample size to achieve $1 - \beta$ power satisfies

$$-z_\alpha + (\delta_1 - \delta) \Big/ \sqrt{Var(\hat{\mu}_{GD1}) + Var(\hat{\mu}_{GD2})} = z_\beta.$$

Using the notations in the above paragraph, the total sample size for two treatment groups is $(1 + \rho)(1 + \gamma)n_1$ with n_1 given as

$$n_1 = \frac{1}{2}DB\left(1 + \sqrt{1 + 8(1 + \rho)D^{-1}C}\right) \qquad (9.25)$$

where $D = \frac{(z_\alpha+z_\beta)^2}{(\delta_1-\delta)^2}$. For the case of testing for equivalence with a significance level α, consider the local alternative hypothesis that $H_a: \mu_1 - \mu_2 = \delta_1$ with $|\delta_1| < \delta$. The required sample size to achieve $1 - \beta$ power satisfies

$$-z_\alpha + (\delta - \delta_1) \Big/ \sqrt{Var(\hat{\mu}_{GD1}) + Var(\hat{\mu}_{GD2})} = z_\beta.$$

Thus, the total sample size for two treatment groups is $(1 + \rho)(1 + \gamma)n_1$ with n_1 given

$$n_1 = \frac{1}{2}EB\left(1 + \sqrt{1 + 8(1 + \rho)E^{-1}C}\right) \qquad (9.26)$$

where $E = \frac{(z_\alpha+z_{\beta/2})^2}{(\delta-|\delta_1|)^2}$.

Note that following similar idea as described above, statistical tests and formulas for sample size calculation for testing hypotheses of non-inferiority, superiority, and equivalence can be obtained.

9.5.2   Binary response

Lu et al. (2009) consider the case where the study endpoint is a discrete variable such as a binary response. Suppose that the study duration of the first stage is cL and the study duration of the second stage is L with $0 < c < 1$. Assume that the response is determined by an underlying lifetime t, and the corresponding lifetime distribution of t for the test treatment is $G_1(t,\theta_1)$ while for the control is $G_2(t,\theta_2)$. If there are n_1 and m_1 randomly selected individuals in the first and second stages for the test treatment, respectively, let r_1 and s_1 be the numbers of respondents observed in the first and second stages for the test treatment, respectively. Similarly, for the control treatment, there are n_2 and m_2 randomly selected individuals for the control treatment. Let r_2 and s_2 be the numbers of respondents observed in the first and second stages, respectively. Based on these observed data, the likelihood functions $L(\theta_i)$ for the test treatment and the control treatment are

$$L(\theta_i) = G_i^{r_i}(cL, \theta_i)\left[1 - G_i(cL, \theta_i)\right]^{n_i - r_i} G_i^{s_i}(L, \theta_i)\left[1 - G_i(L, \theta_i)\right]^{m_i - s_i}$$

for $i = 1, 2$; where $i = 1$ represents the test treatment and $i = 2$ represents the control treatment. Assume that the lifetimes under test and control treatments are exponentially distributed with parameters λ_1 and λ_2, respectively. Thus, $G_1(t; \theta_1) = G(t, \lambda_1)$ and $G_2(t; \theta_2) = G(t, \lambda_2)$. Then the likelihood functions become

$$L(\lambda_i) = \left(1 - e^{-\lambda_i cL}\right)^{r_i} e^{-(n_i - r_i)\lambda_i cL} \left(1 - e^{-\lambda_i L}\right)^{s_i} e^{-(m_i - s_i)\lambda_i L}. \qquad (9.27)$$

Let $\hat{\lambda}_i$ be the maximum likelihood estimate (MLE) of λ_i. Then, for $i = 1, 2$, $\hat{\lambda}_i$ can be found by solving the following likelihood equation

$$\frac{r_i c}{e^{\lambda_i cL} - 1} + \frac{s_i}{e^{\lambda_i L} - 1} - (n_i - r_i)c - (m_i - s_i) = 0, \qquad (9.28)$$

which is obtained by setting the first order partial derivative $L(\lambda_i)$ with respect to λ_i to zero. Note that the MLE of λ_i exist if and only if r_i/n_i and s_i/m_i do not equal 0 or 1 at the same time. Based on the asymptotic normality of MLE (under suitable regularity conditions), $\hat{\lambda}_i$ asymptotically follows a normal distribution. In particular, as n_i and m_i tend to infinity, the distribution of $(\hat{\lambda}_i - \lambda_i)\big/\sigma_i(\lambda_i)$ converges to the standard normal distribution where

$$\sigma_i(\lambda_i) = L^{-1}\left(n_i c^2(e^{\lambda_i cL} - 1)^{-1} + m_i(e^{\lambda_i L} - 1)^{-1}\right)^{-1/2}.$$

Let $\sigma_i(\hat{\lambda}_i)$ be the MLE of $\sigma_i(\lambda_i)$. Based on the consistency of MLE, by the Slutsky's Theorem, $(\hat{\lambda}_i - \lambda_i)\big/\sigma_i(\hat{\lambda}_i)$ follows a standard normal distribution asymptotically. Consequently, an approximate $(1-\alpha)$ confidence interval of λ_i is given as $\left(\hat{\lambda}_i - z_{\alpha/2}\sigma_i(\hat{\lambda}_i), \ \hat{\lambda}_i + z_{\alpha/2}\sigma_i(\hat{\lambda}_i)\right)$, where $z_{\alpha/2}$ is the $(1-\alpha/2)$-quartile of a standard normal distribution. Under an exponential model, comparison of two treatments usually focuses on the hazard rate λ_i. For the comparison of two treatments in pharmaceutical applications, namely, control vs. treatment, it is often of interest to study the hypotheses testing of equality, superiority, non-inferiority, and equivalence of two treatments. Furthermore, to facilitate the planning of a clinical study, researchers are also interested to determine the required sample size which would allow the corresponding tests to achieve a given level of power (Chow, Shao and Wang, 2003). For illustration purposes, consider testing the following hypotheses for equality

$$H_0 : \lambda_1 = \lambda_2 \ vs. \ H_a: \lambda_1 \neq \lambda_2 \ . \tag{9.29}$$

Let $m_i = \rho n_i$ and $n_2 = \gamma n_1$, $i = 1, 2$. Then the total sample size N_T for two treatments is $(1 + \rho)(1 + \gamma)n_1$, where

$$n_1 = \frac{(z_{\alpha/2} + z_\beta)^2(\tilde{\sigma}_1^2(\lambda_1) + \tilde{\sigma}_2^2(\lambda_2))}{(\lambda_1 - \lambda_2)^2}, \tag{9.30}$$

$$\tilde{\sigma}_1^2(\lambda_1) = L^{-2} \left(c^2(e^{\lambda_1 cL} - 1)^{-1} + \rho(e^{\lambda_1 L} - 1)^{-1}\right)^{-1},$$

and

$$\tilde{\sigma}_2^2(\lambda_2) = L^{-2}\gamma^{-1} \left(c^2(e^{\lambda_2 cL} - 1)^{-1} + \rho(e^{\lambda_2 L} - 1)^{-1}\right)^{-1}.$$

Note that following similar idea as described above, statistical tests and formulas for sample size calculation for testing hypotheses of non-inferiority, superiority, and equivalence can be obtained.

9.5.3 Time-to-event data

Following similar idea, Lu et al. (2010, 2011) studied the case where the study endpoint is time-to-event data. Let t_{ijk} denote the length of time of a patient from entering the trial to the occurrence of some events of interest for the kth subject at the jth stage in the ith treatment, where $k = 1, 2, \ldots, n_{ij}$, $j = 1, 2, i = T$ and R. Assume that the study durations for the 1st and the 2nd stage are different, which are given by cL and L respectively, where $c < 1$. Furthermore, assume that t_{ijk} follows a distribution with $G(t, \theta_i)$ and $g(t, \theta_i)$ as the cumulative distribution function and probability density function with parameter vector θ_i, respectively. Then, the data collected from the study can be represented by (x_{ijk}, δ_{ijk}), where $\delta_{ijk} = 1$ indicates that the event of interest is observed and that $x_{ijk} = t_{ijk}$ while $\delta_{ijk} = 0$ means that the event is not observed during the study, i.e., x_{ijk} is censored and that $x_{ijk} < t_{ijk}$. In clinical trials, it is not uncommon to observe censored data due to drop-out, loss to follow-up, or *survival* at the end of the trials. In this article, for simplicity, we will only consider the case where censoring is due to survival at the end of trials. Given the observed data, the likelihood function for the test treatment and the control treatment can be obtained as follows

$$L(\theta_i) = \prod_{j=1}^{2} \prod_{k=1}^{n_{ij}} g^{\delta_{ijk}}(x_{ijk}, \theta_i) \left[1 - G(x_{ijk}, \theta_i)\right]^{1-\delta_{ijk}} \tag{9.31}$$

for $i = T, R$. In particular, suppose that the observed time-to-event data are assumed to follow a Weibull distribution. Denote the cumulative distribution function (cdf) of a Weibull distribution with λ, $\beta > 0$ by $G(t; \lambda, \beta)$ where $G(t; \lambda, \beta) = 1 - e^{-(t/\lambda)^\beta}$. Suppose that $G(t; \theta_T) = G(t; \lambda_T, \beta_T)$ and $G(t; \theta_R) = G(t; \lambda_R, \beta_R)$, i.e., t_{ijk} follows the Weibull distribution with cdf $G(t; \lambda_i, \beta_i)$. Then the likelihood function in (9.31) becomes

$$L(\lambda_i, \beta_i) = \left(\beta_i \lambda_i^{-\beta_i} \right)^{\sum\limits_{j=1}^{2} \sum\limits_{k=1}^{n_{ij}} \delta_{ijk}} e^{- \sum\limits_{j=1}^{2} \sum\limits_{k=1}^{n_{ij}} \tilde{x}_{ijk}} \prod\limits_{j=1}^{2} \prod\limits_{k=1}^{n_{ij}} x_{ijk}^{(\beta_i - 1)\delta_{ijk}}, \tag{9.32}$$

where $\tilde{x}_{ijk} = (x_{ijk}/\lambda_i)^{\beta_i}$. Let $l(\lambda_i, \beta_i) = \log(L(\lambda_i, \beta_i))$ be the log-likelihood function. Based on the log-likelihood function, the maximum likelihood estimators (MLEs) of β_i and λ_i (denoted by $\hat{\beta}_i$ and $\hat{\lambda}_i$) can be obtained. Under the assumption of asymptotic normality of MLE, it can be shown that $\hat{\lambda}_i$ and $\hat{\beta}_i$ are asymptotically normally distributed. Thus, formulas for sample size calculation/allocation can be similarly obtained. For illustration purposes, consider testing the following hypotheses of equality between medians:

$$H_0 : M_T = M_R \ vs. \ H_a : \ M_T \neq M_R , \tag{9.33}$$

where M_i is the median of $G(t; \lambda_i, \beta_i)$, $i = T, R$. Let $\hat{M}_i$ be the MLE of M_i and v_i be the variance of M_i. We first consider the one treatment case, i.e., the following hypotheses is considered,

$$H_0 : M_T = M_0 \ v.s. \ H_a : M_T \neq M_0. \tag{9.34}$$

Based on the asymptotic normality of MLE $\hat{M}_T$, we can then reject the null hypothesis at an approximate α level of significance if $|\hat{M}_T - M_0| \big/ \sqrt{n_{T1}^{-1}\hat{v}_T} > z_{\alpha/2}$. Since $(\hat{M}_T - M_T) \big/ \sqrt{n_{T1}^{-1}\hat{v}_T}$ approximately follows the standard normal distribution, the power of the above test under H_a can be approximated by $\Phi\left(|M_T - M_0| \big/ \sqrt{n_{T1}^{-1}v_T} - z_{\alpha/2} \right)$, where Φ is the distribution function of the standard normal distribution. Hence, in order to achieve a power of $1 - \beta$, the required sample size satisfies $|M_T - M_0| \big/ \sqrt{n_{T1}^{-1}v_T} - z_{\alpha/2} = z_\beta$. If $n_{T2} = \rho \, n_{T1}$, the required total sample size N for the two phases is given as $N = (1 + \rho)n_{T1}$ where n_{T1} is given by

$$n_{T1} = \frac{(z_{\alpha/2} + z_\beta)^2 v_T}{(M_1 - M_0)^2}. \tag{9.35}$$

Following the above idea, the corresponding sample size to achieve a prespecified power of $1 - \beta$ with significance level α can be determined. Hence, the corresponding required sample size for testing hypotheses in (9.33) satisfies the following equation,

$$|M_T - M_R| \big/ \sqrt{n_{T1}^{-1}v_T + n_{R1}^{-1}v_R} - z_{\alpha/2} = z_\beta.$$

Let $n_{i2} = \rho_i n_{i1}$ and $n_{R1} = \gamma n_{T1}$. It can be easily derived that the total sample size N_T for the two treatment groups in two stages is $n_{T1}[1 + \rho_T + (1 + \rho_R)\gamma]$ with n_{T1} given as

$$n_{T1} = \frac{(z_{\alpha/2} + z_\beta)^2(v_T + \gamma^{-1}v_R)}{(M_T - M_R)^2}. \tag{9.36}$$

Note that following a similar idea as described above, statistical tests and formulas for sample size calculation for testing hypotheses of non-inferiority, superiority, and equivalence can be obtained.

9.5.4 Remarks

In the previous sections, as indicated, formulas for sample size calculation/allocation for testing equality, non-inferiority, superiority, and equivalence for continuous, discrete, and time-to-event data can be derived assuming that (i) there is a well-established relationship between different study endpoints at different stages, and (ii) the study objectives for both stages are the same (see also, Pong and Chow, 2010). In practice, however, such a relationship (i.e., one study endpoint is predictive of the other study endpoint) may not exist. Thus, it is suggested that the relationship be validated based on historical data or the data observed from study. When the study objectives are different at different stages (e.g., dose finding at the first stage and efficacy confirmation at the second stage), the above derived formulas are necessary for controlling the overall type I error rate at α and for achieving the desired powers at both stages.

9.6 Analysis for Seamless Design with Different Objectives/Endpoints

In this section, we will focus on statistical inference for the scenario where the study objectives at different stages are different (e.g., dose selection vs. efficacy confirmation) and study endpoints at different stages are different (e.g., biomarker or surrogate endpoint vs. regular clinical study endpoint) based on statistical method proposed by Cheng and Chow (2011).

As indicated earlier, one of major concerns when applying adaptive design methods in clinical trials is probably how to control the overall type I error rate at a pre-specified level of significance. It is also a concern how the data collected from both stages should be combined for the final analysis. Besides, it is of interest to know how the sample size calculation/allocation should be done for achieving individual study objectives originally set for the two stages (separate studies). In this article, a multiple-stage transitional seamless trial design with different study objectives and different study endpoint and with and without adaptations is proposed. The impact of the adaptive design methods on the control of the overall type I error rate under the proposed trial design is examined. Valid statistical tests and the corresponding formulas for sample size calculation/allocation are derived under the proposed trial design.

As indicated earlier, a two-stage seamless trial design that combines two independent studies (e.g., a phase II study and a phase III study) is often considered in clinical research and development. Under such a trial design, the investigator may be interested in having one planned interim analysis at each stage. In this case, the two-stage seamless trial design becomes a four-stage trial design if we consider the time point at which the planned interim analysis will be conducted as the end of the specific stage. In this article, we will refer to such a trial design as a multiple-stage transitional seamless design to emphasize the importance of smooth transition from stage to stage. In what follows, we will focus on the proposed multiple-stage transitional seamless design with (adaptive version) and without (non-adaptive version) adaptations.

9.6.1   Non-adaptive version

Consider a clinical trial comparing k treatment groups, $E_1, ..., E_k$ with a control group C. One early surrogate endpoint and one subsequent primary endpoint are potentially available for assessing the treatment effect. Let θ_i and ψ_i, $i = 1, ..., k$ be the treatment effect comparing E_i with C measured by the surrogate endpoint and the primary endpoint, respectively. The ultimate hypothesis of interest is

$$H_{0,2} : \psi_1 = \cdots = \psi_k, \tag{9.37}$$

which is formulated in terms of the primary endpoint. However, along the way, the hypothesis

$$H_{0,1} : \theta_1 = \cdots \theta_k, \tag{9.38}$$

in terms of the short term surrogate endpoint will also be assessed. Cheng and Chow (2011) assumed that ψ_i is a monotone increasing function of the corresponding θ_i. The trial is conducted as a group sequential trial with the accrued data analyzed at 3 stages (i.e., stage 1, stage 2a, stage 2b, and stage 3) with four interim analyses, which are briefly described below. For simplicity, consider the case where the variances of the surrogate endpoint and the primary outcomes, denoted as σ^2 and τ^2 are known.

At *Stage 1* of the study, $(k + 1)n_1$ subjects will be randomized equally to receive either one of the k treatments or the control. As the result, there are n_1 subjects in each group. At the first interim analysis, the most promising treatment will be selected and used in the subsequent stages based on the surrogate endpoint. Let $\hat{\theta}_{i,1}$, $i = 1, ..., k$ be the pair-wise test statistics, and $S = \arg\max_{1 \leq i \leq k} \hat{\theta}_{i,1}$, then if $\hat{\theta}_{S,1} \leq c_1$ for some c_1, then the trial is stopped and $H_{0,1}$ is accepted. Otherwise, if $\hat{\theta}_{S,1} > c_{1,1}$, then the treatment E_S is recommended as the most promising treatment and will be used in all the subsequent stages. Note that only the subjects receiving either the promising treatment or the control will be followed formally for the primary endpoint. The treatment assessment on all other subjects will be terminated, and the subjects will receive standard care and undergo necessary safety monitoring.

At *Stage 2a*, $2n_2$ additional subjects will be equally randomized to receive either the treatment E_S or the control C. The second interim analysis is scheduled when the short-term surrogate measures from these $2n_2$ Stage 2 subjects and the primary endpoint measures from those $2n_1$ Stage 1 subjects who receive either the treatment E_S or the control C become available. Let $T_{1,1} = \hat{\theta}_{S,1}$ and $T_{1,2} = \hat{\psi}_{S,1}$ be the pair-wise test statistics from Stage 1 based on the surrogate endpoint and the primary endpoint, respectively, and $\hat{\theta}_{S,2}$ be the statistic from Stage 2 based on the surrogate. If

$$T_{2,1} = \sqrt{\frac{n_1}{n_1 + n_2}}\hat{\theta}_{S,1} + \sqrt{\frac{n_2}{n_1 + n_2}}\hat{\theta}_{S,2} \le c_{2,1},$$

then stop the trial and accept $H_{0,1}$. If $T_{2,1} > c_{2,1}$ and $T_{1,2} > c_{1,2}$, then stop the trial and reject both $H_{0,1}$ and $H_{0,2}$. Otherwise, if $T_{2,1} > c_{2,1}$ but $T_{1,2} \le c_{1,2}$, then we will move on to Stage 2b.

At *Stage 2b*, no additional subjects will be recruited. The third interim analysis will be performed when the subjects in (Stage 2a) complete their primary endpoints. Let

$$T_{2,2} = \sqrt{\frac{n_1}{n_1 + n_2}}\hat{\psi}_{S,1} + \sqrt{\frac{n_2}{n_1 + n_2}}\hat{\psi}_{S,2},$$

where $\hat{\psi}_{S,2}$ is the pair-wise test statistic from stage 2b. If $T_{2,2} > c_{2,2}$, then stop the trial and reject $H_{0,2}$. Otherwise, we move on to (Stage 3).

At *Stage 3*, the final stage, $2n_3$ additional subjects will be recruited and followed to their primary endpoints. For the fourth interim analysis, define

$$T_3 = \sqrt{\frac{n_1}{n_1 + n_2 + n_3}}\hat{\psi}_{S,1} + \sqrt{\frac{n_2}{n_1 + n_2 + n_3}}\hat{\psi}_{S,2} + \sqrt{\frac{n_1}{n_1 + n_2 + n_3}}\hat{\psi}_{S,3},$$

where $\hat{\psi}_{S,3}$ is the pair-wise test statistic from stage 3. If $T_3 > c_3$, then stop the trial and reject $H_{0,2}$; otherwise, accept $H_{0,2}$. The parameters in the above designs, $n_1, n_2, n_3, c_{1,1}, c_{1,2}, c_{2,1}, c_{2,2}$, and c_3 are determined such that the procedure will have a controlled type I error rate of α and a target power of $1 - \beta$. The determination of these parameters will be given in next section.

In the above design, the surrogate data in the first stage are used to estimate the most promising treatment rather than assessing $H_{0,1}$. This means that upon completion of Stage 1 a dose does not need to be significant in order to be recommended to the subsequent stages. This feature is important since it does not suffer from any lack of power due to limited sample sizes.

There are two sets of hypotheses to be tested, namely $H_{0,1}$ and $H_{0,2}$. To claim efficacy, $H_{0,2}$ has to be rejected hence is the hypothesis of primary interest. However, to ensure appropriate control of the type I error rate associated with the sequential design with change of endpoints, $H_{0,1}$ has to be assessed along the way according to the closed testing principle. The proposed two-stage seamless design is attractive due to it efficiency (e.g., reduce the lead time between a phase II trial and a phase III study) and flexibility (e.g., allow to make decision early and take appropriate actions such as stop the trial early or delete/add dose groups). At the first stage, with limited number of subjects, the goal is to detect any signals for safety and/or evidence for early efficacy. With limited number of subjects, there will not be any power for detecting a small clinically meaningful difference. This justifies the use of precision analysis for achieving statistical significance as a criterion for dose selection.

9.6.2   Adaptive version

The proposed design approach in the previous section is a group sequential procedure with treatment selection. There is no adaptation involved in the above procedure. Tsiatis and Mehta (2003) and Jennison and Turnbull (2006) argue that adaptive designs typically suffer from loss of efficiency and hence are typically not recommended in regular practice. However, as pointed out by Proschan, Lan, and Wittes (2006), in some scenarios, particularly when there is not enough primary outcome information available, it is appealing to use an adaptive procedure as long as it is statistically justified. For the trials we are considering, since the primary outcome takes a much longer time to observe compared to its surrogate, we feel that an adaptive procedure is useful in our setting. And the transitional feature of our proposed design makes it possible to modify the design adaptively upon completion of the second interim analysis (i.e., Stage 2a). One possible adaptation is the correlation between the surrogate endpoint and the primary outcome. As a nuisance parameter, it plays an important role in the power calculation of the procedure. This nuisance parameter can be estimated using the first stage patients who are followed for their primary outcomes.

Another possible modification is to re-calibrate the treatment effect of the primary outcome by exploring the relationship between the surrogate endpoint and the primary outcome. Specifically, assuming there is a local linear relationship between ψ and θ, a reasonable assumption when focusing only on their values at a neighborhood of the most promising treatment E_S, then at the end of Stage 2a, the treatment effect in terms of the primary endpoint can be re-estimated as

$$\hat{\delta}_S = \frac{\hat{\psi}_{S,1}}{\hat{\theta}_{S,1}} T_{2,1}.$$

Then we could re-estimate the Stage 3 sample size based on a modified treatment effect of the primary outcome $\delta = \max\{\delta_S, \delta_0\}$, where δ_0 is a minimally clinically relevant treatment effect agreed upon prior to the trial. The reason we choose the modified treatment this way is to ensure the clinical relevance of the test procedure. Let m be the re-estimated Stage 3 sample size based on δ. If $m \leq n_3$, then there is no modification for the procedure. If $m > n_3$, then m (instead of the originally planned n_3) patients per arm will be recruited at Stage 3. The justification of the above adaptation can be found in Cheng and Chow (2011).

9.6.3 An example – a hepatitis C virus trial

A pharmaceutical company is interested in conducting a clinical trial utilizing a two-stage seamless adaptive design for evaluation of safety (tolerability) and efficacy of a test treatment for patients with hepatitis C infection. The trial will combine two independent studies (one for dose selection and the other one for efficacy confirmation) into a single study. The study will consist of two stages at which the first stage is for dose selection and the second stage is for establishment of non-inferiority of the selected dose from the first stage as compared to the standard of care therapy (control). The primary objectives of the study then contain study objectives at both stages. For the first stage, the primary objective is to select the optimal dose as compared to the standard of care therapy, while the primary objective of the second stage is to establish non-inferiority of the selected dose as compared to the standard of care therapy. The treatment duration is 48 weeks of treatment followed by a 24 weeks follow-up.

The primary study endpoint is the sustained virologic response (SVR) at week 72, which is defined as an undetectable HCV RNA level (< 10 IU/mL) at week 72. The proposed two-stage seamless adaptive design is briefly outlined below: Stage 1: This stage is a five-arm randomized evaluation of four active dose levels of the test treatment. Qualified subjects will be randomly assigned to one of the five treatment groups at a 1:1:1:1:1 ratio. After all Stage 1 subjects have completed Week 12 of the study, an interim analysis was performed. Based upon the safety results of this analysis as well as virologic response at Weeks 12 and 24, Stage 1 subjects who have not yet completed the study protocol will continue with their assigned therapies for the remainder of the planned 48 weeks, with final follow-up at Week 72. An optimal dose will be selected based on the interim analysis results of the 12-week early virologic response (EVR), which is defined as 2-log10 reduction in HCV RNA level at Week 12, assuming that the 12-week EVR is predictive of 72 week SVR. The 12-week EVR is considered as a surrogate endpoint for the primary endpoint of 72-week SVR. Under this assumption, an optimal dose will be selected using precision analysis under some pre-specified selection criteria. In other words, the dose group with highest confidence level for achieving statistical significance (i.e., the observed difference is not by chance alone) will be selected. The selected dose will then proceed to testing for non-inferiority compared to standard of care in Stage 2. Stage 2: This stage will be a non-inferiority comparison of the selected dose from Stage 1. A separate cohort of subjects will be randomized to receive either the selected dose from Stage 1 or the standard of care treatment as given in Stage 1 in a 1:1 ratio. A second interim analysis will be performed when all Stage 2 subjects have completed Week 12 and 50% of the subjects (Stage 1 and Stage 2 combined) have completed 48 weeks of treatment and a follow-up of 24 weeks. Depending on the results of this analysis, including the virologic response at Weeks 12 and 24, sample size re-estimation will be performed to whether additional subjects are needed in order for achieving the desired power for establishment of non-inferiority for the selected dose.

In both stages, subjects who do not meet the study criteria for virologic response at Weeks 12 and 24, and those who do meet these criteria but then relapse at any later time through study Week 72, will discontinue study treatment and will be offered treatment, off protocol, with standard of care. For the two planned interim analyses, the incidence of EVR as well as safety data, will be reviewed by an independent data safety monitoring board (DSMB). The commonly used O'Brien-Fleming boundaries will be applied for controlling the overall type I error rate at 5% (O'Brien, and Fleming, 1979). Adaptations such as stopping the trial early, discontinuing selected treatment arms, and re-estimating the sample size may be applied as recommended by the DSMB. Stopping rules for the study will be designated by the DSMB, based on their on-going analyses of the data as per their charter.

9.7   Concluding Remarks

As indicated earlier, in practice, statistical methods for a standard group sequential trial design with one planned interim analysis is often applied to the two-stage seamless adaptive design regardless of whether the study objectives and/or the study endpoints at different stages are the same. It is then a concern whether the obtained p-value and confidence interval for assessment of the treatment effect are correct or reliable. Sample size needed for achieving a desired power that obtained under a standard group sequential design may not be sufficient for achieving the study objectives under the two-stage seamless adaptive trial design especially when the study objectives and/or study endpoints at different stages are different.

In its recent draft guidance on adaptive clinical trial design, the FDA classifies adaptive designs as either *well-understood designs* or *less well-understood designs* depending upon the nature of adaptations either blinded or unblinded (FDA, 2010). In practice, however, most of the seamless adaptive designs described in this chapter are considered less well-understood designs. As a result, one of the major challenges is not only the development of a set of criteria for choosing a good design among these less well understood designs, but also the development of appropriate statistical methods under the selected less well-understood designs for valid statistical inference of the test treatment under investigation (Cheng and Chow, 2010).

Chapter 10

Adaptive Treatment Switching

For evaluation of the efficacy of a test treatment for progressive disease such as cancer or HIV, a parallel-group active-control randomized clinical trial is often conducted. Under the study design, qualified patients are randomly assigned to receive either an active control (a standard therapy or a treatment currently available in the marketplace) or the test treatment under investigation. Patients are allowed to switch from one treatment to another due to ethical consideration such as lack of response or there is evidence of disease progression. In practice, it is not uncommon that up to 80 % of patients may switch from one treatment to another. This certainly has an impact on the evaluation of the efficacy of the test treatment. Despite allowing a switch between two treatments, many clinical studies are to compare the test treatment with the active control agent as if no patients had ever switched. Sommer and Zeger (1991) referred to the treatment effect among patients who complied with treatment as *biological efficacy*. In practice, the survival time of a patient who switched from the active control to the test treatment might be on the average longer than his/her survival time would have been if he/she had adhered to the original treatment (either the active control or the test treatment), if switching is based on prognosis to optimally assign patients' treatments over time. We refer to the difference caused by treatment switch as *switching effect*. The purpose of this chapter is to discuss some models for treatment switch with switching effect and methods for statistical inference under these models.

The remainder of this chapter is organized as follows. In the next section, the latent event times model under the parametric setting is described. In Section 10.2, the concept of latent hazard rate is considered by incorporating the switching effect in the latent hazard functions. Statistical inference is also derived using Cox's regression with some additional covariates and parameters in this section. A simulation study is carried out in Section 10.3 to examine

189

the performance of the method as compared two other methods, where the one ignoring the switching data and the one including the switching data but ignoring the switching effect. A mixed exponential model is considered to assess the total survival time in Section 10.4. Some concluding remarks are given in the last section of this chapter.

10.1 Latent Event Times

Suppose that patients are randomly assigned to two treatment groups: a test treatment and an active control. Consider the case where there is no treatment switch and the study objective is to compare the efficacy of the two treatments. Let $T_1, .., T_n$ be independent non-negative survival times and $C_1..., C_n$ be independent non-negative censoring times that are independent of survival times. Thus, the observations are $Y_i = min(T_i, C_i)$, $i = 1$ if $T_i \leq C_i$, and $i = 0$ if $T_i > C_i$. Assume that the test treatment acts multiplicatively on a patient's survival time, i.e., an accelerated failure time model applies. Denote the magnitude of this multiplicative effect by $e^{-\beta}$, where β is an unknown parameter. Assume further that the survival time distribution under the active control has a parametric form $F_\theta(t)$, where θ is an unknown parameter vector and $F_\theta(t)$ is a known distribution when θ is known. Let k_i be the treatment indicator for the ith patient, i.e. $k_i = 1$ for the test treatment and $k_i = 0$ for the active control. Then, the distribution of the survival time is given by

$$P\left(T_i \leq t\right) = F_\theta\left(e^{\beta k_i} t\right), \quad t > 0. \tag{10.1}$$

If F_θ has a density f_θ , then the density of T_i is given by $e^{\beta k_i}$, $t > 0$.

Consider the situation where patients may switch their treatments and the study objective is to compare the biological efficacy. Let $S_i > 0$ denote the ith patient's switching time. Branson and Whitehead (2002) introduced the concept of *latent event time* in the simple case where only patients in the control group may switch. We define the latent event time in the general case as follows. For a patient with no treatment switch, the latent event time is the same as his/her survival time. For patient i who switches at time S_i, the latent event time $\tilde{T}_i$ is an abstract quantity defined to be the patient's survival time that would have been if this patient had not switched the treatment. For patients who switch from the active control group to the test treatment group, Branson and Whitehead (2002) suggested the following model conditional on S_i:

$$\tilde{T}_i \overset{d}{=} S_i + e^{\beta}\left(T_i - S_i\right), \tag{10.2}$$

where d denotes equality in distribution. That is, the survival time for a patient who switched from the active control to the test treatment could be back-transformed to the survival time that would have been if the patient had not switched. For the case where patients may switch from either groups, model (10.2) can be modified as follows

$$\tilde{T}_i \stackrel{d}{=} S_i + e^{\beta(1-2k_i)}(T_i - S_i), \tag{10.3}$$

where k_i is the indicator for the original treatment assignment, not for the treatment after switching.

Model (10.2) or (10.3), however, does not take into account for the fact that the treatment switch is typically based on prognosis and/or investigator's judgment. For example, a patient in one group may switch to another because he/she does not respond to the original assigned treatment. This may result in a somewhat optimal treatment assignment for the patient and a survival time longer than those patients who did not switch. Ignoring such a switching effect will lead to a biased assessment of the treatment effect. Consider the following model conditional on S_i:

$$\tilde{T}_i \stackrel{d}{=} S_i + e^{\beta(1-2k_i)} w_{k,\eta}(S_i)(T_i - S_i), \tag{10.4}$$

where η is an unknown parameter vector and $w_{k,\eta}(S)$ are known functions of the switching time S when and k are given. Typically, $w_{k,\eta}(S)$ should be close to 1 when S is near 0, i.e. the switching effect is negligible if switching occurs too early. Note that

$$\lim_{S \downarrow 0} w_{k,\eta}(S) = 1.$$

An example is

$$w_{k,\eta}(S) = exp\left(\eta_{k,0}S + \eta_{k,1}S^2\right),$$

where $\eta_{k,l}$ are unknown parameters.

Under model (10.1) and model (10.4), the distributions of the survival times for patients who switched treatments are given by (conditional on S_i)

$$
\begin{aligned}
P(T_i \le t) &= P\left(\tilde{T}_i \le S_i + e^{\beta(1-2k_i)} w_{k,\eta}(S_i)(t - S_i)\right) \\
&= F_\theta\left(e^{\beta k_i}\left[S_i + e^{\beta(1-2k_i)} w_{k,\eta}(S_i)(t - S_i)\right]\right) \\
&= F_\theta\left(e^{\beta k_i} S_i + e^{\beta(1-k_i)} w_{k,\eta}(S_i)(t - S_i)\right)
\end{aligned}
$$

for $k_i = 0, 1$. The distributions for patients who never switch are

$$F_\theta\left(e^{\beta k_i} t\right), k_i = 0, 1.$$

Assume that F has a density f_θ. For convenience's sake, we denote $S_i = \infty$ for patient i who never switch. Then, the conditional likelihood function given S_i is

$$L\left(\theta,\beta,\eta\right)$$

$$= \prod_{i:S_i=\infty} \left[e^{\beta k_i} f_y\left(e^{\beta k_i} Y_i\right)\right]^{\delta_i} \left[1 - F_\theta\left(e^{\beta k_i} Y_i\right)\right]^{1-\delta_i}$$

$$\times \prod_{i:S_i<\infty} \left[e^{\beta(1-k_i)} w_{k,\eta}\left(s_i\right) f_\theta\left(e^{\beta k_i} S_i + e^{\beta(1-k_i)} w_{k,\eta}\left(S_i\right)\left(Y_i - S_i\right)\right)\right]^{\delta_i}$$

$$\times \left[1 - F_\theta\left(e^{\beta k_i} S_i + e^{\beta(1-k_i)} w_{k,\eta}\left(S_i\right)\left(Y_i - S_i\right)\right)\right]^{\delta_i}.$$

Let $\gamma = (\theta, \beta, \eta)$. The parameter vector can be estimated by solving the following likelihood equation

$$\frac{\partial \log L\left(\gamma\right)}{\partial \gamma} = 0. \tag{10.5}$$

Under some regularity conditions, the estimate of γ is asymptotically normal with mean vector 0 and covariance matrix

$$\left[E\frac{\partial^2 \log L\left(\gamma\right)}{\partial \gamma \partial \gamma'}\right]^{-1} Var\left[E\frac{\partial \log L\left(\gamma\right)}{\partial \gamma}\right]\left[E\frac{\partial^2 \log L\left(\gamma\right)}{\partial \gamma \partial \gamma'}\right]^{-1}, \tag{10.6}$$

which can be estimated by substituting with its estimate. Statistical inference can then be obtained based on the asymptotic results.

Branson and Whitehead (2002) proposed an iterative parameter estimation (IPE) method for statistical analysis of data with treatment switch. The idea of the method is to relate the distributions of the survival times of the two treatments under a parametric model. Thus, under model (10.2), IPE can be described as follows. First, an initial estimate $\hat{\beta}$ of β is obtained. Then, latent event times are estimated as

$$\hat{T}_i = S_i + b^{\hat{\beta}}\left(T_i - S_i\right)$$

for patients who switched their treatments. Next, a new estimate of β is obtained by using the estimated latent event times as if they were the observed data. Finally, the previously described procedure is iterated until the estimate of β converges.

Note that although a similar IPE method can be applied under model (10.4), it is not recommended for the following reason. If initial estimates of model parameters are obtained by solving the likelihood equation given in (10.5), then iteration does not increase the efficiency of estimates and hence adds unnecessary complexity for computation. On the other hand, if initial estimates are not solutions of the likelihood equation given in (10.5), then they are typically not efficient and the estimates obtained by IPE (if they converge) may not be as efficient as the solutions of the likelihood equation (10.5). Thus, directly solving the likelihood equation (10.5) produces estimates that are either more efficient or computationally simpler than the IPE estimates.

10.2 Proportional Hazard Model with Latent Hazard Rate

The above parametric approach for latent event times is useful. However, statistical analysis under such a parametric model may not be robust against model mis-specifications. For survival data in clinical trials, alternatively, we may consider the following Cox's proportional hazard model, which is a semi-parametric model.

Let $F(t)$ be the distribution of the survival time and $f(t)$ be its corresponding density. Then, the hazard rate at time t is defined as

$$\lambda(t) = f(t)/[1 - F(t)].$$

The Cox's proportional hazard model is then given by

$$\lambda_{k_i}(t) = \lambda_0(t) e^{\beta k_i}, \tag{10.7}$$

where k_i is the treatment indicator and $\lambda_0(t)$ is left unspecified. In a more general setting, we can replace k_i in (10.7) by a covariate vector associated with the ith patient and β by a parameter vector. Under model (10.7), if there is no treatment switch, an estimator of β can be obtained by maximizing the following partial likelihood function

$$L(\beta) = \prod_i \left(\frac{e^{\beta k_i}}{\sum_{j \in R_i} e^{\beta k_j}} \right)^{\delta_i}, \tag{10.8}$$

where R_i is the set of patients who are alive and observed just before time T_i. When there is treatment switch but the switching effect is ignored (i.e. patients switch treatments at random), model (10.7) can be modified by replacing k_i by the time-dependent covariate $k_i(t)$ as follows

$$k_i(t) = \begin{cases} 1 - k_i, & t \geq S_i \\ k_i & t < S_i \end{cases}$$

where S_i is the switching time for the ith patient and $0 \leq t < \infty$. Note that by definition, $S_i = \infty$ if the ith patient never switch. This reduces to a special case of the proportional hazard model with time-dependent covariates (see, e.g., Kalbfleisch and Prentice, 1980; Cox and Oakes, 1984).

Consider the case where the switching effect $w_{k,\eta}(S_i)$ may depend on prognosis and/or investigator's assessment, which is an unknown parameter vector.

Instead of including the switching effect in the model as latent event times (10.4), we include it in the proportional hazard model as follows:

$$\lambda_{k_i}(t) = \lambda_0(t) e^{\beta k_i(t)} w_{k,\eta}(t, S_i), \tag{10.9}$$

where

$$w_{k,\eta}(t, S_i) = \begin{cases} w_{k,\eta}(S_i), & t \geq S_i \\ 1, & t < S_i \end{cases}.$$

We refer to this model as the latent hazard rate model since $\lambda_{ki}(t)$ in (10.9) corresponds to a latent event time and hence can be treated as a latent hazard rate. Under the latent hazard rate model (10.9), the partial likelihood is given by

$$L(\beta, \eta) = \prod_{i:S_i=\infty} \left[e^{\beta k_i} w_{k,\eta}(T_i, S_i) \left(\sum_{j \in R_i} e^{\beta k_j} w_{k,\eta}(T_i, S_i) \right)^{-1} \right]^{\delta_i}. \tag{10.10}$$

Estimators of β and η can be obtained by solving

$$\frac{\partial \log L(\gamma)}{\partial \gamma} = 0,$$

where $\gamma = (\beta, \eta)$. Under some regularity conditions, these estimators are asymptotically normal with mean vector 0 and covariance matrix as given in (10.6). Based on the asymptotic results, statistical inference can be obtained.

If $\log w_{k,\eta}(s)$ is linear in η such as

$$w_{k,\eta}(s) = e^{\eta_{k,0} S + \eta_{k,1} S^2},$$

then model (10.9) is another special case of the proportional hazard model with time-dependent covariates since the switching effect term can be written as

$$w_{k,\eta}(t, S_i) = e^{\eta_{k_i,0} S_i(t) + \eta_{k_i,1} S_i^2(t)}, \tag{10.11}$$

where

$$S_i(t) = \begin{cases} S_i, & t \geq S_i \\ 0 & t < S_i \end{cases},$$

which can be treated as another time-dependent covariate. That is, model (10.9) is the proportional hazard model with time-dependent covariates $k_i(t)$ and $S_i(t)$, where $S_i(t)$ is additional time-independent covariate. Thus, the parameter vector is given by

$$\gamma = (\beta, \eta_{0,0}, \eta_{0,1}, \eta_{1,0}, \eta_{1,1})$$

and it can be estimated by solving

$$\sum_i \delta_i \left(z_{ii} - \frac{\sum_{j \in R_i} Z_{ij} e^{\gamma' Z_{ij}}}{\sum_{j \in R_i} e^{\gamma' Z_{ij}}} \right) = 0,$$

where

$$Z_{ij} = \left(k_j\left(T_i\right), (1 - k_j)S_j\left(T_i\right), (1 - k_j) S_j^2\left(T_i\right), k_j S_j\left(T_i\right), k_j S_j^2\left(T_i\right) \right).$$

The resulting estimator, denoted by $\hat{\gamma}$, is asymptotically normal with mean 0 and a covariance matrix that can be estimated by

$$\hat{B}^{-1} \hat{A} \hat{B}^{-1},$$

where

$$\hat{A} = \sum_i \delta_i \left(z_{ii} - \frac{\sum_{j \in R_i} Z_{ij} e^{\hat{\gamma}' Z_{ij}}}{\sum_{j \in R_i} e^{\hat{\gamma}' Z_{ij}}} \right) \left(z_{ii} - \frac{\sum_{j \in R_i} Z_{ij} e^{\hat{\gamma}' Z_{ij}}}{\sum_{j \in R_i} e^{\hat{\gamma}' Z_{ij}}} \right)',$$

and

$$\hat{B} = \sum_i \delta_i \left(\frac{\sum_{j \in R_i} Z_{ij} e^{\hat{\gamma}' Z_{ij}}}{\sum_{j \in R_i} e^{\hat{\gamma}' Z_{ij}}} \right) \left(\frac{\sum_{j \in R_i} Z_{ij} e^{\hat{\gamma}' Z_{ij}}}{\sum_{j \in R_i} e^{\hat{\gamma}' Z_{ij}}} \right)'$$
$$- \sum_i \delta_i \frac{\sum_{j \in R_i} Z_{ij} Z_{ij}' e^{\hat{\gamma}' Z_{ij}}}{\sum_{j \in R_i} e^{\hat{\gamma}' Z_{ij}}}.$$

The above results can be easily extended to the case where there are some other time-independent and/or time-dependent covariates in model (10.9). The latent event times approach described in the previous section coincides with the latent hazard rate model when the survival time distribution is exponential, i.e.,

$$F(t) = 1 - e^{-t/\theta}$$

with an unknown parameter $\theta > 0$. However, for other types of survival time distributions, the two approaches are different. If we apply the latent event times model (10.4) under the semi-parametric approach in which Cox's proportional hazard model is used for data without treatment switch, then the resultant latent hazard model for $\log \lambda_{k_i}(t)/\lambda_0(t)$ depends on t is rather complicated. Statistical inference under such models could be very difficult.

Simulation Results

In this section, we studied the finite sample performance of the Cox's proportional hazard model with switching effect through simulation. Consider a clinical trial comparing a test treatment with an active control agent. Suppose 300 patients per treatment group is planned. The survival time was generated according to the exponential distribution with hazard rate 0.0693 for the active control group (mean=14.43 months) and 0.0462 for the treatment group (mean=21.65 months). For both treatment groups, the random censoring time was generated according to the uniform distribution over the range of 15–20 months. This results in the censoring percentage of 24.6% for the active control group and 34.6% for the treatment group. On the other hand, the patient treatment switch time was generated according to the exponential distribution with a mean of 7.22 months for the active control group and a mean of 10.82 months for the treatment group. The switching rate is about 67% for both the active control group and the treatment group. This choice of switching rate is within the range of 60–80% practical experience of patients who switch from one treatment to another.

For each combinations of parameters (β and $\eta_{k,j}$), 1,000 simulation runs were done. The results are summarized in Table 10.2.1. As it can be seen from Table 10.2.1, the estimators based on the method of latent hazard rate perform well. The relative bias is within 3% in all cases. The performance of the estimator of β (the treatment effect) is generally better than that of the estimators of η's (switching effects) in terms of both relative bias and the coefficient of variation. We note that the estimated standard deviation has very little bias. Furthermore, the coverage probability of the asymptotic confidence interval is close to the nominal level of 95%.

In the simulation, two other methods were also considered for the purpose of comparison. One method is to estimate β under model (10.7) with $w_{k,\eta}(t; S_i) \equiv 1$, (i.e., ignoring the switching effect), which is clearly biased. The other method is to estimate β under model (10.7) based on data from patients who adhered to their original randomized treatments (i.e., ignoring data from patients who switched). Simulation results indicated that this method has little bias in estimating β. However, the estimator from this method has larger standard deviation (less efficiency). The efficiency gain in using data from patients who switched is about 15% under the switching rate of 67%. This gain is not as large as what is hoped for, because of the fact that the proposed method estimates four additional parameters $\eta_{k,j}$. However, a 15% gain in efficiency in terms of standard deviation amounts to approximately a 32% of reduction in sample size. For example, suppose that a sample size 100 is required in the case of no switching. If the switching rate is 67% and we ignore data from patients who switched, then approximately we need a sample size 300 in order to retain the efficiency. On the other hand, with the same switching rate and the proposed method, the sample size required to retain the same efficiency is 228.

Table 10.2.1: Simulation Results Based on 1000 Simulation Runs

Parameter	Proposed method					Other*	Other†
	β	$\eta_{0,0}$	$\eta_{0,1}$	$\eta_{1,0}$	$\eta_{1,1}$	β	β
True value	-0.406	0.100	0.009	0.080	0.010	-0.406	-0.406
Mean of estimates	-0.396	0.098	0.009	0.082	0.010	-0:393	0.033
SD of estimates	0.128	0.052	0.004	0.049	0.004	0.147	0.094
Mean of estimated SD	0.129	0.053	0.004	0.049	0.004	0.148	0.093
Coverage probability	0.951	0.951	0.949	0.952	0.956	0.951	0.003

*The method that ignores data from patients who switched.

†The method that ignores switching effect, i.e., uses model with $w_{k_i,\eta}\,(t;S_i) \equiv 1$.

10.3   Mixed Exponential Model

As indicated earlier, treatment switch is a common and flexible medical practice in cancer trials due to ethical considerations. Treatment switch is in fact a response-adaptive switch. Due to the treatment switch, however, the treatment effect can only be partially observed, and the effects of different treatments are difficult to separate from each other. In this case, the commonly used exponential models with a single parameter may not be appropriate. Alternatively, a mixed exponential model (MEM) with multiple parameters is more flexible and hence suitable for a wide range of applications (see, e.g., Mendenhal and Hader, 1985; Susarla and Pathala, 1965; Johnson et al., 1994).

In clinical trials, the target patient population often consists of two or more subgroups based on heterogeneous baseline characteristics (e.g., the patients could be a mixture of the second-line and the third-line oncology patients). The median survival time of the third-line patients is usually shorter than that of the second-line patients. If the survival times of the two subgroup populations are modeled by exponential distributions with hazard rates λ_1 and λ_2, respectively, then the survival distribution of the total population in the trial is a mixed exponential distribution with a probability density function of

$$P_1\lambda_1 e^{-\lambda_1 t} + P_2\lambda_2 e^{-\lambda_2 t}(t > 0),$$

where t is the survival time and P_1 and P_2 (fixed or random) are the proportions of the two sub-populations. Following a similar idea of Mendenhal and Hader's (1958), the maximum likelihood estimates of the parameters λ_i and P_i can be obtained. In clinical trials, a patient's treatment is switched in the middle of the study often because there is a biomarker, such as disease progression, indicating the failure of the initial treatment regimen. If the test drug is more effective than the control, then the majority of patients in the control group will switch to the test drug. In this case, the response or survival difference between the two treatment groups will be dramatically reduced in comparison to the case without treatment switching. Moreover, if the test drug is much more effective in treating a patient after disease progression than before disease progression, it could lead to an erroneous conclusion that the test drug is inferior to the control without considering the switching effect, but in fact it is not. This biomarker-based treatment switch is obviously not a random switch but a response-adaptive treatment switch. In what follows, we will focus on the application of mixed exponential model to a clinical trial with biomarker response-adaptive treatment switching (Chang, 2005a).

Biomarker based Survival Model

In cancer trials, there are often some signs/symptoms (or more generally biomarkers) that indicate the state of the disease and the ineffectiveness or failure of a treatment. A cancer patient often experiences several episodes of progressed disease before death. Therefore, it is natural to construct a survival model based on the disease mechanism. In what follows, we consider a mixed exponential model, which is derived from the more general mixed Gamma model. Let τ_i be the time from the $(i-1)^{th}$ disease progression to the ith disease progression, where $i = 1, .., n$. τ_i is assumed to be mutually independent with probability density function of $f_i(\tau_i)$. The survival time t for a subject can be written as follows

$$t = \sum_{i=1}^{n} \tau_i. \tag{10.13}$$

Note that the nth disease progression is death. The following lemma regarding the distribution of linear combination of two random variables is useful.

Lemma   Given $x \sim f_x(x)$ and $y \sim f_y(y)$. Define $z = ax + by$. Then, the probability density function of z is given by

$$f_z(z) = \frac{1}{a} \int_{-\infty}^{\infty} f(\frac{z - by}{a}, y)dy. \tag{10.14}$$

Proof.

$$F_z(z) = P(Z \le z) = \iint_{ax+by \le z} f(x, y)dxdy = \int_{-\infty}^{\infty} \int_{-\infty}^{\frac{z-by}{a}} f(x, y)dxdy. \tag{10.15}$$

Take the derivative with respect to z and exchange the order of the two limit processes, (10.14) is immediately obtained. ∎

Corollary   When x and y are independent, then

$$f_z(z) = \frac{1}{a} \int_{-\infty}^{\infty} f_x(\frac{z - by}{a})f_Y(y)dy. \tag{10.16}$$

Theorem   If n independent random variables τ_i, $i = 1, ..., n$ are exponentially distributed with parameter λ_i, i.e.,

$$\tau_i \sim f_i(\tau_i) = \lambda_i e^{-\lambda_i \tau_i}, (\tau_i \geq 0),$$

then the probability density function of random variable $t = \sum_{i=1}^{n} \tau_i$ is given by

$$f(t; n) = \sum_{i=1}^{n} \frac{\lambda_i e^{-\lambda_i t}}{\prod_{\substack{k=1 \\ k \neq i}}^{n}(1 - \frac{\lambda_i}{\lambda_k})}, \quad t > 0, \tag{10.17}$$

where $\lambda_i \neq \lambda_k$ if $k \neq i$ for i, $k \in m_0 \leq n$ and m_i is the number of replicates for λ_i with the same value.

Proof. By mathematical induction, when n=2, Lamma (10.14) gives ($\lambda_i \neq \lambda_k$ if $i \neq k$)

$$f(t; 2) = \lambda_1 \lambda_2 \int_0^t \exp(-\lambda_1 t - (\lambda_2 - \lambda_1)\tau_2)d\tau_2 = \frac{\lambda_1 e^{-\lambda_1 t}}{1 - \frac{\lambda_1}{\lambda_2}} + \frac{\lambda_2 e^{-\lambda_2 t}}{1 - \frac{\lambda_2}{\lambda_1}}.$$

Therefore, (10.17) is proved for $n = 2$.

Now assume (10.17) hold for any $n \geq 2$, and it will be proven that (10.17) also hold for $n + 1$. From (10.17) and corollary (10.16), we have

$$f(t; n + 1) = \int_0^t f(t - \tau_{n+1}; n)f_{n+1}(\tau_{n+1})d\tau_{n+1}$$

$$= \int_0^t \sum_{i=1}^{n} \frac{\lambda_i e^{-\lambda_i(t-\tau_{n-1})}}{\prod_{\substack{k=1 \\ k \neq i}}^{n}(1 - \frac{\lambda_i}{\lambda_k})} \lambda_{n+1}e^{-\lambda_{n+1}\tau_{n+1}}d\tau_{n+1}$$

$$= \sum_{i=1}^{n} \frac{1}{\prod_{\substack{k=1 \\ k \neq i}}^{n}(1 - \frac{\lambda_i}{\lambda_k})} \left[\frac{\lambda_i e^{-\lambda_i t}}{1 - \frac{\lambda_i}{\lambda_{n+1}}} + \frac{\lambda_{n+1}e^{-\lambda_{n+1}t}}{1 - \frac{\lambda_{n+1}}{\lambda_i}} \right]$$

$$= \sum_{i=1}^{n+1} \frac{\lambda_i e^{-\lambda_i t}}{\prod_{\substack{k=1 \\ k \neq i}}^{n+1}(1 - \frac{\lambda_i}{\lambda_k})}.$$

This completes the proof. ■

For the exponential distribution $f_i(\tau_i) = \lambda_i e^{-\lambda_i \tau}$, by the above theorem, the probability density function of t , which is a mixed Gamma distribution, is given by

$$f(t; n) = \{ \sum_{i=1}^{n} w_i \lambda_i e^{-\lambda_i t}, \quad t > 0; \quad \lambda_i \neq \lambda_k \text{ if } k \neq i, \tag{10.18}$$

where $\lambda_i \neq \lambda_k$ if $k \neq i$ for i, $k \leq m_0 \leq n$, m_i is the number of replicates for λ_i with the same value, and

$$\prod_{\substack{k=1 \\ k \neq i}}^{1}(1 - \frac{\lambda_i}{\lambda_k}) = 1.$$

For disease progression, it is usually true that $\lambda_i > \lambda_k$ for $i > k$. Note that $f(t; n)$ does not depend on the order of λ_i in the sequence, and

$$f(t; n)_{\lambda_n \to +\infty} = f(t; n - 1).$$

The survival function $S(t)$ can be easily obtained from (10.18) by integration and the survival function is given by

$$S(t; n) = \sum_{i=1}^{n} w_i e^{-\lambda_i t}; \ t > 0, \ n \geq 1, \tag{10.19}$$

where the weight is given by

$$w_i = \left[\prod_{k=1, k \neq i}^{n} \left(1 - \frac{\lambda_i}{\lambda_k}\right) \right]^{-1}. \tag{10.20}$$

The mean survival time and its variance are given by

$$\mu = \sum_{i=1}^{n} \frac{w_i}{\lambda_i} \quad \text{and} \quad \sigma^2 = \sum_{i=1}^{n} \frac{w_i}{\lambda_i^2}, \tag{10.21}$$

respectively. When $n = 1$, $w_1 = 1$, (10.19) reduces to the exponential distribution. It can be shown that the weights have the properties of $\sum_{i=1}^{n} w_i = 1$ and $\sum_{i=1}^{n} w_i \lambda_i = 0$.

Effect of Patient Enrollment Rate

In this section, we will examine the effect of the accrual duration on the survival distribution. Let N be the number of patients enrolled and let $(0, t_0)$ be the patient enrollment period defined as the time elapsed from the first patient enrolled to the last patient enrolled. Also, let t denote the time elapsed from the beginning of the trial. Denote $f_d(t)$ and $f_e(\tau_e)$, where $\tau_e \epsilon [0, T_0]$, the probability density function of failure (death) and the patient enrollment rate, respectively. The failure function (or the probability of death before time t) can be expressed as

$$F(t) = \int_0^t f_d(\tau) d\tau = \int_0^t \int_0^{\min(\tau, t_0)} f(\tau - \tau_e) f_e(\tau_e) d\tau_e d\tau. \tag{10.22}$$

For a uniform enrollment rate,

$$f_e(\tau_e) = \begin{cases} \frac{N}{t_0}, & \tau_e \epsilon [0, t_0] \\ 0, & \text{otherwise}, \end{cases}$$

and probability density function (10.18), (10.22) becomes

$$F(t) = \int_0^t \int_0^{\min(\tau,t_0)} \sum_{i=1}^n w_i \frac{\lambda_i e^{-\lambda_i(\tau-\tau_e)}}{t_0} d\tau_e d\tau.$$

After the integration, we have

$$F(t) = \begin{cases} \frac{1}{t_0}\{t + \sum_{i=1}^n \frac{w_i}{\lambda_i}\left[e^{-\lambda_i t} - 1\right]\}, & t \le t_0 \\ \frac{1}{t_0}\{t_0 + \sum_{i=1}^n \frac{w_i}{\lambda_i}\left[e^{-\lambda_i t} - e^{-\lambda_i(t-t_0)}\right]\} & t > t_0 \end{cases}. \tag{10.23}$$

Differentiating it with respect to t, it can be obtained that

$$f(t) = \begin{cases} \frac{1}{t_0}\left(1 - \sum_{i=1}^n w_i e^{-\lambda_i t}\right), & t \le t_0 \\ \frac{1}{t_0}\sum_{i=1}^n w_i \left[e^{-\lambda_i(t-t_0)} - e^{-\lambda_i t}\right], & t > t_0 \end{cases}. \tag{10.24}$$

The survival function is then given by

$$S(t) = 1 - F(t), \tag{10.25}$$

and the number of deaths among N patients can be written as

$$D(t) = NF(t). \tag{10.26}$$

Note that (10.23) is useful for sample size calculation with a nonparametric method. For $n = 1$, (10.26) reduces to the number of deaths with the exponential survival distribution, i.e.,

$$D = \begin{cases} R(t - \frac{1}{\lambda}e^{-\lambda t}), & t \le t_0 \\ R\left[t_0 - \frac{1}{\lambda}(e^{\lambda t_0} - 1)e^{-\lambda t}\right], & t > t_0 \end{cases},$$

where the uniform enrollment rate $R = \frac{N}{t_0}$.

Parameter Estimate It is convenient to use the paired variable $(\hat{t}_j, \delta_j)$ defined as $(\hat{t}_j, 1)$ for a failure time $\hat{t}_j$ and $(\hat{t}_j, 0)$ for a censored time $\hat{t}_j$. The likelihood then can be expressed as

$$L = \prod_{j=1}^N \left[f(\hat{t}_j)\right]^{\delta_j} \left[S(\hat{t}_j)\right]^{1-\delta_j}, \tag{10.27}$$

where the probability density function $f(t)$ and survival function $S(t)$ are given by (10.18) and (10.19), respectively, for instantaneous enrollment, but (10.24) and (10.25) otherwise. Note that for an individual whose survival time is censored at $\hat{t}_j$, the contribution to the likelihood is given by the probability of surviving beyond that point in time, i.e., $S(\hat{t}_j)$. To reduce the number of parameters in the model, we can assume that the hazard rates take the form of a geometric sequence, i.e., $\lambda_i = a\lambda_{i-1}$ or $\lambda_i = a^i\lambda_0$; $i = 1, 2, ..., n$. This leads to a two-parameter model regardless of n, the number of progressions. The maximum likelihood estimates of λ and a can be easily obtained through numerical iterations.

Example 10.3.1   To illustrate the mixed exponential model for obtaining the maximum likelihood estimates with two parameters of λ_1 and λ_2, independent x_{1j} and x_{2j}, $j = 1, .., N$ from two exponential distributions with λ_1 and λ_2, respectively were generated. Let $\tau_j = x_{1j} + x_{2j}$. Then τ_j has a mixed exponential distribution with parameters λ_1 and λ_2. Let $\hat{t}_j = \min(\tau_j, T_s)$, where T_s is the duration of the study. Now, we have the paired variables $(\hat{t}_j, \delta_j)$, $j = 1, ..., N$, which were used to obtain the maximum likelihood estimators $\hat{\lambda}_1$ and $\hat{\lambda}_2$. Using (10.21) and the invariance principle of maximum likelihood estimators, the maximum likelihood estimate of mean survival time, $\hat{\mu}$, can be obtained as

$$\hat{\mu} = \sum_{j=1}^{2} \frac{\hat{w}_j}{\hat{\lambda}_j} = \frac{1}{\hat{\lambda}_1} + \frac{1}{\hat{\lambda}_2}. \tag{10.28}$$

For each of the three scenarios (i.e., $\lambda_1 = 1, \lambda_2 = 1.5$; $\lambda_1 = 1, \lambda_2 = 2$; $\lambda_1 = 1, \lambda_2 = 5$), $5,000$ simulation runs were done. The results of the means and coefficients of variation of the estimated parameters are summarized in Table 10.3.1.   As it can be seen from Table 10.3.1, the mixed exponential model performs well, which gives an excellent estimate of mean survival time for all three cases with virtually no bias and a less than 10% coefficient of variation. The maximum likelihood estimate of λ_1 is reasonably good with a bias less than 6%. However, there are about 5% to 15% over-estimates for λ_2 with large coefficients of variation ranging from 30% to 40%. The bias increases as the percentage of the censored observations increases. Thus, it is suggested that the maximum likelihood estimate of mean survival time rather than the maximum likelihood estimate of the hazard rate be used to assess the effect of a test treatment.

Table 10.3.1: Simulation Results with Mixed Exponential Model

	λ_1	λ_2	μ	λ_1	λ_2	μ	λ_1	λ_2	μ
True	1.00	1.50	1.67	1.00	2.00	1.50	1.00	5.00	1.20
Mean*	1.00	1.70	1.67	1.06	2.14	1.51	1.06	5.28	1.20
CV*	0.18	0.30	0.08	0.20	0.37	0.08	0.18	0.44	0.09
PDs (%)		93			96			96	
Censors (%)		12			8			5	

Note: Study duration $T = 3.2$ with quick enrollment. Number of subjects $N = 100$.
*Mean and coefficient of variation of the estimates from 5,000 runs for each scenario.

Hypothesis Test and Power Analysis

In a two-arm clinical trial comparing treatment difference in survival, the hypotheses can be written as

$$H_0 : \mu_1 \geq \mu_2 \tag{10.29}$$
$$H_a : \mu_1 < \mu_2.$$

Note that hazard rates for the two treatment groups may change over time. In practice, the proportional hazard rates do not generally hold for a mixed exponential model. In what follows, we will introduce two different approaches for hypotheses testing: nonparametric and simulation methods.

Nonparametric Method In most clinical trials, there are some censored observations. In this case, the parametric method is no longer valid. Alternatively, nonparametric methods such as the logrank test (Marubini and Valsecchi, 1995) are useful. Note that procedure for sample size calculation using the logrank test under the assumption of an exponential distribution is available in the literature (see, e.g., Marubini and Valsecchi, 1995; Chang and Chow, 2005). In what follows, we will derive a formula for sample size calculation under the mixed exponential distribution based on logrank statistic. The total number of deaths required for a one-sided logrank test for the treatment difference between two equal-sized independent groups is given by

$$D = \left[z_{1-\alpha} + 2z_{1-\beta} \frac{\sqrt{\theta}}{1+\theta} \right]^2 \left(\frac{1+\theta}{1-\theta} \right)^2, \tag{10.30}$$

where the hazard ratio is

$$\theta = \frac{\ln F_1(T_s)}{\ln F_2(T_s)}, \tag{10.31}$$

T_s is trial duration, and $F_k(T_s)$ is the proportion of patients with the event in the kth group. The relationship between $F_k(T_s)$ and t_0 and T_s and hazard rates is given by (10.23). From (10.23) and (10.26), the total number patients required for the case where the enrollment is uniformly distributed can be obtained as follows

$$N = \frac{\left[z_{1-\alpha} + 2z_{1-\beta} \frac{\sqrt{\theta}}{1+\theta} \right]^2 \left(\frac{1+\theta}{1-\theta} \right)^2}{F_1 + F_2}, \tag{10.32}$$

where t_0 is the duration of enrollment.

Example 10.3.2 Assume a uniform enrollment with a duration of $t_0 = 10$ months and trial duration $T_s = 14$ months. At the end of the study, the proportions of failures are $F_1 = 0.8$ and $F_2 = 0.75$ for the control (group 1) and the active drug (group 2), respectively. Choose a power of 90% and one-sided $\alpha = 0.025$. The hazard ratio is calculated using (10.31) as $\theta = 1.29$. From (10.32), the total number of patients required is $N = 714$. If hazard rates are given instead of the proportions of failures, we may use (10.23) to calculate the proportion of failures first.

Simulation Method   The computer simulation is a very useful tool, which can be directly applied to almost all hypotheses testing problems and power analysis for sample size calculations. It can be used with or without censoring. It can also be easily applied to a trial with treatment switching. The following is the simulation algorithm:

Step 1: Generate simulation data under H_0.   Generate x_i and y_i independently from a mixed exponential distribution with parameters λ_{11} and λ_{12}, the hazard rates under the null hypothesis H_o, using the method as described in the previous section.

Step 2: Find the distribution of test statistic T under H_0.   For each set of data, calculate the test statistic T as defined (e.g., the maximum likelihood estimate of mean difference). By repeating step 1 M times, M values of the test statistic T, and its distribution can be obtained. The precision of the distribution will increase as the number of replications, M, increases.

Step 3: Calculate p-value.   Sort the Ts obtained from step 2, and calculate the test statistic $\hat{T}$ based on the observed value from the trial. The p-value is the proportion of the simulated Ts whose values are larger (less) than $\hat{T}$.

Step 4: Calculate test statistic under H_a.   For the power calculation, data under H_a must be generated (i.e., generate x_i, $i = 1, ..., N$ from a mixed exponential distribution with parameters λ_{11} and λ_{12}, and y_i, $i = 1, ..., N$ from another mixed exponential distribution with parameters λ_{21} and λ_{22}). Calculate the test statistic as in step 2.

Step 5: Calculate the power of test.   Repeat step 4 M times to form the distribution of the test statistic under H_a. The power of the test with N subjects per group is the proportion of the simulated test statistic T with its value exceeding the critical value T_c.

Note that steps 4 and 5 are for power analysis for sample size calculations. For hypotheses testing, only the distribution of the test statistic under H_0 is required. However, for power and sample size calculation, distributions under both H_0 and H_a are required. This simulation approach is useful in dealing with adaptive treatment switching.

Application to Trials with Treatment Switch

As indicated earlier, it is not uncommon to switch a treatment when there is evidence of lack of efficacy or disease progression. Due to the natural course of the disease, most patients will have disease progression during the trial. When this happens, the clinician often gives an alternative treatment. Patients who were initially treated with the standard therapy are often switched to the test drug, but patients who were initially treated with the test drug are not necessarily switched to the standard therapy; rather, they could be switched to a different drug that has a similar effect as the control.

For a typical patient in the kth group who experiences disease progression then dies, the time to disease progression is assumed to be an exponential distribution with a hazard rate of λ_{k1}, and the time from the progression to death is another exponential distribution with a hazard rate of λ_{k2}. Due to treatment switching, a patient in treatment 1 will have a hazard rate of $\lambda_{12}^* = \lambda_{22}$ after switching to treatment 2, and a patient in treatment 2 will have a hazard rate of $\lambda_{22}^* = \lambda_{12}$ after switching to treatment 1. Further, assume all patients eventually have progressive disease and will switch treatment if the trial lasts long enough. Under these conditions, the probability density function and survival function for the kth group are given by

$$f_k^* = w_{k1}^* \lambda_{k1} e^{-\lambda_{k1}t} + w_{k2}^* \lambda_{k2}^* e^{-\lambda_{k2}^*t} \tag{10.33}$$

and

$$S_k^* = w_{k1}^* e^{-\lambda_{k1}t} + w_{k2}^* e^{-\lambda_{k2}t}, \tag{10.34}$$

respectively, where

$$w_{k1}^* = \left[1 - \frac{\lambda_{k1}}{\lambda_{k2}^*}\right]^{-1},$$

and

$$w_{k2}^* = \left[1 - \frac{\lambda_{k2}^*}{\lambda_{k1}}\right]^{-1}.$$

The likelihood for kth group is similar to (10.27), i.e.,

$$L_k^* = \prod_{j=1}^{N} \left[f_k^*(\hat{t}_j)\right]^{\delta_j} \left[S_k^*(\hat{t}_j)\right]^{1-\delta_j}. \tag{10.35}$$

The likelihood for the two groups combined is given by

$$L^* = L_1^* L_2^*.$$

Under the assumption that all patients will eventually switch treatment, maximizing L^* is equivalent to maximizing both L_1^* and L_2^*. After obtaining the maximum likelihood estimates of $\hat{\lambda}_{11}$, $\hat{\lambda}_{22}$, $\hat{\lambda}_{21}$ and $\hat{\lambda}_{12}$ using (10.35), one can calculate the mean survival times $\hat{\mu}_1$ and $\hat{\mu}_2$ for the two groups using

$$\hat{\mu}_k = \left(\frac{1}{\hat{\lambda}_{k1}} + \frac{1}{\hat{\lambda}_{k2}}\right). \tag{10.36}$$

$\hat{\mu}_k$ is called the estimator of latent survival time μ_k. The latent survival time can be interpreted as (i) the survival time that would have been observed if the patient had not switched the treatment, or (ii) overall survival benefit of the drug in treating patients with different baseline severities (e.g., second-line and third-line oncology patients). In the first interpretation, it is assumed that the drug has that magnitude of re-treatment effect, which implies that the investigator should not switch treatment at all. The second interpretation is appropriate regardless of the re-treatment effect of the drug. For the hypotheses testing

$$H_o : \mu_1 \geq \mu_2 \quad \text{vs.} \quad H_a : \mu_1 < \mu_2,$$

the test statistic is defined as

$$T = \hat{\mu}_2 - \hat{\mu}_1.$$

Example 10.3.3 Suppose that a clinical trial comparing two parallel treatment groups was conducted to demonstrate that the test drug (group 2) is better than the control (group 1) in survival. The study duration was 3.2 years and the enrollment was quick (i.e., $t_0 = 0$). The trial protocol allowed the investigator to switch a patient's treatment if his/her disease progression was observed. Suppose that $\lambda_{11} = 1$, $\lambda_{12} = 5$, $\lambda_{21} = 0.7$, and $\lambda_{22} = 1.5$. The latent mean survival times for the two groups calculated using (10.21) are $\mu_1 = 1.2$ and $\mu_2 = 2.095$ for the control and test groups, respectively. The latent survival times indicate that the test drug is better than the control in survival. However, if the treatment switch is not taken into account, the mean survival will be calculated as follows:

$$\mu_1 = \frac{1}{\lambda_{11}} + \frac{1}{\lambda_{22}} = 1.667$$

and

$$\mu_2 = \frac{1}{\lambda_{21}} + \frac{1}{\lambda_{12}} = 1.629,$$

which could lead to a wrong conclusion that the control is better than the test drug. Therefore, it is critical to consider the switching effect in the statistical analysis.

Note that the nonparametric method may not be appropriate for trials with treatment switching. In this case, it is suggested that the method of computer simulation be used. Table 10.3.2 presents results of computer simulation. The results indicate that under H_0, the critical point T_c for rejecting the null hypothesis is 0.443 for the test statistic (the observed mean survival difference). Using $T_c = 0.443$ to run the simulation under H_a with $N = 250$ patients per group shows that the trial has 86% power for detecting the difference. The distributions of the test statistic under H_0 and H_a are plotted in Figure 10.3.1. Under H_a, there is about a 3% over-estimate of μ_1 and a 3% under-estimate of μ_2. There is about a 13% under-estimate in mean difference $\mu_2 - \mu_1$ with a standard deviation of 0.34. The expected standard deviation for mean survival difference

$$\sigma = \sqrt{\sigma_1^2 + \sigma_2^2} = 1.88,$$

where σ_1^2 and σ_2^2 are calculated from (10.21). We can see that the method of computer simulation improves the precision at the cost of accuracy.

Table 10.3.2: Simulation Results with Treatment Switching

	λ_{11}	λ_{12}	μ_1	λ_{21}	λ_{22}	μ_2	$\mu_2 - \mu_1$
	Under H_0 condition						
True	1	5	1.2	1	5	1.2	0.00
Mean*	1.03	5.17	1.20	1.02	5.13	1.20	0.004
SD*	0.11	1.63	.12	0.11	1.60	.12	0.22
PDs (%)	96			96			
Censors (%)	5			5			
	Under H_a condition						
True	1	5	1.2	0.7	1.5	2.10	0.90
Mean*	1.00	5.25	1.24	0.71	1.64	2.06	0.82
SD*	0.14	1.81	0.17	0.07	0.42	0.20	0.34
PDs (%)	96			89			
Censors (%)	11			12			

*Mean and standard deviation of the estimates (5,000 runs).

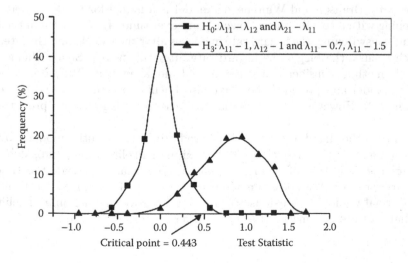

Figure 10.3.1: Distribution of Test Statistic with n=250 (5,000 runs).

Remarks For patients who are never switch regardless of treatment failure or other reasons, the probability density function and survival function are given by (10.18) and (10.19), respectively. Denote P_s the proportion of patients who are willing to switch. Then, the distribution of survival time for a typical patient in the trial is given by

$$\tilde{f}_k(t) = P_s f_k^* + (1 - P_s) f_k,$$

which is the unconditional distribution. For patients who already switched and for patients who did not switch at a certain time, the conditional distributions will be different. This case will not be studied here. It is assumed that re-treatment of a patient with same drug after disease progression is not an option, and all patients will eventually develop progressed disease and switch their treatments at the time of disease progression if the trial lasts long enough. In the simulation, the sample size N has been adjusted several times in order to meet the power requirement. Note that every time N changes, the critical point also changes due to the nature of the test statistic.

10.4   Concluding Remarks

Branson and Whitehead's method considered the use of latent event times to model a patient's observed survival time after switching and the survival time that would have been observed if this patient had not switched treatment. Their model does not take into account the fact that a treatment switch is often based on the observed effect of the current treatment. For example, the survival time of a patient who switches from the active control to the test treatment might be longer than his survival time if he had adhered to the original treatment. Therefore, Branson and Whitehead's model is a model for random treatment switching with a constant latent hazard rate over time. In fact, even in the case of random switching, the hazard rate increases after the switch, and the later the switch occurs, the bigger the hazard rate after the switch. Shao, Chang, and Chow's method considered a generalized time-dependent Cox's proportional hazard model and provided the maximum likelihood estimates (MLE) of the parameters. However, the method for hypothesis testing was not provided.

On the other hand, the biomarker-based mixed exponential model provides a great flexibility for modeling. The maximum likelihood estimate does not require the collection of biomarker data in the trial. Instead, the time to biomarker response can be estimated using one of the hazard rates in the mixed exponential model. One can use the data to improve the maximum likelihood estimates of the parameters if the biomarker response data are available.

Chapter 11

Bayesian Approach

As pointed out by Woodcock (2005), Bayesian approaches to clinical trials are of great interest in the medical product development community because they offer a way to gain valid information in a manner that is potentially more parsimonious of time, resources and investigational subjects than our current methods. The need to streamline the product development process without sacrificing important information has become increasingly apparent. Temper (2005) also indicated that FDA's reviewers have already used some of the thinking processes that involve Bayesian approaches, although the Bayesian approaches are not implemented. In a Bayesian paradigm, initial beliefs concerning a parameter of interest (discrete or continuous) are expressed by a prior distribution. Evidence from further data is then modeled by a likelihood function for the parameter. The normalized product of the prior and the likelihood forms a so-called posterior distribution. Based on the posterior distribution, conclusions regarding the parameter of interest can then be drawn. The possible use of Bayesian methods in clinical trials have been studied extensively in the literature in recent years. See, for example, Brophy and Joseph (1995), Lilford and Braunholtz (1996), Berry and Stangl (1996), Gelman, Carlin and Rubin (2003), Spiegelhalter, Abrams, and Myles (2004), Goodman (1999, 2005), Louis (2005), Berry (2005), and Berry et al. (2011).

Bayesian approaches for dose-escalation trials have been discussed in Chapter 5. In this chapter, our focus will be placed on the use of different utilities of Bayesian approaches in clinical trials. In the next section, some basic concepts of Bayesian approach such as Bayes rule and Bayesian power are given. Section 11.2 discusses the determination of prior distribution. In Section 11.3, Bayesian approaches to multiple-stage design for a single-arm trial is discussed. Section 11.4 introduces the use of Bauesian optimal adaptive designs in clinical trials. Some concluding remarks are given in the last section of this chapter.

11.1   Basic Concepts of Bayesian Approach

In this section, basic concepts of a Bayesian approach such as Bayes rule and Bayesian power are briefly described.

Bayes Rule

Let θ be the parameter of interest. Denote the prior distribution of θ as $\pi(\theta)$. Also let $f(x|\theta)$ be the sampling distribution of X given θ. Basically, a Bayesian approach involve the following four elements:

- The joint distribution of (θ, X), which is given by

$$\varphi(\theta, x) = f(x|\theta)\,\pi(\theta)\,;   \tag{11.1}$$

- The marginal distribution of X, which can be obtained as

$$m(x) = \int \varphi(\theta, x)\, d\theta = \int f(x|\theta)\,\pi(\theta)\, d\theta;   \tag{11.2}$$

- The posterior distribution of θ, which can be obtained by Bayes' formula

$$\pi(\theta|x) = \frac{f(x|\theta)\,\pi(\theta)}{m(x)};   \tag{11.3}$$

- The predictive probability distribution, which is given by

$$P(y|x) = \int P(x|y, \theta)\,\pi(\theta|x)\, d\theta.   \tag{11.4}$$

To illustrate the use of a Bayesian approach, the following examples are useful. We first consider the case where the study endpoint is discrete.

Example 11.1.1   Assume that x follows a binomial distribution with the probability of success p, i.e., $X \sim B(n, p)$. Also, assume that the parameter of interest p follows a beta distribution with parameters α and β, i.e., $p \sim Beta(\alpha, \beta)$. Thus, the prior distribution is given by

$$\pi(p) = \frac{1}{B(\alpha, \beta)} p^{\alpha-1} (1-p)^{\beta-1},\ 0 \leq p \leq 1,   \tag{11.5}$$

where

$$B(\alpha, \beta) = \frac{\Gamma(\alpha)\,\Gamma(\beta)}{\Gamma(\alpha + \beta)}.$$

Furthermore, the sampling distribution of X given p is given by

$$f(x|p) = \binom{n}{x} p^x (1-p)^{n-x}, \quad x = 0, 1, ..., n. \tag{11.6}$$

Thus, the joint distribution of (p, X) is given by

$$\varphi(p, x) = \frac{\binom{n}{x}}{B(\alpha, \beta)} p^{\alpha+x-1} (1-p)^{n-x\beta-1}. \tag{11.7}$$

and the marginal distribution of X is given by

$$m(x) = \frac{\binom{n}{x}}{B(\alpha, \beta)} B(\alpha + x, n - x + \beta). \tag{11.8}$$

As a result, the posterior distribution of p given X can be obtained as

$$\pi(p|x) = \frac{p^{\alpha+x-1}(1-p)^{n-x\beta-1}}{B(\alpha+x, \beta+n-x)} = Beta(\alpha+x, \beta+n-x). \tag{11.9}$$

For another example, consider the case where the study endpoint is a continuous variable.

Example 11.1.2 Assume that x follows a normal distribution with mean θ and variance σ^2/n, i.e., $X \sim N(\theta, \sigma^2/n)$. Also, assume that the parameter of interest θ follows a normal distribution with mean μ and variance σ^2/n_0, i.e., $\theta \sim N(\mu, \sigma^2/n_0)$. Thus, we have

$$\pi(\theta|X) \propto f(X|\theta)\pi(\theta).$$

As a result, the posterior distribution of θ given X can be obtained as

$$\pi(\theta|X) = Ce^{-\frac{(X-\theta)^2 n}{2\sigma^2}} e^{-\frac{(\theta-\mu)^2 n_0}{2\sigma^2}}, \tag{11.10}$$

where C is a constant with θ. It can be verified that (11.10) is a normal distribution wit h mean $\theta \frac{n_0\mu+nx}{n_0+n}$ and variance $\frac{\sigma^2}{n_0+n}$, i.e.,

$$\theta|X \sim N\left(\theta\frac{n_0\mu+nX}{n_0+n}, \frac{\sigma^2}{n_0+n}\right).$$

Now, based on (11.10), we can make predictions concerning future values of x by taking into account for the uncertainty about its mean θ. For this purpose, we rewrite $X = (X - \theta) + \theta$ so that X is the sum of two independent quantities, i.e., $(X - \theta) \sim N(0, \sigma^2/n)$ and $\theta \sim N(\mu, \sigma^2/n_0)$. As a result, the predictive probability distribution can be obtained as (see, e.g., Spiegelhalter, Abrams, and Rubin, 2004)

$$X \sim N\left(\mu, \sigma^2\left(\frac{1}{n} + \frac{1}{n_0}\right)\right). \tag{11.11}$$

Note that if we observe the first n_1 observations (i.e., the mean of the first n_1 observations, x_{n_1} is known), then the predictive probability distribution is given by

$$X|x_{n_1} \sim N\left(\frac{n_0\mu + n_1 x_{n_1}}{n_0 + n_1}, \ \sigma^2\left(\frac{1}{n_0 + n_1} + \frac{1}{n}\right)\right). \tag{11.12}$$

The above basic Bayesian concepts can be easily applied to some classical designs in clinical trials. However, it may affect the power and consequently sample size calculation. For illustration purposes, we consider the following example.

Example 11.1.3   Consider a two-arm parallel-group design comparing a test treatment and a standard therapy or an active control agent. Under the two-arm trial, it can be verified that the power is a function of effect size of ε (see, e.g., Chow, Shao and Wang, 2003). That is,

$$\text{power}(\varepsilon) = \Phi_0\left(\frac{\sqrt{n}\varepsilon}{2} - z_{1-\alpha}\right), \tag{11.13}$$

where Φ_0 is cumulative distribution function of the standard normal distribution. Suppose the prior distribution of the uncertainty ε is $\pi(\varepsilon)$. Then the expected power is given by

$$P_{\exp} = \int \Phi_0\left(\frac{\sqrt{n}\varepsilon}{2} - z_{1-\alpha}\right) \pi(\varepsilon)\, d\varepsilon. \tag{11.14}$$

In practice, a numerical integration is usually employed for evaluation of (11.14). To illustrate the implication of (11.14), we assume a one-sided $\alpha = 0.025$ (i.e., $z_{1-\alpha} = 1.96$) and the following prior for ε

$$\pi(\varepsilon) = \begin{cases} 1/3, & \varepsilon = 0.1, 0.25, 0.4 \\ 0, & \text{otherwise.} \end{cases} \tag{11.15}$$

Conventionally, we use the mean (median) of the effect size $\bar{\varepsilon} = 0.25$ to design the trial and perform sample size calculation assuming that $\bar{\varepsilon} = 0.25$ is the true effect size. For the two-arm balanced design with $\beta = 0.2$ or *power* $= 80\%$, the classical approach gives the following sample size

$$n = \frac{4(z_{1-\alpha} + z_{1-\beta})^2}{\varepsilon^2} = \frac{4(1.96 + 0.842)^2}{0.25^2} = 502. \tag{11.16}$$

On the other hand, the Bayesian approach based on the expected power from (11.14) yields

$$
\begin{aligned}
& P_{\exp} \\
& = \frac{1}{3}[\Phi_0(\frac{0.1\sqrt{n}}{2} - z_{1-\alpha}) + \Phi_0(\frac{0.25\sqrt{n}}{2} - z_{1-\alpha}) + \Phi_0(\frac{0.4\sqrt{n}}{2} - z_{1-\alpha})] \\
& = \frac{1}{3}[\Phi_0(\frac{0.1\sqrt{502}}{2} - 1.96) + \Phi_0(\frac{0.25\sqrt{502}}{2} - 1.96) + \Phi_0(\frac{0.4\sqrt{502}}{2} - 1.96)] \\
& = \frac{1}{3}[\Phi_0(-0.839\,73) + \Phi_0(0.840\,67) + \Phi_0(2.521\,1)] \\
& = \frac{1}{3}(0.2005 + 0.7997 + 0.9942) = 0.664\,8 = 66\%.
\end{aligned}
\tag{11.17}
$$

As it can be seen from the above, the expected power is only 66%, which is lower than the desired power of 80%. As a result, in order to reach the same power, the sample size is necessarily increased.

If $\pi(\varepsilon)$ follows a normal distribution as $N(\mu, \sigma^2/n_0)$, then the expected power can be obtained using the predictive distribution by evaluating the chance that the critical event occurs, i.e.,

$$
P(X > \frac{1}{\sqrt{n}} z_{1-\alpha}\sigma).
$$

This gives

$$
P_{\exp} = \Phi\left(\sqrt{\frac{n_0}{n_0 + n}}\left(\frac{\mu\sqrt{n}}{\sigma} - z_{1-\alpha}\right)\right).
\tag{11.18}
$$

As indicated earlier, the total sample size required for achieving the desired power is a function of the effect size ε, i.e.,

$$
n(\varepsilon) = \frac{4(z_{1-a} + z_{1-\beta})^2}{\varepsilon^2}.
\tag{11.19}
$$

Thus, the expected total sample size can be obtained as

$$
n_{\exp} = \int \frac{4(z_{1-a} + z_{1-\beta})^2}{\varepsilon^2} \pi(\varepsilon)\, d\varepsilon.
\tag{11.20}
$$

For a given flat prior, i.e., $\pi(\varepsilon) \sim \frac{1}{b-a}$, where $a \leq \varepsilon \leq b$, we have

$$
\begin{aligned}
n_{\exp} &= \int_a^b \frac{4(z_{1-a} + z_{1-\beta})^2}{\varepsilon^2} \frac{1}{b-a}\, d\varepsilon \\
&= \frac{4}{ab}(z_{1-a} + z_{1-\beta})^2.
\end{aligned}
\tag{11.21}
$$

This gives the following sample size ratio

$$
R_n = \frac{n_{\exp}}{n} = \frac{\varepsilon^2}{ab}.
$$

As it can be seen from the above, if $\varepsilon = 0.25$, $\alpha = 0.025$, $\beta = 0.8$, $n = 502$, $a = 0.1$, $b = 0.4$ (note that $(a + b)/2 = \varepsilon$), then

$$R_n = \frac{0.25^2}{(0.1)(0.4)} = 1.56.$$

This indicates that the frequentist approach could substantially underestimate the sample size required for achieving the desired power.

Bayesian Power

For testing the null hypothesis that $H_0 : \theta \le 0$ against an alternative hypothesis that $H_a : \theta > 0$, we defined the Bayesian significance as

$$P_B = P(\theta < 0 | data) < \alpha_B.$$

Note that the Bayesian significance can be easily found based on the posterior distribution. For the case where the data and the prior both follow a normal distribution, the posterior distribution is given by

$$\pi(\theta|x) = N\left(\frac{n_0\mu + nx}{n_0 + n}, \frac{\sigma^2}{n_0 + n}\right). \tag{11.22}$$

Thus, Bayesian significance can be calculated if the parameter estimate X satisfies

$$X > \frac{\sqrt{n_0 + n}z_{1-\alpha}\sigma - n_0\mu}{n}. \tag{11.23}$$

Note that the Bayesian power is then given by

$$P_B(n) = \Phi\left(\frac{\mu\sqrt{n_0 + n}\sqrt{n_0}}{\sigma\sqrt{n}} - \sqrt{\frac{n_0}{n}}z_{1-\alpha}\right). \tag{11.24}$$

Example 11.1.4 For illustration purpose, consider a phase II hypotension study comparing a test treatment with an active control agent. Suppose the primary endpoint is the reduction in systolic blood pressure (SBP). Assume that the estimated treatment effect is normally distributed, i.e.,

$$\theta \sim N\left(\mu, \frac{2\sigma^2}{n_0}\right).$$

The design is targeted to achieve the Bayesian power at $(1-\beta_B)$ at the Bayesian significance level of $\alpha_B = 0.2$. For the sample size, the sample mean difference

$$\hat{\theta} \sim N\left(0, \frac{2\sigma^2}{n}\right),$$

where n is the sample size per group. For large sample size, we can assume that σ is known. In this case, the sample size n is the solution of the following equation

$$\Phi\left(\frac{\mu\sqrt{n_0 + n}\sqrt{n_0}}{\sigma\sqrt{2n}} - \sqrt{\frac{n_0}{n}}z_{1-\alpha_B}\right) = 1 - \beta_B. \tag{11.25}$$

This leads to

$$\frac{\mu\sqrt{n_0 + n}\sqrt{n_0}}{\sqrt{2n}} - \sqrt{\frac{n_0}{n}}z_{1-\alpha_B} = z_{1-\beta_B}. \tag{11.26}$$

The above can be rewritten as follows

$$An + B\sqrt{n} + C = 0, \tag{11.27}$$

where

$$\begin{cases} A = z_{1-\beta_B}^2 - \mu^2 n_0, \\ B = 2\, z_{1-\beta_B} z_{1-\alpha}\sqrt{2n_0}, \\ C = 2z_{1-\alpha}^2 n_0 - \mu^2 n_0^2. \end{cases} \tag{11.28}$$

As a result, we can solve (10.27) for n, which is given by

$$n = \left(\frac{-B + \sqrt{B^2 - 4AC}}{2A}\right)^2. \tag{11.29}$$

11.2 Multiple-Stage Design for Single-Arm Trial

As indicated in Chapter 6, in phase II cancer trials, it is undesirable to stop a study early when the test drug is promising and it is desirable to terminate the study as early as possible when the test treatment is not effective due to ethical consideration. For this purpose, a multiple-stage design single-arm trial is often employed to determine whether the test treatment is promising for further testing. For a multiple-stage single-arm trial, the classical method and the Bayesian approach are commonly employed. In this section, these two methods are briefly described.

Classical Approach for Two-stage Design

The most commonly used two-stage design in phase II cancer trials is probably Simon's optimal two-stage design (Simon, 1989). The concept of Simon's optimal two-stage design is to permit early stopping when a moderately long sequence of initial failure occurs. Thus, under a two-stage trial design, the hypotheses of interest are given below:

$$H_0 : p \leq p_0 \quad \text{vs.} \quad H_a : p \geq p_1,$$

where p_0 is the undesirable response rate and p_1 is the desirable response rate ($p_1 > p_0$). If the response rate of a test treatment is at the undesirable level, one may reject it as an ineffective treatment with a high probability, and if its response rate is at the desirable level, one may not reject it as a promising compound with a high probability. Note that under the above hypotheses, the usual type I error is the false positive in accepting an ineffective drug and the type II error is the false negative in rejecting a promising compound.

Let n_1 and n_2 be the number of subjects in the first and second stage, respectively. Under a two-stage design, n_1 patients are treated at the first stage. If there are fewer than r_1 responses, then stop the trial. Otherwise, additional n_2 patients are recruited and tested at the second stage. A decision regarding whether the test treatment is promising is then made based on the response rate of the $n = n_1 + n_2$ subjects. Note that the rejection of H_0 (or H_a) means that further (or not further) study if the test treatment should be carried out. Simon (1989) proposed selecting the optimal two-stage design that achieves the minimum expected sample size under the null hypothesis. Let $n_{\exp}$ and P_{et} be the expected sample size and the probability of early termination after the first stage. Thus, we have

$$n_{\exp} = n_1 + (1 - P_{et})n_2.$$

At the end of the first stage, we would terminate the trial early and reject the null hypothesis if r_1 or fewer responses are observed. As a result, P_{et} is given by

$$P_{et} = B_c(r_1; n_1, p),$$

where $B_c(r_1; n_1, p)$ denotes the cumulative binomial distribution that $X \leq r_1$. Thus, we reject the test treatment at the end of the second stage if r or fewer responses are observed. The probability of rejecting the test treatment with success probability p is then given by

$$B_c(r_1; n_1, p) + \sum_{x=r_1+1}^{\min(n_1, r)} B(x; n_1, p)B_c(r - x; n_2, p),$$

where $B(x; n_1, p)$ denotes the binomial probability density function. For specifies values of p_0, p_1, α, and β, Simon's optimal two-stage design can be obtained as the two-stage design that satisfies the error constraints and minimizes the expected sample size when the response rate is p_0.

Example 11.3.1 Assume the undesirable and desirable response rates under the null hypothesis and the alternative hypothesis are given by 0.05 and 0.25, respectively. For a given one-sided $\alpha = 0.05$ with a desired power of 80%, we obtain the sample size and the operating characteristics as follows. The sample size required at stage 1 is $n_1 = 9$. The cumulative sample size at stage 2 is $n = 17$. The actual overall α and the actual power are given by 0.047 and

0.812, respectively. The stopping rules are specified as follows. At stage 1, stop and accept the null hypothesis if the response rate is less than or equal to $0/9$. Otherwise, continue to stage 2. The probability of stopping for futility is 0.63 when H_0 is true and 0.075 when H_a is true. At stage 2, stop and accept the null hypothesis if the response rate is less than or equal to $2/17$. Otherwise, stop and reject the null hypothesis.

Bayesian's Approach

Assume that $X \sim B(n,p)$ and $p \sim Beta(a,b)$. At the first stage with n_1 subjects, the posterior distribution of p given X is given by

$$\pi_1(p|x) = Beta(a+x, b+n_1-x). \tag{11.30}$$

Similarly, at the end of the second stage with n subjects, the posterior distribution of p given X is

$$\pi(p|x) = Beta(a+x, b+n-x). \tag{11.31}$$

As a result, the cutoff point for stopping the trial is chosen in such a way that the Bayesian power at the first stage is $(1-\beta_1)$ at Bayesian significance level of α_{B1}. Similarly, the n is chosen such that the Bayesian power at the second stage is $(1-\beta)$ at Bayesian significance level α_B. Based on (11.30) and (11.31), conditional power and predictive power can be derived. Given X out of n_1 patients who respond at the first stage, the probability (or conditional power) of having at least y additional responses out of the n_2 additional patients at the second stage is given by

$$P(y|x, n_1, n_2) = \sum_{i=y}^{n_2} \binom{n_2}{i} \left(\frac{x}{n_1}\right)^i (1 - \frac{x}{n_1})^{n_2-i}. \tag{11.32}$$

However, the Bayesian approach provides a different look. Assume that the prior follows a binomial prior distribution $p \in [0,1]$. Thus, the sampling distribution of X given p is given by

$$P(X = x|p) = \binom{n_1}{x} p^x (1-p)^{n_1-x}.$$

Since

$$P(a < p < b \cap X = x) = \int_a^b \binom{n_1}{x} p^x (1-p)^{n_1-x} dp,$$

and

$$P(X = x) = \int_0^1 \binom{n_1}{x} p^x (1-p)^{n_1-x} dp,$$

The posterior distribution of p given X can be obtained as

$$P(a < p < b \mid X = x) = \frac{\int_a^b \binom{n_1}{x} p^x (1-p)^{n_1-x} dp}{\int_0^1 \binom{n_1}{x} p^x (1-p)^{n_1-x} dp}$$

$$= \frac{\int_a^b p^x (1-p)^{n_1-x} dp}{B(x+1, n_1-x+1)},$$

where

$$B(x+1, n_1-x+1) = \frac{\Gamma(x+1)\Gamma(n_1-x+1)}{\Gamma(n_1+2)}.$$

Thus, the posterior distribution of p conditionally on $X = x$ responses out of n_1 is a *Beta* distribution, i.e.,

$$\pi(p|x) = \frac{p^x (1-p)^{n_1-x}}{B(x+1, n_1-x+1)}. \tag{11.33}$$

As a result, the predictive power (which is different from the frequentist's conditional power) or the predictive probability of having at least y responders out of additional m patients, given the observed response rate of x/n_1 at the first stage, is given by

$$P(y|x, n_1, n_2) = \int_0^1 P(X \ge k|p, n_2) \pi(p|x) \, dp$$

$$= \int_0^1 \sum_{i=y}^{n_2} \binom{n_2}{i} p^i (1-p)^{n_2-i} \frac{p^x (1-p)^{n_1-x}}{B(x+1, n_1-x+1)} dp. \tag{11.34}$$

Carrying out the integration, we have

$$P(y|x, n_1, n_2) = \sum_{i=y}^{n_2} \binom{n_2}{i} \frac{B(x+i+1, n_2+n_1-x-i+1)}{B(x+1, n_1-x+1)}.$$

Note that the above results follow directly from the fact that

$$\int_0^1 p^a (1-p)^b \, dp = B(a+1, b+1). \tag{11.35}$$

As a result, the conditional and/or predictive power can be used to design the sequential or other adaptive designs.

11.3 Bayesian Optimal Adaptive Designs

In practice, different adaptations and choices of priors with many possible probabilistic outcomes (good or bad) could lead to different types of adaptive designs. How to select an efficient adaptive design among these designs has become an interesting question to the investigators. In this section, we propose to evaluate so-called utility index for choosing a Bayesian optimal adaptive design. The utility index is an indicator of patients' health outcomes. Bayesian optimal design is a design that has maximum expected utility under financial, time, and other constraints.

For illustration purpose, we apply the approach for choosing a Bayesian optimal design among the three commonly considered two-arm designs in pharmaceutical research and development. The three commonly considered two-arm trial designs include a classical approach of two separate two-arm designs (i.e., a two-arm phase II design followed by a two-arm phase III design) and two different seamless phase II/III designs, which are group sequential designs with O'Brien-Fleming boundary and Pocock boundary, respectively. For each design, we calculate the utility index and weight it by its prior probability to obtain the expected utility for the design. For a given design, the Bayesian optimal design is the one with maximum utility. For convenience's sake, we consider three scenarios of prior knowledge, which are given in Table 11.3.1

Table 11.3.1: Prior Knowledge

Scenario	Effect Size	Prior Prob.
1	0	0.2
2	0.1	0.2
3	0.2	0.6

Assume that there is no dose selection issue (i.e., the dose has been determined by the toxicity and biomarker response in early studies). For the classical approach of two separate two-arm designs, we consider a phase IIb and a phase III (assuming that one phase III study is sufficient for regulatory approval). For the phase II study, we assume $\delta = 0.2$, one-sided $\alpha = 0.1$ and power=0.8. Thus, the total sample size required is $n_1 = 450$. For the phase III trial, we assume

$$\delta = 0.2(0) + 0.2(0.1) + 0.6(0.2)$$
$$= 0.14,$$

which was calculated from Table 11.3.1. Furthermore, assuming that $\alpha = 0.025$ (one-sided) and power=0.9, the total sample size required is $n = 2144$. If the phase II study didn't show any statistical significance, we will not conduct the phase III trial. Note that the rule is not always followed in practice. The probability that continues to phase III is the weighted continual probability given in Table 11.3.2, i.e.,

$$P_c = \Sigma_{i=1}^3 P_c(i)\pi(i)$$
$$= 0.2(0.1) + 0.2(0.4) + 0.6(0.9)$$
$$= 0.64.$$

Thus, the expected sample size for phase II and phase III trials as a whole is given by

$$\bar{N} = (1 - P_c)n_1 + P_c n$$
$$= (1 - 0.62)(450) + 0.62(2144)$$
$$= 1500.$$

The overall expected power is then given by

$$\bar{P} = \Sigma_{i=1}^3 P_c(i)\pi(i)P_3(i)$$
$$= (0.2)(0.1)(0.025) + (0.2)(0.4)(0.639) + (0.6)(0.9)(0.996)$$
$$= 0.59$$

Table 11.3.2: Characteristics of Classic Phase II and III Designs

Scenario, i	Effect Size	Prior Prob. π	Prob. of Continue to Phase III, P_c	Phase III Power, P_3
1	0	0.2	0.1	0.025
2	0.1	0.2	0.4	0.639
3	0.2	0.6	0.9	0.996

In conclusion, the classical approach for separate phase II and phase III designs (i.e., a phase II design followed by a phase III design) has an overall power of 59% with expected total (combined) sample size of 1500. On the other hand, for seamless phase II/III designs, we assume (i) $\delta = 0.14$, (ii) one-sided $\alpha = 0.025$, (iii) power =0.90, (iv) O'Brien-Fleming efficacy stopping boundary, and (v) symmetrical futility stopping boundary. Suppose there is one planned interim analysis when 50% of patients are enrolled. Thus, this design has one interim analysis and one final analysis. Thus, we have

- The sample sizes for the two analyses are 1,085, and 2,171, respectively.

- The sample size ratio between the two groups is 1.

- The maximum sample size for the design is 2,171.

- Under the null hypothesis, the expected sample size is 1,625.

- Under the alternative hypothesis, the expected sample size is 1,818.

The decision rules are specified as follows. At stage 1, accept the null hypothesis if $z_1 < 0$. We would reject the null hypothesis if $z_1 \geq 2.79$; otherwise, continue. At stage 2, accept the null hypothesis if $z < 1.974$ and reject the null hypothesis if $z \geq 1.97$. The stopping probabilities at the first stage are given by

- Stopping for H_0 when H_0 is true is 0.5000,

- Stopping for H_a when H_0 is true is 0.0026,

- Stopping for H_0 when H_a is true is 0.0105,

- Stopping for H_a when H_a is true is 0.3142.

The operating characteristics are summarized in Table 11.3.3.

Table 11.3.3: Characteristics of Seamless Phase II/III Design with OB Boundary

Scenario, i	Effect Size	Prior Prob. π	N_{exp}	Power
1	0	0.2	1600	0.025
2	0.1	0.2	1712	0.46
3	0.2	0.6	1186	0.98

Furthermore, the average total expected sample size can be obtained as

$$\Sigma \pi (i) N_{exp} (i) = 0.2(1600) + 0.2(1712) + 0.6(1186)$$
$$= 1374.$$

and the average power is given by

$$\Sigma \pi (i) N_{exp} (i) Power (i) = 0.2(0.025) + 0.2(0.46) + 0.6(0.98)$$
$$= 0.69.$$

Now, consider another type of seamless phase II/III adaptive trial design using Pocock's efficacy stopping boundary and the symmetric futility stopping boundary. Based on the same parameter specifications, i.e., $\alpha = 0.025$, power $= 0.9$, mean difference $= 0.14$, and standard deviation $= 1$, we have

- The sample sizes for the two analyses are 1,274 and 2,549, respectively.

- The sample size ratio between the two groups is 1.

- The maximum sample size for the design is 2,549.

- Under the null hypothesis, the expected sample size is 1,492.

- Under the alternative hypothesis, the expected sample size is 1,669.

The decision rules are specified as follows. At stage 1, accept the null hypothesis if the p-value > 0.1867 (i.e., $z_1 < 0.89$). We would reject the null hypothesis if p-value ≤ 0.0158 (i.e., $z_1 \geq 2.149$); otherwise, continue. At stage 2, accept the null hypothesis if the p-value > 0.0158 (i.e., $z = 2.149$) and reject the null hypothesis if the p-value ≤ 0.0158. The stopping probabilities at the first stage are given by

- Stopping for H_0 when H_0 is true is 0.8133,

- Stopping for H_a when H_0 is true is 0.0158,

- Stopping for H_0 when H_a is true is 0.0538,

- Stopping for H_a when H_a is true is 0.6370.

Other operating characteristics are summarized in Table 11.3.4.

Table 11.3.4: Characteristics of Seamless Phase II/III
Design with Pocock Boundary

Scenario, i	Effect Size	Prior Prob. π	N_{exp}	Power
1	0	0.2	1492	0.025
2	0.1	0.2	1856	0.64
3	0.2	0.6	1368	0.996

Furthermore, the average total expected sample size can be obtained as

$$\Sigma\pi\,(i)\,N_{exp}\,(i) = 0.2(1492) + 0.2(1856) + 0.6(1368)$$
$$= 1490,$$

and the average power is given by

$$\Sigma\pi\,(i)\,N_{exp}\,(i)\,Power\,(i) = 0.2(0.025) + 0.2(0.64) + 0.6(0.996)$$
$$= 0.73.$$

In addition, we may compare these designs from the financial perspective. Assume that the pre-patient cost of the trial is about \$50K and the value of regulatory approval before deducting the cost of the trial is \$1B. For simplicity, potential time savings are not included in the calculation. We consider the following expected utility

$$\text{Expected utility} = (\text{average power})(\$80M) - (\text{average } N_{\text{exp}})(\$50K).$$

Table 11.3.5 summarizes the comparison of the classical separate phase II and phase III design and the two seamless phase II/III designs using O'Brien-Fleming boundary and Pocock boundary.

Table 11.3.5: Comparison of Classic and Seamless Designs

Design	N_{max}	Average N_{exp}	Average Power	Expected utility
Classic	1500	0.59		$0.515B
OB	1374	0.69		$0.621B
Pocock	1490	0.73		$0.656B

As it can be seen from Table 11.3.5, the Pocock's design is the best among the three designs based on power or the expected utility.

11.4 Concluding Remarks

The Bayesian approach has several advantages in pharamceutical development. First, it provides the opportunity to continue updating the information/knowledge regarding the test treatment under study. Second, the Bayesian approach is a decision-making process that specifically ties to a particular trial, a clinical development program, and a company's portfolio for pharmaceutical development. In practice, regulatory agencies require the type I error rate to be controlled with many externally mandated restrictions when implementing a Bayesian design, which might decrease the application of Bayesian methods in clinical trials. In essence, once Bayesian methods become more familiar to clinical scientists, they will face fewer externally mandated restrictions.

In the past several decades, the process of pharamceutical development has been criticized for not being able to bring promising and safe compounds to the marketplace in a timely fashion. As a result, there is increasing demand from political bodies and consumer groups to make drug development more efficient, safer, and yet faster. However, it is a concern that we may abandon fundamental scientific principles for pharmaceutical (clinical) research and development. Alternatively, it is suggested that a Bayesian approach be used because it will lead to more rapid and more economical drug development without sacrificing good science. However, the use of Bayesian approach in pharmaceutical development is not widely accepted by the regulatory agencies such as the U.S. FDA although it has been used more in certain therapeutic areas of medical device development. It should be noted that the Bayesian approach is useful for some diseases such as cancer in which there is a burgeoning number of biomarkers available for modelling the disease's progress. These biomarkers will enable a patient's disease progression to be monitored more accurately. Consequently, a more accurate assessment of the patient's outcome can be made. In recent years, trials in early phases of clinical development (e.g., phases I or II) are becoming increasingly Bayesian, especially in the area of oncology. Moreover, strategic planning and portfolio management such as formal utility assessment and decision-making processes in some pharmaceutical companies are becoming increasingly Bayesian. The use of the Bayesian approach in various phases of pharmaceutical development will become evident to the decision-makers in the near future.

Chapter 12

Biomarker Adaptive Trials

12.1 Introduction

As indicated earlier, on March 16, 2006, the U.S. FDA released a report addressing the recent slowdown in innovative medical therapies submitted to the FDA for approval, "Innovation/Stagnation: Challenge and Opportunity on the Critical Path to New Medical Products." The report describes the urgent need to modernize the medical product development process—the *Critical Path*—to make product development more predictable and less costly. Through this initiative, the FDA encourages a national effort to advance medical product development sciences that can turn discoveries into medical miracles. FDA took the lead in the development of a national Critical Path Opportunities List, to bring concrete focus to these tasks. According to the Critical Path Opportunities Report, biomarker development is considered the most important area for improving medical product development.

Pizzo (2006) indicated that translational medicine can have a much broader definition, referring to the development and application of new technologies, biomedical devices, and therapies in a patient-driven environment such as clinical trials, where the emphasis is on early patient testing and evaluation. Thus, in this chapter, our emphasis will be placed on biomarker development in early clinical development. Since biomarker development is often carried out under an adaptive design setting in early clinical development, we will focus on statistical consideration for the use of biomarker adaptive trial design in early clinical development for translational medicine. Biomarkers, as compared to a true clinical endpoints such as survival, can often be measured earlier, easier, and more frequently, which is often less subject to competing risks and less confounded. The utilization of biomarkers will lead to a better target population with a larger effect size, a smaller sample size required, and faster decision making. With the advancement of proteomic, genomic and genetic technologies, personalized medicine with the right drug for the right patient becomes possible.

Conley and Taube (2004) described the future of biomarker/genomic markers in cancer therapy: "The elucidation of the human genome and fifty years of biological studies have laid the groundwork for a more informed method for treating cancer with the prospect of realizing improved survival. Advances in knowledge about the molecular abnormalities, signaling pathways, influence the local tissue milieu and the relevance of genetic polymorphism offer hope of designing effective therapies tailored for a given cancer in particular individual, as well as the possibility of avoiding unnecessary toxicity." Wang, Hung, and O'Neill (2009) from FDA have pointed out: "Generally, when the primary clinical efficacy outcome in a phase III trial requires a much longer time to observe, a surrogate endpoint thought to be strongly associated with the clinical endpoint may be chosen as the primary efficacy variable in phase II trials. The results of the phase II studies then provide an estimated effect size on the surrogate endpoint, which is supposedly able to help size the phase III trial for the primary clinical efficacy endpoint, where often it is thought to have a smaller effect size."

What exactly is a biomarker? Biomarkers are measurable characteristics that reflect physiological, pharmacological, or disease processes in animals or humans. Thus, the National Institutes of Health Workshop defines *biomarker* as a characteristic that is objectively measured and evaluated as an indicator of normal biologic processes, pathogenic processes, or pharmacological responses to a therapeutic intervention. Biomarkers can reduce uncertainty by proving quantitative predictions about performance of the medical product under development. The existence of predictive biomarkers is important in expediting medical product development because a validated biomarker can provide an accurate and reliable prediction of clinical performance based on the response of the biomarker. This process of predicting clinical performance through a validated biomarker response or based on some non-clinical or animal test results is referred to as the translational process. As a result, translational research can revolutionize medical product development in a disease area. On the other hand, *clinical endpoint* (or outcome) is a characteristic or variable that reflects how a patient feels or functions, or how long a patient survives. *Surrogate endpoint* is a biomarker intended to substitute for a clinical endpoint. Biomarkers can also be classified as classifier, prognostic, and predictive biomarkers.

In the next section, types of biomarkers (i.e., classifier, prognostic biomarker, and predictive biomarker) are briefly described. Also included in this section is the relationship (or translation) among these biomarkers. Adaptive trial designs using classifier, prognosis, and predictive biomarkers are discussed in the subsequent sections. A brief concluding remark is given in the last section of this chapter.

12.2 Types of Biomarkers and Validation

12.2.1 Types of biomarkers

Based on the characteristics of biomarkers, basically, biomarkers can be classified into the categories of classifier biomarker, prognostic biomarker, and predictive biomarker, which are briefly described below.

A *classifier biomarker* is a marker, e.g., a DNA marker, that usually does not change over the course of study. A classifier biomarker can be used to select the most appropriate target population or even for personalized treatment. For example, a study drug is expected to have effects on a population with a biomarker, which is only 20% of the overall patient population. Because the sponsor suspects that the drug may not work for the overall patient population, it may be efficient and ethical to run a trial only for the subpopulations with the biomarker rather than the general patient population. On the other hand, some biomarkers such as RNA markers are expected to change over the course of the study. This type of marker can be either a prognostic or predictive marker.

A *prognostic biomarker* informs the clinical outcomes, independent of treatment. It provides information about natural course of the disease in individuals with or without treatment under study. A prognostic marker does not inform the effect of the treatment. For example, non-small cell lung cancer (NSCLC) patients receiving either EGFR inhibitors or chemotherapy have better outcomes with a mutation than without a mutation. Prognostic markers can be used to separate good and poor prognosis patients at the time of diagnosis. If expression of the marker clearly separates patients with an excellent prognosis from those with a poor prognosis, then the marker can be used to aid the decision about how aggressive the therapy needs to be. The poor prognosis patients might be considered for clinical trials of novel therapies that will, hopefully, be more effective (Conley and Taube, 2004). Prognostic markers may also inform the possible mechanisms responsible for the poor prognosis, thus leading to the identification of new targets for treatment and new effective therapeutics.

A *predictive biomarker* informs the treatment effect on the clinical endpoint. A predictive marker can be population-specific: a marker can be predictive for population A but not population B. A predictive biomarker, as compared to true endpoints like survival, can often be measured earlier, more easily, and more frequently and is less subject to competing risks. For example, in a trial of a cholesterol-lowering drug, the ideal endpoint may be death or development of coronary artery disease (CAD). However, such a study usually requires thousands of patients and many years to conduct. Therefore, it is desirable to have a biomarker, such as a reduction in post-treatment cholesterol, if it predicts the reductions in the incidence of CAD. Another example would be an oncology study where the ultimate endpoint is death. However, when a patient has disease progression, the physician will switch the patient's initial treatment to an alternative treatment. Such treatment modalities will jeopardize the assessment of treatment effect on survival because the treatment switching is response-adaptive rather than random. If a marker, such as time-to-progression

(TTP) or response rate (RR), is used as the primary endpoint, then we will have much cleaner efficacy assessments because the biomarker assessment is performed before the treatment switching occurs.

Note that a classifier biomarker is commonly used in an enrichment process of target clinical trials for personalized medicine. Correlation between biomarker and true endpoint makes a prognostic marker, while correlation between biomarker and true endpoint does not make a predictive biomarker. More details regarding the validation of a biomarker and the relationship (or translation) among different types of biomarkers are given in subseqent sections. In practice, there is a gap between identifying genes that are associated with clinical outcomes and establishing a predictive model between relevant genes and clinical outcomes.

12.2.2   Biomarker validation

In clinical trials, a frequently asked question is whether or not we can use a biomarker as the primary endpoint for late phase confirmatory trials. We will address this question by examining the following scenarios that (i) the treatment has no effect on the true endpoint or the biomarker, (ii) the treatment has no effect on the true endpoint but does affect the biomarker. (iii) the treatment has a small effect on the true endpoint but has a larger effect on the biomarker. Table 12.2.1 summarizes the type I error rates (α) and powers for using the true endpoint and biomarker under different scenarios.

Table 12.2.1: Issues with Biomarker Primary Endpoint

Effect size ratio	Endpoint	Power (alpha)
0.0/0.0	True endpoint	(0.025)
	Biomarker	(0.025)
0.0/0.4	True endpoint	(0.025)
	Biomarker	(0.810)
0.2/0.4	True endpoint	0.300
	Biomarker	0.810

Note: N = 100 per group. Effect size ratio = effect size of true endpoint to effect size of biomarker.

For the first scenario, we can use either the true endpoint or biomarker as the primary endpoint because both control the type I error. For the second scenario, we cannot use the biomarker as the primary endpoint because α will be inflated to 81%. In the third scenario, it is suggested that the biomarker should be used as the primary endpoint from a power perspective. However, before the biomarker is fully validated, we don't know which scenario is true as it is realized that the use of the biomarker as the primary endpoint could lead to a dramatic inflation of the type I error. Thus, it is suggested that the biomarker must be validated before it can be used as primary endpoint. In practice, some commonly used statistical methods for biomarker validation are reviewed below.

For biomarker validation, Prentice (1989) proposed four operational criteria that (i) treatment has a significant impact on the surrogate endpoint; (ii) treatment has a significant impact on the true endpoint; (iii) the surrogate has a significant impact on the true endpoint; and (iv) the full effect of treatment upon the true endpoint is captured by the surrogate endpoint. Note that this method is for a binary surrogate (Molenberghs et al., 2005). Freedman et al. (1992), on the other hand, argued that the last Prentice criterion is difficult statistically because it requires that the treatment effect is not statistically significant after adjustment of the surrogate marker. They further articulated that the criterion might be useful to reject a poor surrogate marker, but it is inadequate to validate a good surrogate marker. Therefore they proposed a different approach based on the proportion of treatment effect on true endpoint explained by biomarkers and a large proportion required for a good marker. However, as noticed by Freedman et al., this method is practically infeasible due to the low precision of the estimation of the proportion explained by the surrogate. Buyse and Molenberghs (1998) proposed the internal validation matrices, which include relative effect (RE) and adjusted association (AA). The former is a measure of association between the surrogate and the true endpoint at an individual level, and the latter expresses the relationship between the treatment effects on the surrogate and the true endpoint at a trial level. The practical use of the Buyse-Molenberghs' method raises a few concerns: (i) a wide confidence interval of RE requires a large sample size; (ii) treatment effects on the surrogate and the true endpoint are multiplicative, which cannot be checked using data from a single trial. Other methods such as external validation using meta-analysis and two-stage validation for fast track programs are also available in the literature. However, these methods also face similar challenges in practice.

Note that Case and Qu (2006) proposed a method for quantifying the indirect treatment effect via surrogate markers, while Alonso et al. (2006) proposed a unifying approach for surrogate marker validation based on Prentice's criteria. Weir and Walley (2006) give an excellent review on biomarker validation.

12.2.3 Translation among biomarker, treatment, and true-endpoint

In clinical trials, the validation of a biomarker is usually referred to as the proof that the biomarker is predictive of the primary clinical endpoint. In other words, the biomarker can be used as a surrogate endpoint for the primary clinical endpoint. Thus, before we discuss biomarker validations, it is of interest to study the three-way relationships among treatment, biomarker, and the true endpoint. It should be noted that the correlations among them are not transitive. In the following example, we will show that it could be the case that there is a correlation (R_{TB}) between treatment and the biomarker and a correlation

(R_{BE}) between the biomarker and the true endpoint, but there is no correlation (R_{TE}) between treatment and the true endpoint (Figures 12.2.1 and 12.2.2).

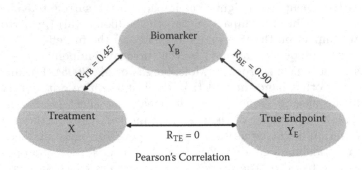

Figure 12.2.1: Treatment-biomarker-endpoint three-way relationship.

The hypothetical example to be discussed is a trial with fourteen patients, seven in the control group and seven in the test group. The biomarker and true endpoint outcomes are displayed in Figure 12.2.2. The results show that the Pearson's correlation between the biomarker and the true endpoint is 1 (perfect correlation) in both treatment groups. If the data are pooled from the two groups, the correlation between the biomarker and the true endpoint is still high, about 0.9. The average response with the true endpoint is 4 for each group, which indicates that the drug is ineffective compared with the control. On the other hand, the average biomarker response is 6 for the test group and 4 for the control group, which indicates that the drug has effects on the biomarker.

Facing the data, what we typically do is to fit a regression model with the data, in which the dependent variable is the true endpoint (Y_T) and the independent variables (predictors) are the biomarker (Y_B) and the treatment (X). After model fitting, we can obtain that

$$Y_T = Y_B - 2X. \tag{12.1}$$

This model fits the data well based on model-fitting p-value and R^2. Specifically, R^2 is equal to 1, p-values for model and all parameters are equal to 0, where the coefficient 2 in model (12.1) is the separation between the two lines. Based on (12.1), we would conclude that both biomarker and treatment affect the true endpoint. However, we know that the treatment has no effect on biomarker at all.

In fact, the biomarker predicts the response in the true endpoint, but it does not predict the treatment effect on the true endpoint, i.e., it is a prognostic marker. Therefore, a prognostic marker could be easily mistakenly treated as a predictive or surrogate marker. This "mis-translation" in an early clinical trial could result in a huge waste in resources for the later phase. It is also explained why there are a limit of validated surrogate makers in clinical trials.

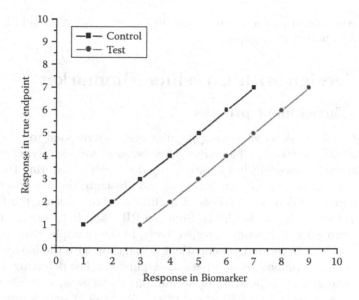

Figure 12.2.2: Correlation vs. prediction.

12.2.4   Multiplicity and false positive rate

Let's further discuss the challenges of biomarker adaptive trials from a multiplicity point of view. In early phase of clinical development, we often have a large number of biomarkers to test. Running hypothesis testing on many biomarkers can be done either with a high false positive rate without multiplicity adjustment or a low power with multiplicity adjustment. Also, if model selection procedures are used without multiplicity adjustment as we commonly see in current practice, the false positive rate could be inflated dramatically. Another source of false positive discovery rate is the so-called publication bias. Last, but not least, the source of false positive finding is due to the multiple testing conducted by different companies or research units. Imagine that 100 companies study the same biomarker, and even if family-wise type I error rate is strictly controlled at a 5% level within each company, there will still be, on average, five companies that have positive findings about the same biomarker just by chance.

12.2.5   Remarks

In reality, there are many possible scenarios: (i) same effective size for the biomarker and true endpoint, but the biomarker response can be measured earlier; (ii) bigger effective size for the biomarker and smaller for the true endpoint; (iii) no treatment effect on the true endpoint, limited treatment effect on the biomarker; and (iv) treatment effect on the true endpoint only occurs after the biomarker response reaches a threshold. Validation of biomarkers is challenging, and the sample size is often insufficient for the full validation. Therefore validations are often performed to a certain degree, and soft validation scientifically (e.g., pathway) is important.

12.3   Design with Classifier Biomarker

12.3.1   Enrichment process

In clinical trials, as different patient populations may respond to a test treatment differently, a classifier biomarker may be used for identifying a patient population that is most likely to respond to the treatment during the enrichment (screening) process of a clinical trial. To illustrate the use of a classifier biomarker in an enrichment process of a clinical trial, consider the following hypothetical example (Table 12.3.1). Suppose RR_+ and RR_- are the response rates with and without treatment, respectively. In the example, there is a treatment effect of 25% in the 10 million patient population with the biomarker, but only 9% in the 50 million general patient population. For detecting a 9% difference in the general population of 50 million, a sample size of 800 subjects is required for achieving an 80% power at the 5% level of significance. On the other hand, a total of 110 subjects are required for achieving an 80% power for detecting a much bigger difference of 25% in a smaller patient population with biomarker positive. As a result, the sponsor faces the dilemma of whether to target the general patient population or to use a biomarker to select a smaller set of patients that are expected to have a much bigger treatment effect.

Table 12.3.1: Response Rate and Sample Size Required

	Population	RR_+	RR_-	Sample Size*
Biomarker (+)	10M	50%	25%	110
Biomarker (-)	40M	30%	25%	
Total	50M	34%	25%	800

Note: *Sample size required for achieving a power of 80%.

Based on the above hypothetical example, we will need to screen 550 subjects in the general population in order to obtain 110 subjects with a biomarker if our goal is to detect a 25% difference in response rate for patients with biomarker positive. In practice, several challenges are arised. First, the estimated effect size for each subpopulation at the design stage is often not reliable. Second, there is a cost associated with screening patients for the biomarker. Third, the test for detecting the biomarker often requires high accuracy, specificity, and sensitivity (in practice, the diagnostic tool may not be available at the time of the clinical trial). Finally, screening patients for the biomarker may cause a burden and consequently has an impact on patient recruitment. These factors must be considered at the planning stage of clinical trial.

12.3.2 Classic design with classifier biomarker

Denote treatment difference between the test and control groups by δ_+, δ_-, and δ, for biomarker-positive, biomarker-negative, and overall patient populations, respectively. The null hypothesis for biomarker-positive subpopulation is

$$H_{01} : \delta_+ = 0. \tag{12.2}$$

The null hypothesis for biomarker-negative subpopulation is

$$H_{02} : \delta_- = 0. \tag{12.3}$$

The null hypothesis for overall population is

$$H_0 : \delta = 0. \tag{12.4}$$

Without loss of generality, assume that the first n patients have the biomarker among N patients and the test statistic for the subpopulation is given by

$$Z_+ = \frac{\sum_{i=1}^{n} x_i - \sum_{i=1}^{n} y_i}{n\sigma} \sqrt{\frac{n}{2}} \sim N(0,1) \text{ under } H_0, \tag{12.5}$$

where x_i, and y_i $(i = 1, ..., n)$ are the responses in treatment A and B.

Similarly, the test statistic for the biomarker-negative group is defined as

$$Z_- = \frac{\left(\sum_{i=n+1}^{N} x_i - \sum_{i=n+1}^{N} y_i\right)}{(N-n)\sigma} \sqrt{\frac{N-n}{2}} \sim N(0,1) \text{ under } H_0. \tag{12.6}$$

The test statistic for overall population is given by

$$Z = \frac{\hat{\delta}}{\sigma} \sqrt{\frac{N}{2}} = T_+ \sqrt{\frac{n}{N}} + T_- \sqrt{\frac{N-n}{N}} \sim N(0,1) \text{ under } H_0. \tag{12.7}$$

We choose the test statistic for the trial as

$$T = \max(Z, Z_+). \tag{12.8}$$

It can be shown that the correlation coefficient between Z and Z_+ is

$$\rho = \sqrt{\frac{n}{N}}. \tag{12.9}$$

Therefore, the stopping boundary can be determined by

$$\Pr(T \geq z_{2,1-\alpha} | H_0) = \alpha, \tag{12.10}$$

where $z_{2,1-\alpha}$ is the bivariate normal $100(1-\alpha)$-equipercentage point under H_0.

The p-value corresponding to an observed test statistic t is given by

$$p = \Pr\left(T \geq t | H_0\right). \qquad (12.11)$$

The power can be calculated using

$$\Pr\left(T \geq z_{2,1-\alpha} | H_a\right) = \alpha. \qquad (12.12)$$

The numerical integration or simulation can be performed to evaluate $z_{2,1-\alpha}$ and the power.

Note that the test statistic for the overall population can be defined as

$$Z = w_1 Z_+ + w_2 Z_-,$$

where w_1 and w_2 are constants satisfying $w_1^2 + w_2^2 = 1$. In such a case, the correlation coefficient between Z and Z_+ is $\rho = w_1$.

More generally, if there are m groups under consideration, we can define a statistic for the gth group as

$$Z_g = \frac{\hat{\delta}_g}{\sigma}\sqrt{\frac{n_g}{2}} \sim N(0,1) \text{ under } H_0. \qquad (12.13)$$

The test statistic for the overall population is given by

$$T = \max\left\{Z_1, ..., Z_g\right\}, \qquad (12.14)$$

where $\{Z_1, ..., Z_m\}$ is asymptotically m-variate standard normal distribution under H_o with expectation $0 = \{0, ..., 0\}$ and correlation matrix R$=\{\rho_{ij}\}$. It can be easily shown that the correlation between Z_i and Z_j is given by

$$\rho_{ij} = \sqrt{\frac{n_{ij}}{n_i n_j}}, \qquad (12.15)$$

where n_{ij} is the number of concordant pairs between the ith and j^{th} groups.

The asymptotic formulation for power calculation with the multiple tests is similar to that for multiple-contrast tests (Bretz and Hothorn, 2002):

$$\Pr\left(T \geq z_{m,1-\alpha} | H_a\right)$$
$$= 1 - \Pr(Z_1 < z_{m,1-\alpha} \cap ... \cap T_m < z_{m,1-\alpha} | H_a$$
$$= 1 - \Phi_m\left((z_{m,1-\alpha} - e)\, diag\left(\frac{1}{v_0}, ..., \frac{1}{v_m}\right); 0; R\right),$$

where $z_{m,1-\alpha} = (z_{m,1-\alpha}, ..., z_{m,1-\alpha})$ stands for the m-variate normal $100(1-\alpha)$-equipercentage point under H_0, $\mathbf{e} = (E_a(T_0), ..., E_a(T_m))$ and $\mathbf{v} = (v_0, ..., v_m) = \left(\sqrt{V_0(T_0)}, \sqrt{V_1(T_1)}, ..., \sqrt{V_1(T_m)}\right)$ are vectorially summarized expectations and standard errors.

The power is given by

$$p = \Pr\left(T \geq z_{m,1-p}\right). \tag{12.16}$$

For other types of endpoints, we can use inverse-normal method, i.e., $Z_g = \Phi\left(1 - p_g\right)$, where p_g is the p-value for the hypothesis test in the gth population group, then (12.15) and (12.16) are still approximately valid.

12.3.3 Adaptive design with classifier biomarker

In the interests of a strong alpha-controlled method, let the hypothesis test for a biomarker-positive subpopulation at the first stage (size $= n_1/\text{group}$) be

$$H_{o1} : \delta_+ \leq 0 \tag{12.17}$$

and the hypothesis test for overall population (size $= N_1/\text{group}$) be

$$H_o : \delta \leq 0 \tag{12.18}$$

with the corresponding stagewise p-values, p_{1+} and p_1, respectively. These stagewise p-values should be adjusted. A conservative way is using the Bonferroni method or a method similar to the Dunnett method that takes the correlation into consideration. For Bonferroni-adjusted p-value and MSP, the test statistic is $T_1 = 2\min\left(p_{1+},\ p_1\right)$ for the first stage. The population with a smaller p-value will be chosen for the second stage and the test statistic for the second stage is defined as $T_2 = T_1 + p_2$, where p_2 is the stagewise p-value from the second stage. This method is implemented in SAS (see Appendix).

12.3.4 An example - biomarker-adaptive design

Suppose in an active-control trial, the estimated treatment difference is 0.2 for the biomarker-positive population (BPP) and 0.1 for the biomarker-negative population (BNP) with a common standard deviation of $\sigma = 1$. Using SAS macros in the appendix at end of this chapter, we can generate the operating characteristics under the global null hypothesis H_0 ($\mu_{0+} = 0$, $\mu_{0-} = 0$), the null configurations H_{01} ($\mu_{0+} = 0$, $\mu_{0-} = 0.1$) and H_{02} ($\mu_{0+} = 0.2$, $\mu_{0-} = 0$), and the alternative hypothesis H_a ($\mu_{0+} = 0.2$, $\mu_{0-} = 0.1$) under a two-stage design and a classic single-stage design (see Tables 12.3.2-12.3.3), respectively.

Table 12.3.2: Simulation Results of Two-Stage Design

Case	FSP	ESP	Power	AveN	pPower	oPower
H_0	0.876	0.009	0.022	1678	0.011	0.011
H_{01}	0.538	0.105	0.295	2098	0.004	0.291
H_{02}	0.171	0.406	0.754	1852	0.674	0.080
H_a	0.064	0.615	0.908	1934	0.311	0.598

H_{01} and H_{02} = no effect for BPP and overall population.

Table 12.3.3: Simulation Results of Classic Single-Stage Design

Case	FSP	ESP	Power	AveN	pPower	oPower
H_0	0.878	0.022	0.022	2400	0.011	0.011
H_{01}	0.416	0.274	0.274	2400	0.003	0.271
H_{02}	0.070	0.741	0.741	2400	0.684	0.056
H_a	0.015	0.904	0.904	2400	0.281	0.623

H_{01} and H_{02} = no effect for BPP and overall population.

Trial monitoring is particularly important for these types of trials. Assume we have decided the sample sizes N_2 per treatment group for overall population at stage 2, of which n_2 (can be modified later) subjects per group are biomarker-positive. Ideally, a decision on whether the trial continues for the biomarker-positive patients or overall patients should be dependent on the expected utility at the interim analysis. The utility is the total gain (usually as a function of observed treatment effect) subtracted by the cost due to continuing the trial using BPP or the overall patient population. For simplicity, we define the utility as the conditional power. The population group with larger conditional power will be used for the second stage of the trial. Suppose we design a trial with $n_{1+} = 260$, $n_{1-} = 520$, $p_{1+} = 0.1$, $p_1 = 0.12$, and stopping boundaries: $\alpha_1 = 0.01, \beta_1 = 0.15$, and $\alpha_2 = 0.1871$. For $n_{2+} = 260$, and $n_{2-} = 520$, the conditional power based on MSP is 82.17% for BPP and 99.39% for the overall population. The calculations are presented as follows:

$$P_c(p_1, \delta) = 1 - \Phi\left(\Phi^{-1}(1 - \alpha_2 + p_1) - \frac{\delta}{\sigma}\sqrt{\frac{n_2}{2}}\right), \ \alpha_1 < p_1 \leq \beta_1.$$

For the biomarker-positive population,

$$\Phi^{-1}(1 - 0.1871 + 0.1) = \Phi^{-1}(0.912\,9) = 1.3588, 0.2\sqrt{260/2} = 2.280\,4,$$

$$P_c = 1 - \Phi(1.3588 - 2.2804) = 1 - \Phi(-0.921\,6) = 1 - 0.1783 = 0.821\,7.$$

For the biomarker-negative population,

$$\Phi^{-1}(1 - 0.1871 + 0.12) = \Phi^{-1}(0.932\,9) = 1.4977,$$

$$0.2\sqrt{(260 + 520)/2} = 3.949\,7,$$

$$P_c = 1 - \Phi(1.4977 - 3.949\,7) = 1 - \Phi(-2.452) = 1 - 0.0071 = 0.992\,9.$$

Therefore, we are interested in the overall population. Of course, different n_2 and N_2 can be chosen at the interim analyses, which may lead to different decisions regarding the population for the second stage.

The following aspects should also be considered during design: power vs. utility, enrolled patients vs. screened patients, screening cost, and the prevalence of biomarkers.

12.4 Adaptive Design with Prognostic Biomarker

12.4.1 Optimal design

A biomarker before it is proved predictive can only be considered as a prognostic marker. In the following example, we discuss how to use a prognostic biomarker (a marker may be predictive) in trial design. The adaptive design proposed permits early stopping for futility based on the interim analysis of the biomarker. At the final analysis, the true endpoint will be used to preserve the type I error. Assume there are three possible scenarios: (1) H_{01}: effect size ratio ESR = 0/0, (2) H_{02}: effect size ratio ESR = 0/0.25, and (3) H_a : effect size ratio ESR = 0.5/0.5, but biomarker response earlier. ESR is the ratio of effect size for true endpoint to the effect size for biomarker. We are going to compare three different designs: classic design and two adaptive designs with different stopping boundaries as shown in Table 12.4.1.

Table 12.4.1: Adaptive Design with Biomarker

Design	Condition	Power	Expected N/arm	Futility boundary
Classic	H_{01}		100	
	H_{02}		100	
	H_a	0.94	100	
Adaptive	H_{01}		75	
	H_{02}		95	$\beta_1 = 0.5$
	H_a	0.94	100	
Adaptive	H_{01}		55	
	H_{02}		75	$\beta_1 = 0.1056$
	H_a	0.85	95	

Based on simulation results (Table 12.4.1), we can see that the two adaptive designs reduce the sample size required under the null hypothesis. However, this comparison is not good enough because it does not consider the prior distribution of each scenario at the design stage.

We have noticed that there are many different scenarios with associated probabilities (prior distribution) and many possible adaptive designs with associated probabilistic outcomes (good and bad). Suppose we have also formed the utility function, the criterion for evaluating different designs. Now let's illustrate how we can use utility theory to select the best design under financial, time, and other constraints.

Table 12.4.2: Prior Knowledge about Effect Size

Scenario	Effect Size Ratio	Prior Probability
H_{01}	0/0	0.2
H_{02}	0/0.25	0.2
H_a	0.5/0.5	0.6

Let's assume the prior probability for each of the scenarios mentioned earlier as shown in Table 12.4.2. For each scenario, we conduct computer simulations to calculate the probability of success and the expected utilities for each design. The results are summarized in Table 12.4.3.

Table 12.4.3: Expected Utilities of Different Designs

Design	Classic	Biomarker-adaptive	
		$\beta_1 = 0.5$	$\beta_1 = 0.1056$
Expected Utility	419	441	411

Based on the expected utility, the adaptive design with the stopping boundary $\beta_1 = 0.5$ is the best. Of course, we can also generate more designs and calculate the expected utility for each design and select the best one.

12.4.2   Prognostic biomarker in designing survival trial

Insufficiently validated biomarkers such as tumor response rate (RR) can be used in oncology trials for interim decision making whether to continue to enroll patients or not to reduce the cost. When the response rate in the test group is lower, because of the correlation between RR and survival, it is reasonable to believe the test drug will be unlikely to have survival benefit. However, even when the trial stopped earlier due to unfavorable results in response rate, the survival benefit can still be tested. We have discussed this for a Non-Hodgkin's Lymphoma (NHL) trial.

12.5   Adaptive Design with Predictive Marker

If a biomarker is proved to be predictive, then we can use it to replace the true endpoint from the hypothesis test point of view. In other words, a proof of treatment effect on predictive marker is a proof of treatment effect on the true endpoint. However, the correlation between the effect sizes of treatment in the predictive (surrogate) marker and the true endpoints is desirable but unknown. This is one of the reasons that follow-up study on the true endpoint is highly desirable in the NDA accelerated approval program.

Changes in biomarkers over time can be viewed as stochastic process (marker process) and have been used in the so-called threshold regression. A predictive marker process can be viewed as an external process that covariates with the parent process. It can be used in tracking progress of the parent process if the parent process is latent or is only infrequently observed. In this way, the marker process forms a basis for predictive inference about the status of the parent process of clinical endpoint. The basic analytical framework for a marker process conceives of a bivariate stochastic process $\{X(t), Y(t)\}$ where the parent process $\{X(t)\}$ is one component process and the marker process $\{Y(t)\}$ is the other. Whitmore, Crowder, and Lawless (1998) investigated the failure inference based on a bivariate. The Wiener model has also been used in this aspect, in which failure is governed by the first-hitting time of a latent degradation process. Lee, DeGruttola, and Schoenfeld (2000) apply this bivariate marker model to CD4 cell counts in the context of AIDS survival. Hommel, Lindig, and Faldum (2005) studied a two-stage adaptive design with correlated data.

12.6 Concluding Remarks

In the previous sections, we have discussed the adaptive designs with classifier, prognostic, and predictive biomarkers. These designs can be used to improve the efficiency by identifying the right population, making decisions earlier to reduce the impact of failure, and delivering the efficacious and safer drugs to market earlier. However, full validation of a biomarker is statistically challenging, and sufficient validation tools may not be available. However, adaptive designs with biomarkers can be beneficial even when the biomarkers are not fully validated. The Bayesian approach is an ideal solution for finding an optimal design, while computer simulation is a powerful tool for the utilization of biomarkers in trial design.

12.7 Appendix

12.7.1 SAS macro for two-stage design and classic single-stage design

Typical SAS macro calls to simulate the global null (H_0) and the alternative (H_a) conditions under a two-stage design are given below, respectively.

```
Title "Simulation under global H0, 2-stage design";
%BMAD(nSims=100000, CntlType="strong", nStages=2, u0p=0,
    u0n=0, sigma=1.414, np1=260, np2=260, nn1=520, nn2=520,
    alpha1=0.01, beta1=0.15,alpha2=0.1871);

Title "Simulations under Ha, 2-stage design";
%BMAD(nSims=100000, CntlType="strong", nStages=2, u0p=0.2,
    u0n=0.1, sigma=1.414, np1=260, np2=260, nn1=520, nn2=520,
```

alpha1=0.01, beta1=0.15,alpha2=0.1871);

For the classic single stage design, we may consider the following SAS macro calls to simulate the global null (H_0) and the alternative (H_a) conditions, respectively.

Title "Simulations under global H_0, single-stage design";
%BMAD(nSims=100000, CntlType="strong", nStages=1, u0p=0,
u0n=0, sigma=1.414, np1=400, np2=0, nn1=800, nn2=0, alpha1=0.025);

Title "Simulations under Ha, single-stage design";
%BMAD(nSims=100000, CntlType="strong", nStages=1, u0p=0.2,
u0n=0.1, sigma=1.414, np1=400, np2=0, nn1=800, nn2=0, alpha1=0.025);

12.7.2   SAS macro for biomarker-adaptive trials with two parallel groups

This SAS Macro is developed for simulating biomarker-adaptive trials with two parallel groups. The key SAS variables are defined as follows: Alpha1 = early efficacy stopping boundary (one-sided), beta1 = early futility stopping boundary, Alpha2 = final efficacy stopping boundary, u0p = response difference in biomarker-positive population, u0n = response in biomarker-negative population, sigma = asymptotic standard deviation for the response difference, assuming homogeneous variance among groups. For binary response, sigma $=\sqrt{r_1(1 - r_1) + r_2(1 - r_2)}$; For Normal response, sigma $= \sqrt{2}\sigma$. np1, np2 = sample sizes per group for the first and second stage for the biomarker-positive population. nn1, nn2 = sample sizes per group for the first and second stage for the biomarker-negative population. cntlType = "strong," for the strong type I error control and cntlType = "weak," for the weak type I error control, AveN = average total sample-size (all arms combined), pPower = the probability of significance for biomarker-positive population, oPower = the probability of significance for overall population.

```
%Macro BMAD(nSims=100000, cntlType="strong", nStages=2,
      u0p=0.2, u0n=0.1, sigma=1, np1=50, np2=50, nn1=100,
      nn2=100, alpha1=0.01, beta1=0.15,alpha2=0.1871);
Data BMAD;
 Keep FSP ESP Power AveN pPower oPower;
 seedx=1736; seedy=6214; u0p=&u0p; u0n=&u0n; np1=&np1;
      np2=&np2; nn1=&nn1; nn2=&nn2; sigma=&sigma;
      FSP=0; ESP=0;Power=0; AveN=0; pPower=0; oPower=0;
 Do isim=1 to &nSims;
      up1=Rannor(seedx)*sigma/Sqrt(np1)+u0p;
      un1=Rannor(seedy)*sigma/Sqrt(nn1)+u0n;
      uo1=(up1*np1+un1*nn1)/(np1+nn1);
      Tp1=up1*np1**0.5/sigma; To1=uo1*(np1+nn1)**0.5/sigma;
```

```
      T1=Max(Tp1,To1); p1=1-ProbNorm(T1);
      If &cntlType="strong" Then p1=2*p1; *Bonferroni;
      If p1>&beta1 Then FSP=FSP+1/&nSims;
      If p1<=&alpha1 Then Do;
          Power=Power+1/&nSims; ESP=ESP+1/&nSims;
          If Tp1>To1 Then pPower=pPower+1/&nSims;
          If Tp1<=To1 Then oPower=oPower+1/&nSims;
      End;
      AveN=AveN+2*(np1+nn1)/&nSims;
      If &nStages=2 And p1>&alpha1 And p1<=&beta1 Then Do;
         up2=Rannor(seedx)*sigma/Sqrt(np2)+u0p;
         un2=Rannor(seedy)*sigma/Sqrt(nn2)+u0n;
         uo2=(up2*np2+un2*nn2)/(np2+nn2);
         Tp2=up2*np2**0.5/sigma; To2=uo2*(np2+nn2)**0.5/sigma;
         If Tp1>To1 Then Do;
            T2=Tp2; AveN=AveN+2*np2/&nSims;
         End;
          If Tp1<=To1 Then Do;
            T2=To2; AveN=AveN+2*(np2+nn2)/&nSims;
         End;
         p2=1-ProbNorm(T2); Ts=p1+p2;
         If .<TS<=&alpha2 Then Do;
           Power=Power+1/&nSims;
           If Tp1>To1 Then pPower=pPower+1/&nSims;
           If Tp1<=To1 Then oPower=oPower+1/&nSims;
         End;
      End;
  End;
 Run;
 Proc Print Data=BMAD (obs=1); Run;
 %Mend BMAD;
```

Chapter 13

Target Clinical Trials

13.1 Introduction

In clinical research, it is of particular interest to clinicians to identify patients with disease targets under study, who are most likely to respond to the test treatment under investigation. In practice, an enrichment process is often employed to identify such a target patient population. Clinical trials utilizing an enrichment design are referred to as target clinical trials. As indicated by several authors, after completion of the human genome project, the disease targets at certain molecular level can be identified and should be utilized for treatment of diseases (see, e.g., Maitournam and Simon, 2005; Casciano and Woodcock, 2006). As a result, diagnostic devices for detection of diseases using biotechnology such microarray, polymerase chain reaction (PCR), mRNA transcript profiling, and others become possible in practice (FDA, 2005a, 2005b, 2007). The treatments specific for the molecular targets could then be developed for those patients who are most likely to benefit. Consequently, personalized medicine could become a reality. A typical example is the clinical development of Herceptin (trastuzumab), which is targeted at the patients with metastatic breast cancer with an over-expression of HER2 (human epidermal growth factor receptor) protein. We will refer to these treatments as the target treatments or drugs. Development of target treatments involves translation from the accuracy and precision of diagnostic devices for the molecular targets to the effectiveness and safety of the treatment modality for the patient population with the targets. Therefore, evaluation of target treatments is much more complicated than that of the traditional drugs. To address the issues of development of the targeted drugs, in April 2005, the U.S. FDA *Drug-Diagnostic Co-development Concept Paper*.

In clinical trials, it is well recognized that subjects with and without disease targets may respond to the treatment differently with different effect sizes. In other words, patients with disease targets may show a much larger effect size, while patients without disease targets may exhibit a relatively small effect size.

In practice, fewer subjects are required for detecting a bigger effect size. Thus, the traditional clinical trials may conclude that the test treatment is ineffective based on the detection of a combined effect size, while the test treatment is in fact effective for those patients with the disease targets. Thus, personalized medicine is possible if we can identify those subjects with the disease targets. As indicated in the FDA's drug-diagnostic co-development concept paper, one of the useful designs for evaluation of the target treatments is the enrichment design (see also Chow and Liu, 2004). Under the enrichment design, the target clinical trials consist of two phases. The first phase is the enrichment phase in which each patient is tested by a diagnostic device for detection of the pre-defined molecular targets. Then patients with a positive result by the diagnostic device are randomized to receive either the target treatment or a concurrent control. However, in practice, no diagnostic test is perfect with 100% positive predicted value (PPV). As a result, some of the patients enrolled in target clinical trials under the enrichment design might not have the specific targets and hence the treatment effects of the drug for the molecular targets could be under-estimated due to misclassification (Liu and Chow, 2008)

Under the enrichment design, following the idea as described in Liu and Chow (2008), Liu, Lin and Chow (2009) proposed using the EM algorithm (Dempster et al., 1977; McLachlan and Krishnan, 1997) in conjunction with the bootstrap technique (Efron and Tibshirani, 1993) for obtaining the inference of the treatment effects. Their method, however, depends upon the accuracy and reliability of the diagnostic device. A poor (i.e., less accurate and reliable) diagnostic device may result in a large proportion of mis-classification which has an impact on the assessment of the true treatment effect. To overcome (correct) the problem of an inaccurate diagnostic device, a Bayesian approach in conjunction with the EM algorithm and bootstrap technique for obtaining a more accurate and reliable estimate of treatment effect may be useful.

In the next section, the potential impact of target clinical trials utilizing an enrichment process is illustrated through the typical example of the clinical development of Herceptin. Section 13.3 discusses statistical methods for evaluation of treatment effects of target clinical trials under a study design recommended by the FDA. Alternative study designs (also recommended by the FDA) and suggested statistical methods are described in Section 13.4. Brief concluding remarks are provided in the last section of this chapter.

13.2   Potential Impact and Significance

To illustrate the potential impact and significance of target clinical trials utilizing an enrichment process, consider the example of Herceptin for treating patients with metastatic breast cancer with and over-expression of HER2 protein using the gene amplification by FISH (fluorescence in situ hybridization) or clinical trial assay (CTA) which is an investigational immunohistochemica (IHC) assay consists of 4-point ordinal score system (0, 1+, 2+, 3+). Table 13.2.1 gives the treatment effects of Herceptin plus chemotherapy as a function of HER2 over-expression. As it can be seen from Table 13.2.1, Herceptin plus chemotherapy provides statistically significantly additional clinical benefits in terms of overall survival over chemotherapy alone for patients with a staining score of 3+, while Herceptin plus chemotherapy fails to provide additional survival benefits for patients with a CTA score of 2+. However, as indicated in the Decision Summary of HercepTest (a commercial IHC assay for overexpression of HER2 protein), the findings of inter-laboratory reproducibility study showed that 12 of 120 samples (10%) had discrepancy results between 2+ and 3+ staining intensity. It follows that some patients tested with a score of 3+ may actually have a score of 2+ and vice versa.

Table 13.2.1: Treatment Effects as a Function of HER2 Over-expression or Amplification

HER2 Assay Result	Number of Patients	Relative Risk for Mortality (95%)
CTA 2+ or 3+	469	0.80(0.64, 1.00)
FISH (+)	325	0.70(0.53, 0.91)
FISH (−)	126	1.06(0.70, 1.63)
CTA 2+	120	1.26(0.82, 1.94)
FISH (+)	32	1.31(0.53, 3.27)
FISH (−)	83	1.11(0.68, 1.82)
CTA 3+	349	0.70(0.51, 0.89)
FISH (+)	293	0.67(0.51, 0.89)
FISH (−)	43	0.88(0.39, 1.98)

Source: From U.S. FDA Annotated Redlined Draft Package Insert for Herceptin, Rockville, Maryland, 2006.

Utilizing the information will allow the clinicians to identify optimal clinical benefit to patients who are most likely to respond to the treatment under investigation through an enrichment process. Target clinical trials under an enrichment design will make personalized medicine possible. Under a valid study design, the methodology proposed by Liu, Lin, and Chow (2009) can be applied not only to different types of study endpoints such as continuous variables, binary responses, and time-to-event data for testing hypotheses of equality, superiority/non-inferiority, and equivalence, but also to various critical diseases across therapeutic areas such as cardiovascular, infectious diseases, and oncology in public health.

13.3 Evaluation of Treatment Effect

Liu, Lin, and Chow (2009) considered the situation where a particular molecular target involved with the pathway in pathogenesis of the disease has been identified and there is a validated diagnostic device available for detection of the identified molecular target. It is assumed that the device is only for detection of the molecular target and is not for prognosis of clinical outcomes of patients. In addition, it is also assumed that the device has been evaluated in the diagnostic effectiveness trial and met the regulatory requirements for diagnostic accuracy.

13.3.1   Study design

Under an enrichment design, one of the objectives of target clinical trials is to evaluate the treatment effects of the molecular targeted test treatment in the patient population with the molecular target. The diagram in the FDA concept paper (FDA, 2005b) for demonstration of this design is reproduced in Figure 13.3.1.

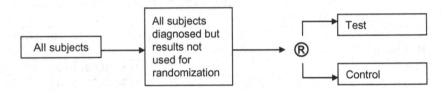

Figure 13.3.1: Target clinical trials under an enrichment design.

Under the enrichment design, Liu, Lin, and Chow (2009) considered a two-group parallel design in which patients with a *positive* result by the diagnostic device are randomized in a 1:1 ratio are randomized to receive the molecular targeted test treatment (T) or a control treatment (C) (see Figure 13.3.2).

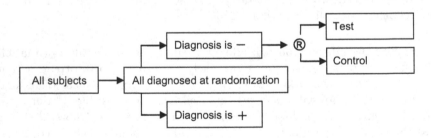

Figure 13.3.2: Enrichment design for patients with positive results.

In other words, only patients with positive diagnosed results are included in the study. For simplicity, Liu, Lin and Chow (2009) assumed that the primary efficacy endpoint is a continuous variable. Let Y_{ij}, be the responses of the jth subject in the ith group, where $j = 1, \ldots, n_i$; $i = $ T,C. Y_{ij} are assumed approximately normality distributed with homogeneous variances between the test and control treatments.

Table 13.3.1: Population Means by Treatment and Diagnosis

Positive diagnosis	True target condition	Indicator of diagnostic	Test group	Control group	Difference
+	+	γ	μ_{T+}	μ_{C+}	$\mu_{T+} - \mu_{C+}$
	−	$1 - \gamma$	μ_{T-}	μ_{C-}	$\mu_{T-} - \mu_{C-}$

Note: γ is the positive predicted value.

Table 13.3.1 gives the expected values of Y_{ij} by treatment and diagnostic result of the molecular target. In Table 13.3.1, μ_{T+}, μ_{C+} (μ_{T-}, μ_{C-}) are the means of test and control groups for the patients with (without) the molecular target. The inference for the treatment effects could be obtained through either estimation or hypothesis testing. For estimation, the parameter of interest is the treatment effects for the patients truly having the molecular target $\theta = \mu_{T+} - \mu_{C+}$. However, this effect may be contaminated due to misclassification, i.e., for those subjects who do not have the molecular target but got positive diagnosed results and those subject who have the molecular target but got negative diagnosed results.

The hypothesis for detection of treatment difference in the patient population truly with the molecular target is the hypothesis of interest:

$$H_0 : \mu_{T+} - \mu_{C+} = 0 \quad vs. \quad H_a : \mu_{T+} - \mu_{C+} \neq 0. \tag{13.1}$$

13.3.2 Statistical methods

Let $\bar{y}_T$ and $\bar{y}_C$ be the sample means of test and control treatments, respectively. Since no diagnostic test is perfect for diagnosis of the molecular target of interest without error, therefore, some patients with a positive diagnostic result may in fact not have the molecular target. It follows that

$$E(\bar{y}_T - \bar{y}_C) = \gamma(\mu_{T+} - \mu_{C+}) + (1 - \gamma)(\mu_{T-} - \mu_{C-}), \tag{13.2}$$

where γ is the positive predicted value. Liu and Chow (2008) indicated that the expected value of the difference in sample means consists of two parts. The first part is the treatment effects of the molecular target drug in patients with a positive diagnosis who truly have the molecular target of interest. The second part is the treatment effects of the patients with a positive diagnosis, but in fact they do not have the molecular target. The reason for developing the targeted treatment is based on the assumption that the efficacy of the targeted treatment is greater than in the patients truly with the molecular target than those without the target. In addition, the targeted treatment is also expected to be more efficacious than the untargeted control in the patient population truly with the molecular targets. It follows that

$$\mu_{T+} - \mu_{C+} > \mu_{T-} - \mu_{C-}.$$

As a result, the difference in sample means obtained under the enrichment design for target clinical trials actually under-estimated the true treatment effects of the molecular target test drug in the patient population truly with the molecular target of interest. As it can be seem from (13.2), the bias of the difference in sample means decreases as the positive predicted value increases. On the other hand, the positive predicted value of a diagnostic test increases as the prevalence of the disease increases (Fleiss, Levin and Paik, 2003). For a disease which is highly prevalent, say greater than 10%, even with a high diagnostic accuracy of 95% sensitivity and specificity for the diagnostic device, the positive predicted value is only about 67.86%. It follows that the downward bias of the traditional difference in sample means could be substantial for estimation of treatment effects of the molecular target drug in patients truly with the target of interest.

The traditional unpaired two-sample t-test approach is to reject the null hypothesis in (13.1) at the at the α level of significance level if

$$t = \left| (\bar{y}_T - \bar{y}_C)/\sqrt{s_p^2(1/n_T + 1/n_C)} \right| \geq t_{\alpha/2, n_T + n_C - 2},$$

where s_p^2 is the pooled sample variance, and $t_{\alpha, n_T + n_C - 2}$ is the αth upper percentile of a central t distribution with $n_T + n_C - 2$ degrees of freedom. Since $\bar{y}_T - \bar{y}_C$ under-estimates $\mu_{T+} - \mu_{C+}$, the planned sample size may not be sufficient for achieving the desired power for detecting the true treatment effects in the patients truly with molecular target of interest. Based on the above t-statistic, the corresponding $(1 - \alpha)$ 100% confidence interval can be obtained as follows

$$(\bar{y}_T - \bar{y}_C) \pm t_{\alpha/2, n_T + n_c - 2} \sqrt{s_p^2 \left(\frac{1}{n_T} + \frac{1}{n_C} \right)}.$$

Although all patients randomized under the enrichment design have a positive diagnosis, the true status of the molecular target for individual patients in the target clinical trials is in fact unknown. It follows that under the assumption of homogeneity of variance, Y_{ij} are independently distributed as a mixture of two normal distributions with mean μ_{i+} and μ_{i-} respectively and common variance σ^2 (McLachlan and Peel, 2000):

$$\varphi(y_{ij}|\mu_{i+}, \sigma^2)^\gamma \varphi(y_{ij}|\mu_{i-}, \sigma^2)^{1-\gamma} \; i = T, C \; ; \; j = 1, \ldots, n_i, \qquad (13.3)$$

where $\varphi(.|.)$ denotes the density of a normal variable.

However, γ is an unknown positive predicted value which is usually estimated from the data. Therefore, the data obtained from the targeted clinical trials are incomplete because the true status of the molecular target of the patients is missing. The EM algorithm is a one of the methods for obtaining the maximum likelihood estimators (MLE) of the parameters for an underlying distribution from a given data set when the data is incomplete or has missing values. On the other hand, the diagnostic device for detection of molecular targets has been validated in diagnostic effectiveness trials for its diagnostic accuracy. Therefore, the estimates of the positive predictive value for the diagnostic device can be obtained from the previously conducted diagnostic effectiveness trials. As a result, we can apply the EM algorithm to estimate the treatment effect for the patients truly with the molecular target by incorporating the estimates of the positive predictive value of the device obtained from the diagnostic effectiveness trials as the initial values.

For each patient, we have a pair of variables (Y_{ij}, X_{ij}), where Y_{ij} is the observed primary efficacy endpoint of patient j in treatment i and X_{ij} is the latent variable indicating the true status of the molecular target of patient j in treatment i; $j = 1, \ldots, n_i$, $i = T, C$. In other words, X_{ij} is an indicator variable with value of 1 for the patients truly with the molecular target and with a value of 0 for the patients truly without the target. In addition, X_{ij} are assumed i.i.d. Bernoulli random variables with probability γ for the molecular target. Let $\Psi = (\gamma, \mu_{T+}, \mu_{T-}, \mu_{C+}, \mu_{C-}, \sigma^2)'$ be the vector containing all unknown parameters and $\mathbf{y}_{obs} = (y_{T1}, \ldots, y_{Tn_T}, y_{C1}, \ldots, y_{Cn_C})'$ be the vector of the observed primary efficacy endpoints from the target clinical trials. It follows that the complete-data log-likelihood function is given by

$$
\log L_c(\Psi) = \sum_{j=1}^{n_T} x_{Tj} \left[\log \gamma + \log \varphi(y_{Tj} | \mu_{T+}, \sigma^2) \right]
$$

$$
+ \sum_{j=1}^{n_T} (1 - x_{Tj}) \left[\log(1 - \gamma) + \log \varphi(y_{Tj} | \mu_{T-}, \sigma^2) \right]
$$

$$
+ \sum_{j=1}^{n_C} x_{Cj} \left[\log \gamma + \log \varphi(y_{Cj} | \mu_{C+}, \sigma^2) \right]
$$

$$
+ \sum_{j=1}^{n_C} (1 - x_{Cj}) \left[\log(1 - \gamma) + \log \varphi(y_{Cj} | \mu_{C-}, \sigma^2) \right]. \quad (13.4)
$$

Furthermore, from the previous diagnostic effectiveness trials, an estimate of the positive predictive value of the device is known. Therefore, at the initial step of the EM algorithm for estimation the treatment effects in the patients truly with the molecular target, the observed latent variable X_{ij} are generated as i.i.d. Bernoulli random variables with the positive predicted value γ estimated by that obtained from the diagnostic effectiveness trial. The procedures for implementation of the EM algorithm in conjunction with the bootstrap procedure for inference of θ in the patient population truly with the molecular target are briefly described below.

At the $(k + 1)st$ iteration, the E-step requires the calculation of the conditional expectation of the complete-data log-likelihood $L_c(\Psi)$, given the observed data $\mathbf{y}_{obs}$, using currently fitting $\hat{\Psi}^{(k)}$ for Ψ.

$$
Q(\Psi; \hat{\Psi}^{(k)}) = E_{\Psi(k)} \left\{ \log L_c(\Psi) | \mathbf{y}_{obs} \right\}
$$

Since $\log L_c(\Psi)$ is a linear function of the unobservable component labeled variables x_{ij}, the E-step is calculated by replacing x_{ij}, by its conditional expectation given y_{ij}, using $\hat{\Psi}^{(k)}$ for Ψ. That is, x_{ij} is replaced by

$$
\begin{aligned}
\hat{x}_{ij}^{(k)} &= E_{\Psi(k)}\{x_{ij}|y_{ij}\} \\
&= \frac{\widehat{\gamma}_i^{(k)}\varphi(y_{ij}|\widehat{\mu}_{i+}^{(k)},(\widehat{\sigma}_i^2)^{(k)})}{\widehat{\gamma}_i^{(k)}\varphi(y_{ij}|\widehat{\mu}_{i+}^{(k)},(\widehat{\sigma}_i^2)^{(k)}) + (1-\widehat{\gamma}_i^{(k)})\varphi(y_{ij}|\widehat{\mu}_{i-}^{(k)},(\widehat{\sigma}_i^2)^{(k)})}, \quad i = T,C,
\end{aligned}
$$

which is the estimate of the posterior probability of the observation y_{ij} with molecular target after the kth iteration. The M-step requires the computation of $\widehat{\gamma}_i^{(k+1)}, \hat{\mu}_{i+}^{(k+1)}, \hat{\mu}_{i-}^{(k+1)}$, and $(\hat{\sigma}_i^2)^{(k+1)}; i = T,C$, by maximizing $\log L_c(\Psi)$. It is equivalent to computing the sample proportion, the weighted sample mean, and sample variance with the weight x_{ij}. Since $\log L_c(\Psi)$ is linear in the x_{ij}, it follows that x_{ij} are replaced by their conditional expectations $\hat{x}_{ij}^{(k)}$. On the $(k+1)th$ iteration, the intent is to choose the value of Ψ, say $\hat{\Psi}^{(k+1)}$, that maximizes $Q(\Psi; \hat{\Psi}^{(k)})$. It follows that on the M-step of the $(k+1)st$ iteration, the current fit for the positive predicted value of test drug group and control group is given by

$$
\widehat{\gamma}_i^{(k+1)} = \frac{\sum_{j=1}^{n_i} \hat{x}_{ij}^{(k)}}{n_i}, \quad i = T,C.
$$

Under the assumption that $n_T = n_C$, it follows that the overall positive predicted value is estimated by

$$
\widehat{\gamma}^{(k+1)} = \left(\widehat{\gamma}_T^{(k+1)} + \widehat{\gamma}_C^{(k+1)}\right)\big/2.
$$

The means of the molecularly target test drug and control can then be estimated respectively as

$$
\hat{\mu}_{T+}^{(k+1)} = \sum_{j=1}^{n_T} \hat{x}_{Tj}^{(k)} y_{Tj}\bigg/ \sum_{j=1}^{n_T} \hat{x}_{Tj}^{(k)}, \quad \hat{\mu}_{T-}^{(k+1)} = \sum_{j=1}^{n_T} (1-\hat{x}_{Tj}^{(k)}) y_{Tj}\bigg/ \sum_{j=1}^{n_T} (1-\hat{x}_{Tj}^{(k)}),
$$

$$
\hat{\mu}_{C+}^{(k+1)} = \sum_{j=1}^{n_C} \hat{x}_{Cj}^{(k)} y_{Cj}\bigg/ \sum_{j=1}^{n_C} \hat{x}_{Cj}^{(k)}, \text{ and } \hat{\mu}_{C-}^{(k+1)} = \sum_{j=1}^{n_C} (1-\hat{x}_{Cj}^{(k)}) y_{Cj}\bigg/ \sum_{j=1}^{n_C} (1-\hat{x}_{Cj}^{(k)}),
$$

with unbiased estimators for the variances of molecularly targeted drug and control given respectively by

$$
(\hat{\sigma}_T^2)^{(k+1)} = \left(\sum_{j=1}^{n} \hat{x}_{Tj}^{(k)}(y_{Tj} - \hat{\mu}_{T+}^{(k)})^2 + \sum_{j=1}^{n}(1-\hat{x}_{Tj}^{(k)})(y_{Tj} - \hat{\mu}_{T-}^{(k)})^2\right)\big/(n_T - 2),
$$

and

$$
(\hat{\sigma}_C^2)^{(k+1)} = \left(\sum_{j=1}^{n} \hat{x}_{Cj}^{(k)}(y_{Cj} - \hat{\mu}_{C+}^{(k)})^2 + \sum_{j=1}^{n}(1-\hat{x}_{Cj}^{(k)})(y_{Cj} - \hat{\mu}_{C-}^{(k)})^2\right)\big/(n_C - 2).
$$

It follows that an unbiased estimate for the pooled variance is given as

$$(\hat{\sigma}^2)^{(k+1)} = \frac{[(n_T - 2) \times (\hat{\sigma}_T^2)^{(k+1)} + (n_C - 2) \times (\hat{\sigma}_C^2)^{(k+1)}]}{(n_T + n_C - 4)}.$$

Therefore, the estimator for the treatment effects in the patients with the molecular target θ obtained from the EM algorithm is given as $\hat{\theta} = \hat{\mu}_{T+} - \hat{\mu}_{C+}$.

Liu, Lin and Chow (2009) proposed to apply the parametric bootstrap method to estimate the standard error of $\hat{\theta}$.

Step 1: Choose a large bootstrap sample size, say B = 1000. For $1 \le b \le B$, generate the bootstrap sample y_{obs}^b according to the probability model in (3). The parameters in (3) for generating bootstrap samples y_{obs}^b are substituted by the estimators obtained from the EM algorithm based on the original observations of primary efficacy endpoints from the target clinical trials.

Step 2: The EM algorithm is applied to the bootstrap sample y_{obs}^b to obtain estimates $\widehat{\theta}_b^*$, b = 1,...,B.

Step 3: An estimator for the variance of $\hat{\theta}$ by the parametric bootstrap procedure is given as $S_B^2 = \sum_{b=1}^{B} (\hat{\theta}_b^* - \bar{\theta}^*)^2/(B - 1)$, where $\bar{\theta}^* = \sum_{b=1}^{B} \hat{\theta}_b^*/B$.

Let $\hat{\theta}$ be the estimator for the treatment effects in the patients truly with the molecular target obtained from the EM algorithm. Nityasuddhi and Böhning (2003) show that the estimator obtained under the EM algorithm is asymptotic unbiased. Let S_B^2 denote the estimator of the variance of $\hat{\theta}$ obtained by the bootstrap procedure. It follows that the null hypothesis is rejected and the efficacy of the molecular targeted test drug is different from that of the control in the patient population truly with the molecular target at the α level if

$$t = \left| \hat{\theta}/\sqrt{S_B^2} \right| \ge z_{\alpha/2}, \tag{13.5}$$

where $z_{\alpha/2}$ is the $\alpha/2$ upper percentile of a standard normal distribution. Thus, the corresponding $(1 - \alpha)100\%$ asymptotic confidence interval for $\theta = \mu_{T+} - \mu_{C+}$ can be constructed as $\hat{\theta} \pm z_{1-\alpha/2}\sqrt{S_B^2}$ (see, e.g., Basford et al., 1997). It should be noted that although the assumption that $\mu_{T+} - \mu_{C+} > \mu_{T-} - \mu_{C-}$ is one of the reasons for developing the targeted treatment, this assumption is not used in the EM algorithm for estimation of θ. Hence, the inference for θ by the proposed procedure is not biased in favor of the targeted treatment.

13.3.3 Simulation results

Liu, Lin and Chow (2009) conducted a simulation study to evaluate the finite sample performance of the proposed method of EM algorithm. In the simulation, μ_{T-}, μ_{C+}, and μ_{C-} are assumed equal and set to be a generic value of 100. To investigate the impact of the positive predictive value, sample size, difference in means, and variability, Liu, Lin and Chow (2009) considered the following specifications of parameters: (i) the positive predicted values are set to be 0.5, 0.7, 0.8, and 0.9 which reflect a range of low, median, and high positive predicted value, and (ii) the range of the standard deviation σ is set as 20, 40, or 60. To investigate the finite sample properties, the sample sizes are set as 50, 100, and 200 per group. The mean differences are chosen a fraction of the standard deviation, from 10% to 60% by 10%; and 75% and 100%. In addition, the size of the proposed testing procedure was investigated at $\mu_{T+} = 100$. For each of 288 combinations, 5,000 random samples were generated and the number of the bootstrap samples was set to be 1,000. The simulation results indicate that the absolute relative bias of the estimator for θ by the current method ranges from 10% to more than 50% and increases as the positive predictive value decreases. On the other hand, most of absolute relative bias of the estimator for θ obtained by the EM algorithm are smaller than 0.05% although it can as high as 10% for few combinations when the difference in means is 2. The variability has little impact on the bias of both methods. However, for the EM procedure, the relative bias tends to decrease as the sample size increases. The bias of the current method with consideration of the true status of molecular target can be as high as 50% when the positive predictive value is low. Consequently, the empirical coverage probabilities of the corresponding 95% confidence interval can be as low as only 0.28% when the positive predictive value is 50%, mean difference is 20, standard deviation is 20, and n is 200. The coverage probability of the 95% confidence interval by the current method is an increasing function of the positive predictive value. On the other hand, only 36 of the 288 coverage probabilities (12.5%) of the 95% confidence intervals by the current method exceed 0.9449 and 24 of them occurred when the positive predictive value is 0.9. On the contrary, only 14.6% of the 288 coverage probabilities of the 95% confidence intervals by the EM method are below 0.9449. However, 277 of the 288 coverage probability of the 95% confidence interval constructed by the EM algorithm are above 0.94. No coverage probability of the EM method is below 0.91. Therefore, the proposed procedures for estimation of the treatment effects in the patients population with the molecular target by the EM algorithm is not only unbiased but also provide sufficient coverage probability.

13.4   Other Study Designs and Models

As indicated above, Liu, Lin, and Chow (2009) proposed statistical methods for assessment of the treatment effect for patients with positive diagnosed results under the enrichment design described in Figure 13.3.2. Their methods suffer from the lack information regarding the proportion of subjects who truly have molecular targets in the patient population and the unknown positive predicted value. Consequently, the conclusion drawn from the collected data may be biased and misleading.

13.4.1 FDA recommended study designs

In addition to the study designs as given in Figure 13.1 and Figure 13.2, the 2005 FDA concept paper also recommended the following study design for different study objectives.

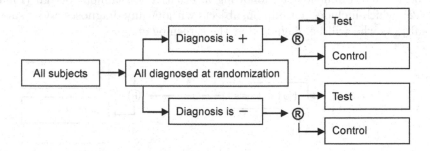

Figure 13.4.1: Enrichment design for patients with and without molecular targets

This study design allows the evaluation of the treatment effect within subpopulations, i.e., the subpopulation of patients with positive or negative results. Similar to Table 13.3.1 for the study design given in Figure 13.3.2, the expected values of Y_{ij} by treatment and diagnostic result of the molecular targets are summarized in Table 13.4.1.

Table 13.4.1: Population Means by Treatment and Diagnosis

Positive diagnosis	True target condition	Indicator of diagnostic	Test group	Control group	Difference
+	+	γ_1	μ_{T++}	μ_{C++}	$\mu_{T++} - \mu_{C++}$
	−	$1 - \gamma_1$	μ_{T+-}	μ_{C+-}	$\mu_{T+-} - \mu_{C+-}$
−	+	γ_2	μ_{T-+}	μ_{C-+}	$\mu_{T-+} - \mu_{C-+}$
	−	$1 - \gamma_2$	μ_{T--}	μ_{C--}	$\mu_{T--} - \mu_{C--}$

Note that: 1. γ_i is the positive predicted value, i=1 (positive diagnosis) and i=2 (negative diagnosis).

2. μ_{ijk} is the mean for subjects in the ith group with kth true target status but with jth diagnosed result.

As a result, it may of interest in estimating the following treatment effects:

$$\theta_1 = \gamma_1(\mu_{T++} - \mu_{C++}) + (1 - \gamma_1)(\mu_{T+-} - \mu_{C+-});$$
$$\theta_2 = \gamma_2(\mu_{T-+} - \mu_{C-+}) + (1 - \gamma_2)(\mu_{T--} - \mu_{C--});$$
$$\theta_3 = \delta\gamma_1(\mu_{T++} - \mu_{C++}) + (1 - \delta)\gamma_2(\mu_{T-+} - \mu_{C-+});$$
$$\theta_4 = \delta\gamma_1(\mu_{T+-} - \mu_{C+-}) + (1 - \delta)\gamma_1(\mu_{T--} - \mu_{C--});$$
$$\theta_5 = \delta[\gamma_1(\mu_{T+-} - \mu_{C+-}) + (1 - \gamma_1)(\mu_{T+-} - \mu_{C+-})]$$
$$+(1 - \delta)[\gamma_2(\mu_{T-+} - \mu_{C-+}) + (1 - \gamma_2)(\mu_{T--} - \mu_{C--})],$$

where δ is the proportion of subjects with positive molecular targets. Following a similar idea as described in the previous section,, estimates of $\theta_1 - \theta_5$ can be obtained. In other words, estimates of θ_1 and θ_2 can be obtained based on data collected from the subpopulations of subjects with and without positive diagnoses who truly have the molecular target of interest. Similarly, the combined treatment effect θ_5 can be assessed. These estimates, however, depend upon both $\gamma_i, i = 1, 2$ and δ. To obtain some information regarding $\gamma_i, i = 1, 2$ and δ, the FDA recommends the following alternative enrichment design (Figure 13.4.2), which includes a group of subjects without any diagnoses and a subset of subjects who will be diagnosed at the screening stage.

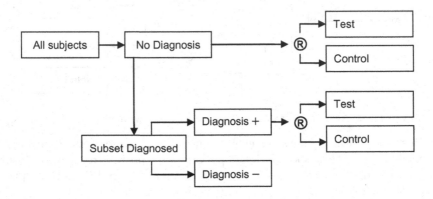

Figure 13.4.2: Alternative enrichment design for target clinical trials.

13.4.2   Statistical methods

As indicated earlier, the method proposed by Liu, Lin and Chow (2009) suffers from the lack of information regarding the uncertainty in accuracy of the diagnostic device. As an alternative, we propose considering a Bayesian approach to incorporate the uncertainty in accuracy and reliability of the diagnostic device for the molecular target into the inference of treatment effects of the targeted drug. For each patient, we have a pair of variables (y_{ij}, x_{ij}), where y_{ij} is the observed primary efficacy endpoint of patient j in treatment I and x_{ij} is the latent variable indicating the true status of the molecular target of patient j in treatment I; $j = 1, \ldots, n_i, i = T, C$. In other words, x_{ij} is an indicator variable with value of 1 for patients with the molecular target and with a value of 0 for patients without the target. x_{ij} are assumed i.i.d. Bernoulli random variables with probability of the molecular target being γ. Thus $x_{ij} = 1$ if $y_{ij} \sim N(\mu_{i+}, \sigma^2)$ and $x_{ij} = 0$ if $y_{ij} \sim N(\mu_{i-}, \sigma^2)$, i=T,C; j=1,..., n_i. The likelihood function is given by

$$L(\Psi|Y_{obs}, x_{ij}) = \prod_{j, x_{Tj}=1} \gamma\varphi(y_{Tj}|\mu_{T+}, \sigma^2) \times \prod_{j, x_{Tj}=0} (1 - \gamma)\varphi(y_{Tj}|\mu_{T-}, \sigma^2)$$
$$\times \prod_{j, x_{Cj}=1} \gamma\varphi(y_{Cj}|\mu_{C+}, \sigma^2) \times \prod_{j, x_{Cj}=0} (1 - \gamma)\varphi(y_{Cj}|\mu_{C-}, \sigma^2),$$

where i=T,C; $j = 1, \ldots, n_i$ and $\varphi(.|.)$ denotes the density of a normal variable. For Bayesian approach, a beta distribution can be employed as the prior distribution for γ, while normal prior distributions can be used for μ_{i+} and μ_{i-}. In addition, a gamma distribution can be used as a prior for σ^{-2}. Under the assumptions of these prior distributions, the conditional posterior distributions of $\gamma, \mu_{i+}, \mu_{i-}, \sigma^{-2}$ can be derived. In other words, assuming that

$$f(\gamma) \sim Beta(\alpha_\gamma, \beta_\gamma),$$
$$f(\mu_{i+}) \sim N(\lambda_{i+}, \sigma_0^2),$$
$$f(\mu_{i-}) \sim N(\lambda_{i-}, \sigma_0^2),$$

and

$$f(\sigma^{-2}) \sim Gamma(\alpha_g, \beta_g),$$

where μ_{i+}, μ_{i-}, and γ are assumed to be independent and $\alpha_\gamma, \beta_\gamma, \alpha_g, \beta_g, \lambda_{i+}, \lambda_{i-}$ and σ_0^2 are assumed to be known. Thus, the conditional posterior distribution of x_{ij} is given by

$$f(x_{ij}|\gamma, \mu_{i+}, \mu_{i-}, Y_{obs}) \sim Bernoulli \left(\frac{\gamma \varphi(y_{ij}|\mu_{i+}, \sigma_0^2)}{\gamma \varphi(y_{ij}|\mu_{i+}, \sigma_0^2) + (1 - \gamma) \varphi(y_{ij}|\mu_{i-}, \sigma_0^2)} \right),$$

where

$$E_\Psi[x_{ij}|\gamma, \mu_{i+}, \mu_{i-}, Y_{obs}] = \frac{\gamma \varphi(y_{ij}|\mu_{i+}, \sigma^2)}{\gamma \varphi(y_{ij}|\mu_{i+}, \sigma^2) + (1 - \gamma) \varphi(y_{ij}|\mu_{i-}, \sigma^2)}, i = T, C; \ j = 1, \ldots,$$

n_i in the EM algorithm. The joint distribution of $\gamma, \mu_{i+}, \mu_{i-}$ and σ^2 is given by

$$f(\gamma, \mu_{i+}, \mu_{i-}, \sigma^2|Y_{obs}, x_{ij})$$
$$= \prod_{j, x_{Tj}=1} \varphi(y_{Tj}|\mu_{T+}, \sigma^2) \times \prod_{j, x_{Tj}=0} \varphi(y_{Tj}|\mu_{T-}, \sigma^2)$$
$$\times \prod_{j, x_{Cj}=1} \varphi(y_{Cj}|\mu_{C+}, \sigma^2) \times \prod_{j, x_{Cj}=0} \varphi(y_{Cj}|\mu_{C-}, \sigma^2)$$
$$\times \varphi(\mu_{T+}|\lambda_{T+}, \sigma_0^2) \times \varphi(\mu_{T-}|\lambda_{T-}, \sigma_0^2)$$
$$\times \varphi(\mu_{C+}|\lambda_{C+}, \sigma_0^2) \times \varphi(\mu_{C-}|\lambda_{C-}, \sigma_0^2)$$
$$\times \frac{\Gamma(\alpha_\gamma + \beta_\gamma)}{\Gamma(\alpha_\gamma)\Gamma(\beta_\gamma)} (\gamma)^{\sum_{j=1}^{n_T} x_{Tj} + \sum_{j=1}^{n_C} x_{Cj} + \alpha_\gamma - 1} (1 - \gamma)^{\sum_{j=1}^{n_T}(1-x_{Tj}) + \sum_{j=1}^{n_C}(1-x_{Cj}) + \beta_\gamma - 1}.$$

Thus, the conditional posterior distribution of $\gamma, \mu_{i+}, \mu_{i-}$, and σ^{-2} can be obtained as follows:

$$f(\gamma|\mu_{i+}, \mu_{i-}, \sigma^{-2}, Y_{obs}, x_{ij})$$
$$\sim Beta \left(\sum_{j=1}^{n_T} x_{Tj} + \sum_{j=1}^{n_C} x_{Cj} + \alpha_\gamma, \sum_{j=1}^{n_T}(1 - x_{Tj}) + \sum_{j=1}^{n_C}(1 - x_{Cj}) + \beta_\gamma \right),$$

$$f(\mu_{i+}|\gamma, \mu_{i-}, \sigma^{-2}, Y_{obs}, x_{ij}) \sim N \left(\frac{\sigma^{-2} \sum_{j=1}^{n_i} x_{ij} y_{ij} + \sigma_0^{-2} \lambda_{i+}}{\sigma^{-2} \sum_{j=1}^{n_i} x_{ij} + \sigma_0^{-2}}, \frac{1}{\sigma^{-2} \sum_{j=1}^{n_i} x_{ij} + \sigma_0^{-2}} \right),$$

$$f(\mu_{i-}|\gamma, \mu_{i+}, \sigma^{-2}, Y_{obs}, x_{ij})$$

$$\sim N\left(\frac{\sigma^{-2}\sum_{j=1}^{n_i}(1-x_{ij})y_{ij} + \sigma_0^{-2}\lambda_{i-}}{\sigma^{-2}\sum_{j=1}^{n_i}(1-x_{ij}) + \sigma_0^{-2}}, \frac{1}{\sigma^{-2}\sum_{j=1}^{n_i}(1-x_{ij}) + \sigma_0^{-2}}\right),$$

$$f(\sigma^{-2}|\gamma, \mu_{i+}, \mu_{i-}, Y_{obs}, x_{ij}) \sim Gamma\left(\frac{n_T + n_C}{2}\right.$$

$$\left. +\sigma_g, \frac{1}{2}\sum_{i=T,C}\left[\sum_{j=1}^{n_i}x_{ij}(y_{ij}-\mu_{i+})^2 + \sum_{j=1}^{n_i}(1-x_{ij})(y_{ij}-\mu_{i-})^2\right] + \beta_g\right),$$

respectively. Consequently, the conditional posterior distribution of $\theta = \mu_{T+} - \mu_{C+}$ can be obtained as follows:

$$f(\hat{\theta}|\gamma, \mu_{i+}, \mu_{i-}, \sigma^2, Y_{obs}, x_{ij}) \sim N\left(\frac{\sigma^{-2}\sum_{j=1}^{n_T}x_{Tj}y_{Tj} + \sigma_0^{-2}\lambda_{T+}}{\sigma^{-2}\sum_{j=1}^{n_T}x_{Tj} + \sigma_0^{-2}}\right.$$

$$\left. +\frac{\sigma^{-2}\sum_{j=1}^{n_C}x_{Cj}y_{Cj} + \sigma_0^{-2}\lambda_{C+}}{\sigma^{-2}\sum_{j=1}^{n_C}x_{Cj} + \sigma_0^{-2}}, \frac{1}{\sigma^{-2}\sum_{j=1}^{n_T}x_{Tj} + \sigma_0^{-2}} + \frac{1}{\sigma^{-2}\sum_{j=1}^{n_C}x_{Cj} + \sigma_0^{-2}}\right).$$

As a result, statistical inference for $\theta = \mu_{T+} - \mu_{C+}$ can be obtained following similar ideas, statistical inferences for the treatment effects (θ_1 through θ_5 as described in Section 13.4.1) can be derived. Note that different priors for γ, μ_{i+}, μ_{i-}, and σ^{-2} may be applied depending upon disease targets across different therapeutic areas. However, different prior assumptions will result in different statistical inference for assessment of treatment effect under study.

13.5   Concluding Remarks

As indicated, in practice, there exists no perfect diagnostic test (i.e., with 100% positive predicted value) for identifying molecular targets. Thus, validated diagnostic devices are necessarily developed in target clinical trials utilizing an enrichment process. Valid statistical methods under the FDA recommended enrichment study designs are necessarily developed for testing hypotheses of equality, superiority/non-inferiority, and equivalence with continuous study endpoints, binary responses, and time-to-event data. A Bayesian approach in conjunction with the EM algorithm or bootstrap technique under the framework of the enrichment process may be useful.

Under the FDA recommended study designs, future research of particular interest to clinicians and biostatisticians include, but are not limited to, (i) the study of the impact of sensitivity and specificity (or misclassification) of the diagnostic device on the derived statistical inference, (ii) the development of valid statistical inferences on treatment effects such as θ_1 through θ_5 under various study designs for target clinical trials as recommended by FDA, (iii) a comparison of the study designs in terms of relative efficiency for evaluation of the effect of the test treatment under investigation, and (iv) the derivation of formulas or procedures for sample size calculation based on the derived valid statistical methods.

Chapter 14

Sample Size and Power Estimation

In clinical trials, power analysis for sample size calculation is often performed under a valid study design for achieving the intended study objectives with a desired power at a pre-specified level of significance. As discussed in previous chapters, most adaptive trial designs are considered less well-understood designs at which valid statistical methods for assessment of treatment effects might have not yet been developed. In this case, explicit formulas for sample size calculation and power estimation are not trackable. However, required sample size for achieving the desired power can still be obtained through clinical trial simulation. In this chapter, we will develop a set of algorithms for K-stage group sequential design (which is considered a well-understood adaptive trial design) based on well-established statistical methods such as the method of the sum of p-values (MSP), the method of the product of p-values (MPP), and the method of inverse-normal p-valuse (MINP). For other less well-understood adaptive designs, sample size required for achieving the desired power at a pre-specified level of significance can be obtained through clinical trial simulation under some framework with clearly specified model and parameter assumptions.

In the next section, a general framework for clinical trial simulation for sample size calculation is briefly described. Also included in this section is stopping rules for early futility or efficacy that are commonly considered in clinical trials. Algorithms for sample size calculation and power estimation for K-stage group sequential design based on the methods of sum of p-values, product of p-values, and inverse-normal p-values are given in Sections 14.3, 14.4., and 14.5, respectively. Section 14.6 describes the algorithm for sample size re-estimation in K-stage group sequential design. A brief summary is provided in the last section of this chapter.

14.1   Framework and Model/Parameter Assumptions

14.1.1   Simulation framework

The framework of clinical trial simulation for sample size calculation and power estimation consists of trial design, study objectives (hypotheses), model/ parameter assumptions, and statistical tests. For the trial design, some critical design characteristics such as (i) a parallel design or a crossover design, (ii) a balanced or unbalanced design, (iii) the number of treatment groups, and (iv) adaptations need to be clearly specified. Under the trial design, hypotheses for testing for equality, superiority, or non-inferiority/equivalence can then be formulated for achieving the study objectives. A valid model with parameters assumptions is necessarily implemented to generate virtual patients for extrapolating (or predicting) clinical outcomes. We can then evaluate the performance of the test treatment through the study of properties of the statistical tests derived under the null hypothesis (for the overall type I error rate) and the alternative hypothesis (for the power of the statistical test).

More specifically, we begin a clinical trial simulation by choosing a statistical model under a valid trial design with various assumptions according to the trial setting. We then simulate the trial by creating virtual patients and generating the clinical outcomes for each virtual patient based on the model specifications under the null hypothesis of H_0 for a large number of times (say m times). For each simulation run, we calculate the test statistic. The m test statistic values constitute a distribution of the test statistic numerically. Similarly, we repeat the process to simulate the trial under the alternative hypothesis of H_a m times. The m test statistic values obtained represent the distribution of the test statistic under the alternative hypothesis. These two distributions can be used to determine the critical region for a given α level of significance, p-value for a given data, and the corresponding power for the given critical region. To provide a better understanding, Figure 14.1.1 provides the flowchart of the general simulation framework.

Note that the computer simulation starts with generating data under the null hypothesis. The data are often generated from a simple distribution such as a normal distribution for continuous variables, a binary distribution for discrete variables, and an exponential distribution for time-to-event data. The generation of simulated data occurs only once per simulation run. The adaptive algorithm is usually applied later for the case of a sequential trial design or an N-adjustable design (sample size re-estimation). In some cases such as response-adaptive randomization, the randomization may have to be generated step-by-step. It should be noted that under the above mentioned framework, other operating characteristics such as stopping boundary, conditional probability can also be obtained.

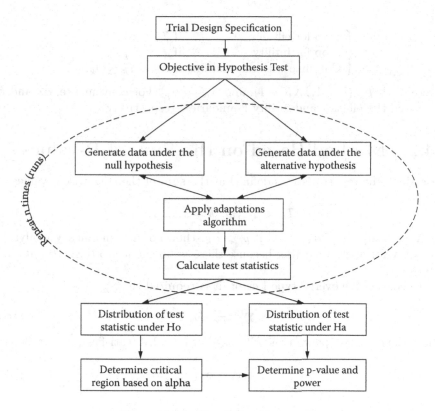

Figure 14.1.1: Simulation Framework

14.1.2 Stopping rules

Consider a clinical trial with K-stage design for evaluation of the efficacy of a test treatment under investigation. Suppose at each stage, a hypothesis test is to be performed followed by some actions that depend on the analysis results from previous stages. In clinical trials, such actions could be an early futility or an efficacy stopping, sample size re-estimation, modification of randomization, or other adaptations. The objective of the trial (i.e., a hypothesis testing for efficacy of the test treatment under investigation) can be formulated as follows:

$$H_0 \text{ vs. } H_a, \tag{14.1}$$

where H_0 is the null hypothesis of no treatment effect, while H_a is the alternative of treatment effect. Thus, we wish to reject H_0 and conclude H_a for efficacy. Generally, the test statistics T_k at the kth stage is a function $\eta(p_1, p_2, ..., p_k)$, where p_i is the one-sided p-value from the ith stage subsample and $\eta(p_1, p_2, ..., p_k)$ is strictly increasing function of all p_i ($i = 1, 2, ...k$). Thus, commonly considered stopping rules are given by

$$\begin{cases} \text{Stop for efficacy} & \text{if } T_k \le \alpha_k, \\ \text{Stop for futility} & \text{if } T_k > \beta_k, \\ \text{Continue with adaptations if } \alpha_k < T_k \le \beta_k, \end{cases} \qquad (14.2)$$

where $\alpha_k < \beta_k$ $(k = 1, ..., K - 1)$, and $\alpha_K = \beta_K$. For convenience, α_k and β_k are called the efficacy and futility boundaries, respectively.

14.2 Method Based on the Sum of P-values

For MSP, the test statistic is defined as the sum of the stagewise p-values:

$$T_k = \Sigma_{i=1}^k p_i, \ \ k = 1, ..., K. \qquad (14.3)$$

If we setup $\alpha_k > \alpha_{k-1}$ and if $p_i > \alpha_k$, then no interim efficacy analysis is necessary for stage $i + 1$ to k because there is no chance to reject H_0 at these stages.

To control the overall type I error, it is required that

$$\Sigma_{i=1}^K \pi_i = \alpha, \qquad (14.4)$$

where the error π_i spent at the kth stage $(k = 1, 2, 3)$ satisfies (Chang, 2007)

$$\pi_1 = \alpha_1, \qquad (14.5)$$

$$\pi_2 = \frac{1}{2} (\alpha_2 - \alpha_1)^2, \qquad (14.6)$$

$$\pi_3 = \alpha_1 \alpha_2 \alpha_3 + \frac{1}{3}\alpha_2^3 + \frac{1}{6}\alpha_3^3 - \frac{1}{2}\alpha_1\alpha_2^2 - \frac{1}{2}\alpha_1\alpha_3^2 - \frac{1}{2}\alpha_2^2\alpha_3. \qquad (14.7)$$

The error spent π_i can be predetermined or specified as error spending function $\pi_k = f(k)$. The stopping boundary can be solved through numerical iterations. Specifically, (i) determine π_i $(i = 1, 2, ..., K)$; (ii) from $\pi_1 = \alpha_1$, solve for α_1; from $\pi_2 = \frac{1}{2}(\alpha_2 - \alpha_1)^2$, obtain α_2; from $\pi_K = \pi_K(\alpha_1, ..., \alpha_{K-1})$, obtain α_K.

To obtain power for group sequential design using MSP, Monte Carlo simulation can be used. Algorithm 14.2.1 is developed for this purpose. To obtain efficacy stopping boundaries, one can let $\delta = 0$, then the power from the simulation output is numerically equal to α. Using trial-and-error method, to adjust $\{\alpha_i\}$ until the output power $= \alpha$. The final set of $\{\alpha_i\}$ is the efficacy stopping boundary.

Algorithm 14.2.1: K-Stage Group Sequential with MSP (large n)

Objective: return power for a two-group K-stage adaptive design.
Note: the mean difference has distribution $N(\delta, 2\sigma^2)$.

Input treatment difference δ and common σ, one-sided α, $\delta_{\min}$, stopping boundaries $\{\alpha_i\}$ and $\{\beta_i\}$, stagewise sample size $\{n_i\}$, number of stages K, nRuns.
   power:= 0
  For $iRun := 1$ **To** nRuns
    $T := 0$
    For $i := 1$ **To** K
      Generate $\hat{\delta}_i$ from $N\left(\delta, 2\sigma^2\right)$
      $p_i := 1 - \Phi\left(\hat{\delta}_i\sqrt{n_i/2}/\sigma\right)$
      $T := T + p_i$
      If $T > \beta_i$ **Then Exitfor**
      If $T \le \alpha_i$ **Then** power := power+1/nRuns
    Endfor
  Endfor
  Return power

§

14.3   Method Based on Product of P-values

The method based on product of p-values is referred to as MPP. The test statistic in this method is based on the product (Fisher's combination) of the stagewise p-values from the subsamples (Bauer & Köhne, 1994; Bauer & Röhmel 1995), defined as

$$T_k = \Pi_{i=1}^k p_i, \ k = 1, ..., K. \tag{14.8}$$

For non-futility boundary, choose $\beta_1 = 1$. It is interesting to know that when $p_1 < \alpha_2$, there is no point in continuing the trial because $p_1 p_2 < p_1 < \alpha_2$ and efficacy should be claimed. Therefore it is suggested that we should choose $\beta_1 > \alpha_2$ and $\alpha_1 > \alpha_2$. In general, if $p_k \le \max(a_k, ...\alpha_n)$, stop the trial. In other words, α_k should monotonically decrease in k. The relationships between error-spent π_i and stopping boundary α_i at the ith stage are given up to three stages:

$$\pi_1 = \alpha_1, \tag{14.9}$$

$$\pi_2 = \alpha_2 \ln \frac{1}{\alpha_1}, \tag{14.10}$$

$$\pi_3 = \alpha_3 \left(\ln \alpha_2 - \frac{1}{2}\ln \alpha_1\right)\ln \alpha_1. \tag{14.11}$$

Algorithm 14.3.1 is a Monte Carlo simulation algorithm for K-stage group sequential design. To obtain efficacy stopping boundaries, one can let $\delta = 0$, then the power from the simulation output is numerically equal to α. Using trial-and-error method, to adjust $\{\alpha_i\}$ until the output power $= \alpha$. Then the final set of $\{\alpha_i\}$ is the efficacy stopping boundary.

Algorithm 14.3.1: K-Stage Group Sequential with MPP (large n)

Objective: Return power for atwo-group K-stage adaptive design.
Note: the mean difference has distribution $N(\delta, 2\sigma^2)$.
Input treatment difference δ and common σ, one-sided α, $\delta_{\min}$, stopping boundaries $\{\alpha_i\}$ and $\{\beta_i\}$, stagewise sample size $\{n_i\}$, number of stages K, nRuns.

    power:= 0
  For $iRun := 1$ **To** nRuns
     $T := 1$
     For $i := 1$ **To** K
        Generate $\hat{\delta}_i$ from $N\left(\delta, 2\sigma^2\right)$
        $p_i = 1 - \Phi\left(\hat{\delta}_i \sqrt{n_i/2}/\sigma\right)$
        $T := T \cdot p_i$
        If $T > \beta_i$ **Then Exitfor**
        If $T \leq \alpha_i$ **Then** power := power+1/nRuns
     Endfor
  Endfor
  Return power

§

14.4   Method with Inverse-Normal P-values

Let z_k be the stagewise normal test statistic at the kth stage. In general, $z_i = \Phi^{-1}(1 - p_i)$, where p_i is the stagewise p-value from the ith stage subsample. The test statistic can be expressed as

$$T_k^* = \sum_{i=1}^{k} w_{ki} z_i, \tag{14.12}$$

where the prefixed weights satisfy the equality $\sum_{i=1}^{k} w_{ki}^2 = 1$ and the stagewise statistic z_i is based on the subsample for the ith stage.

Note that when w_{ki} is fixed, the standard multi-variate normal distribution of $\{T_1^*, ..., T_k^*\}$ will not change regardless of adaptations as long as z_i ($i = 1, ..., k$) has the standard normal distribution. To be consistent with the unified formations, in which the test statistic is on p-scale, we use the transformation $T_k = 1 - \Phi(T_k^*)$ such that

$$T_k = 1 - \Phi\left(\sum_{i=1}^{k} w_{ki} z_i\right), \tag{14.13}$$

where Φ = the standard normal c.d.f.

The stopping boundary and power can be obtained using Algorithm 14.4.1.

Algorithm 14.4.1: K-Stage Group Sequential with MINP (large n)

Objective: Return power for K-stage adaptive design.
Input treatment difference δ and common σ, one-sided α, $\delta_{\min}$, stopping boundaries $\{\alpha_i\}$ and $\{\beta_i\}$, stagewise sample size $\{n_i\}$, weights $\{w_{ki}\}$, number of stages K, nRuns.

    power:= 0
    For $iRun := 1$ **To** nRuns
        $T := 1$
        For $i := 1$ **To** K
            Generate $\hat{\delta}_i$ from $N\left(\delta, 2\sigma^2\right)$
            $z_i = \hat{\delta}_i \sqrt{n_i/2}/\sigma$
        Endfor
        For $k := 1$ **To** K
            $T_k^* := 0$
            For $i := 1$ **To** k
                $T_k^* := T_k^* + w_{ki} z_i$
            Endfor
            $T_k; = 1 - \Phi\left(T_k^*\right)$
            If $T_k > \beta_k$ **Then Exitfor**
            If $T_k \le \alpha_k$ **Then** power := power+1/nRuns
        Endfor
    Endfor
    Return power

§

Chang (2007) has implemented Algorithms 14.1-14.3 using SAS and R for normal, binary, and survival endpoints.

The operating characteristics such as average sample size, futility stopping probability, and efficacy stopping probabilities are important to evaluate an adaptive design. Algorithm 14.4.2 provides simulation algorithm for obtain those characteristics.

Algorithm 14.4.2: Operating Characteristics of Group Sequential Design

Objective: return power, average sample size per group (AveN), futility stopping probability (FSP_i), and efficacy stopping probability (ESP_i) for a two-group K-stage adaptive design with MSP
Note: the mean difference has distribution $N\left(\delta, 2\sigma^2\right)$.
Input treatment difference δ and common σ, one-sided α, stopping boundaries $\{\alpha_i\}$ and $\{\beta_i\}$, stagewise sample size $\{n_i\}$, number of stages K, nRuns.

    power:= 0
    For $iRun := 1$ **To** nRuns

$T := 0$
For $i := 1$ **To** K
    $FSP_i := 0$
    $ESP_i := 0$
Endfor
    For $i := 1$ **To** K
        Generate $\hat{\delta}_i$ from $N\left(\delta, 2\sigma^2\right)$
        $p_i := 1 - \Phi\left(\hat{\delta}_i\sqrt{n_i/2}/\sigma\right)$
        $T := T + p_i$
        If $T > \beta_i$ **Then**
            $FSP_i := FSP_i + 1/\text{nRuns}$
            Exitfor
        Endif
        If $T \leq \alpha_i$ **Then**
            $ESP_i := ESP_i + 1/\text{nRuns}$
            power $:=$ power$+1/\text{nRuns}$
            Exitfor
        Endif
    Endfor
Endfor
$aveN := 0$
For $i := 1$ **To** K
    $aveN := aveN + (FSP_i + ESP_i)n_i$
Endfor
Return $\{\text{power}, aveN, \{FSP_i\}, \{ESP_i\}\}$
§

14.5   Sample Size Re-estimation

The statistical method for the adjustment can be based on observed effect
size or the conditional power. For a two-stage sample size re-estimation (SSR),
the sample size for the second stage can be calculated based on the target
conditional power:

$$
\begin{cases}
\quad n_2 = \frac{2\hat{\sigma}^2}{\hat{\delta}^2}\left(z_{1-\alpha_2+p_1} - z_{1-cP}\right)^2, & \text{for MSP} \\
\quad n_2 = \frac{2\hat{\sigma}^2}{\hat{\delta}^2}\left(z_{1-\alpha_2/p_1} - z_{1-cP}\right)^2, & \text{for MPP} \quad, \\
n_2 = \frac{2\hat{\sigma}^2}{\hat{\delta}^2}\left(\frac{z_{1-\alpha_2}}{w_2} - \frac{w_1}{w_2}z_{1-p_1} - z_{1-cP}\right)^2, & \text{for MINP}
\end{cases}
\tag{14.14}
$$

where, for the purpose of calculation, $\hat{\delta}$ and $\hat{\sigma}$ are taken to be the observed
treatment effect and standard deviation at stage 1; cP is the target conditional
power.

For a general K-stage design, the sample-size rule at the kth stage can be
based on the observed treatment effect in comparison with the initial assessment:

$$n_j = \min\left(n_{j,\max}, \left(\frac{\delta}{\bar{\delta}}\right)^2 n_j^0\right), j = k, k+1, ..., K, \qquad (14.15)$$

where n_j^0 is original sample size for the jth stage, δ is the initial assessment for the treatment effect.

We now can develop algorithms for sample size re-estimation using MSP, MPP and MINP. As samples, Algorithms 14.5.1 and 14.5.2 are provided for two-stage SSR based on conditional power using MSP and MPP, respectively, and Algorithm 14.5.3 is provided for K-stage SSR using MINP. The algorithms return power as simulation outputs.

Algorithm 14.5.1: Two-Stage Sample-Size Re-estimation with MSP

Objective: Return power for two-stage adaptive design.
Input treatment difference δ and common σ, stopping boundaries $\alpha_1, \alpha_2, \beta_1$, n_1, n_2, target conditional power cP for SSR, and nRuns.
    power := 0
    For $iRun$:= 1 **To** nRuns
        Generate $\hat{\delta}_1$ from $N\left(\delta, 2\sigma^2\right)$
        $p_1 := 1 - \Phi\left(\hat{\delta}_1\sqrt{n_1/2}/\sigma\right)$
        If $p_1 > \beta_1$ **Then Exitfor**
        If $p_1 \leq \alpha_1$ **Then** power := power+1/nRuns
        If $\alpha_1 < p_1 \leq \beta_1$ **Then**
            $n_2 := \frac{2\sigma^2}{\hat{\delta}_1^2}\left(z_{1-\alpha_2+p_1} - z_{1-cP}\right)^2$
            Generate $\hat{\delta}_2$ from $N\left(\delta, 2\sigma^2\right)$
            $p_2 := 1 - \Phi\left(\hat{\delta}_2\sqrt{n_2/2}/\sigma\right)$
            $T := p_1 + p_2$
            If $T \leq \alpha_2$ **Then** power := power+1/nRuns
      Endif
    Endfor
    Return power
    §

Algorithm 14.5.1 can be easily modified for MPP as shown below.

Algorithm 14.5.2: Two-Stage Sample-Size Re-estimation with MPP

Objective: Return power for two-stage adaptive design
Input treatment difference δ and common σ, stopping boundaries $\alpha_1, \alpha_2, \beta_1$, n_1, n_2, target conditional power cP for SSR, and nRuns.
    power := 0
    For $iRun$:= 1 **To** nRuns
        Generate $\hat{\delta}_1$ from $N\left(\delta, 2\sigma^2\right)$

$$p_1 := 1 - \Phi\left(\hat{\delta}_1\sqrt{n_1/2}/\sigma\right)$$

If $p_1 > \beta_1$ **Then Exitfor**

If $p_1 \leq \alpha_1$ **Then** power := power+1/nRuns

If $\alpha_1 < p_1 \leq \beta_1$ **Then**

$$n_2 := \frac{2\sigma^2}{\hat{\delta}_1^2}\left(z_{1-\alpha_2/p_1} - z_{1-cP}\right)^2$$

Generate $\hat{\delta}_2$ from $N\left(\delta, 2\sigma^2\right)$

$$p_2 := 1 - \Phi\left(\hat{\delta}_2\sqrt{n_2/2}/\sigma\right)$$

$$T := p_1 p_2$$

If $T \leq \alpha_2$ **Then** power := power+1/nRuns

Endif

Endfor

Return power

§

Algorithm 14.5.3: K-Stage Sample-Size Re-estimation with MINP (large sample size)

Objective: Return power for K-stage adaptive design

Note: sample size re-estimation will potentially increase the overall sample size only by the subsample size for the last stage n_K.

Input treatment difference δ and common σ, one-sided α, stopping boundaries $\{\alpha_i\}$ and $\{\beta_i\}$, stagewise sample size $\{n_i\}$, sample size limits $\{n_{i,\max}\}$, number of stages K, weights $\{w_{ki}\}$, and nRuns.

power:= 0

For $iRun := 1$ **To** nRuns

    For $i := 1$ **To** K

        Generate $\hat{\delta}_i$ from $N\left(\delta, 2\sigma^2\right)$

$$z_i = \hat{\delta}_i\sqrt{n_i/2}/\sigma$$

    Endfor

    For $k := 1$ **To** K

$$T_k^* := 0$$

        For $i := 1$ **To** k

$$T_k^* := T_k^* + w_{ki} z_i$$

$$\bar{\delta} = \bar{\delta} + w_{ki}^2 \hat{\delta}_i$$

        Endfor

$$T_k; := 1 - \Phi\left(T_k^*\right)$$

        If $T_k > \beta_k$ **Then Exitfor**

        If $T_k \leq \alpha_k$ **Then** power := power+1/nRuns

        If $\alpha_k < T_k \leq \beta_k$ **Then**

            For $j := k$ **To** K

$$n_j := \min\left(n_{j,\max}, \left(\frac{\delta}{\bar{\delta}}\right)^2 n_j^0\right)$$

            Endfor

        Endif

Endfor
Endfor
Return power
§

14.6 Summary

In this chapter, we have introduced the uniform formulations for hypothesis-based adaptive design and provided sample algorithms for well-understood k-stage group sequential designs. For sample size and power estimation of some less well-understood adaptive trial designs such as two-stage seamless adaptive designs (e.g., phase i/ii design or phase ii/iii design) with different study objectives and/or different study endpoints at different stages, some formulas for sample size calculation/allocation are provided in Chapter 9 (see also Pong and Chow, 2010).

Readers develop algorithms for obtaining other less well-understood adaptive design operating characteristics in a similar way using various adaptive design methods. Implementation of these algorithms are straightforward using any computer language such as C+, Visual Basic, Java, PHP, SAS, R, etc.

Note that for sample size and power estimation of various adaptive designs, several commercial software packages such as EAST and ExpDesign Studio are available. More details regarding the availability and application of these software packages are given in the next chapter.

Chapter 15

Clinical Trial Simulation

15.1 Introduction

Clinical trial simulation is a process that uses computers to mimic the conduct of a clinical trial by creating virtual patients and extrapolate (or predict) clinical outcomes for each virtual patient based on the pre-specified models (Li and Lai, 2003). The primary objective of clinical trial simulation is multi-fold. First, it is to monitor the conduct of the trial, project outcomes, anticipate problems and recommend remedies before it is too late. Second, it is to extrapolate (or predict) the clinical outcomes *beyond* the scope of previous studies from which the existing models were derived using the model techniques. Third, it is to study the validity and robustness of the trial under various assumptions of study designs. Clinical trial simulation is often conducted to verify (or confirm) the models depicting the relationships between the inputs such as dose, dosing time, patient characteristics, and disease severity and the clinical outcomes such as changes in the signs and symptoms or adverse events within the study domain. In practice, clinical trial simulation is often considered to predict potential clinical outcomes under different assumptions and various design scenarios at the planning stage of a clinical trial for a better planning of the actual trial.

Clinical trial simulation is a powerful tool in pharmaceutical development (Chang 2010). The concept of clinical trial simulation is very intuitive and easy to implement. In practice, clinical trial simulation is often considered to be a useful tool for evaluation of the performance of a test treatment under a model with complicated situations. It can achieve the goal with minimum assumptions by controlling type I error rate effectively. It can also be used to visualize the dynamic trial process from patient recruitment, drug distribution, treatment administration, and pharmacokinetic processes to biomarker development and clinical responses.

As indicated earlier, more adaptations give the investigator more flexibility in identifying best clinical benefits of the test treatment under investigation. However, a multiple adaptive design with more adaptations could be very

271

complicated and consequently appropriate statistical methods for assessment of the treatment effect may not be available and are difficult, if not impossible, to obtain. Thus, one of the major obstacles for implementing adaptive design methods in clinical trials is that appropriate statistical methods are not well established with respect to various adaptations. Current software packages such as SAS cannot be applied directly and hence are not helpful. Although there are some software packages available in the marketplace such as ExpDesign Studio (CTriSoft Intl, 2002), EastSurvAdapt (East, 2010), and ADDPLAN (http://www.addplan.com), which cover certain types of adaptive trial designs, new software packages for adaptive design methods in clinical trials are necessarily developed to assist in implementing adaptive trial designs in clinical trials (Pong and Chow, 2010). An overview of software available for group sequential and adaptive designs can be found in Wassmer and Vandemeulebroecke (2006).

In this chapter, we will review the application of clinical trial simulations in both early and late phases of pharmaceutical development through the demonstration of ExpDesign Studio. In the next section, the application of ExpDesign Studio is briefly described. Applications in early phase development and late phase development are discussed in Sections 15.3 and 15.4, respectively. Examples are given whenever possible. Some concluding remarks are given in the last section of this chapter.

15.2   Software Application of ExpDesign Studio

In this section, we will introduce the application of clinical trial simulation using the software of ExpDesign Studio^M developed by CTriSoft Intl. Other well-known software such as East$^{®}$ developed by Cytel will not be discussed here. Readers can visit their website for more information.

15.2.1   Overview of ExpDesign Studio

ExpDesign Studio (ExpDesign) is an integrated environment for designing experiments or clinical trials. It is a powerful and user-friendly statistical software product that has seven integrated main components: classical design (CD), sequential design (SD), multistage design (MSD), dose-escalation design (DED), adaptive design (AD), adaptive trial monitoring (ATM), and dose-escalation trial monitoring (DTM) modules. In addition, the ExpDesign randomizor can generate random variates from a variety of distributions. The ExpDesign toolkit provides features for distributional calculation, confidence intervals, and function and data plotting.

Classical trials are the most commonly used in practice. ExpDesign provides nearly 150 methods for sample-size calculations in CD for different trial designs. It includes methods for single-, two-, and multiple-group designs, and for superiority, noninferiority, and equivalence designs with various endpoints. Group sequential trials are advanced designs with multiple analyses. A group sequential trial is usually a cost-effective design compared to a classical design.

SD covers a broad range of sequential trials with different endpoints and different types of stopping boundaries. A multistage design is an exact method for group sequential trials with a binary response, whereas group sequential design uses an asymptotic approach. MSD provides three optimal designs among others: MinMax, MinExp, and MaxUtility, which minimize the maximum sample size, minimize the expected sample size, and maximize the utility index, respectively. A dose-escalation trial in aggressive disease areas such as oncology has unique characteristics. Due to the toxicity of the testing drug, researchers are allowed to use fewer patients to obtain as much information as possible about the toxicity profi le or maximum tolerable dose. By means of computer simulations, DED provides researchers with an efficient way to search for an optimal design for dose-escalation trials with a variety of criteria. It includes traditional escalation rules, restricted escalation rules, and two-stage design.

ExpDesign Studio covers many statistical tools required for designing a trial. It is helpful to get familiar with the functions of the icons on the toolbar. The black-white icons on the left-hand side of the toolbar are standard for all word processors. The first group of the four color icons is the starting point to launch the four different types of designs: *Conventional Trial Design*, *Sequential Trial Design*, *Multi-Stage Trial Design*, and *Dose-Escalation Trial Design* (see Figure 15.2.1). Alternatively, one may click one of the four buttons in the ExpDesignTM Studio to start the corresponding design. The next set of three color icons are for launching *Design Example*, *Computing Design Parameters*, and generating *Design Report*. Following these are four color icons for the toolkits including *Graphic Calculator*, *Distribution Calculator*, *Confidence Interval Calculator* and *TipDay*. One can move the mouse over any icon on the toolbar to see the Tiptext, which describes what the icon is for.

15.2.2 How to design a trial with ExpDesign Studio

To get started, we first double click on ExpDesign Studio icon. Then, on the ExpDesign start window, select the trial design one wishes to implement.

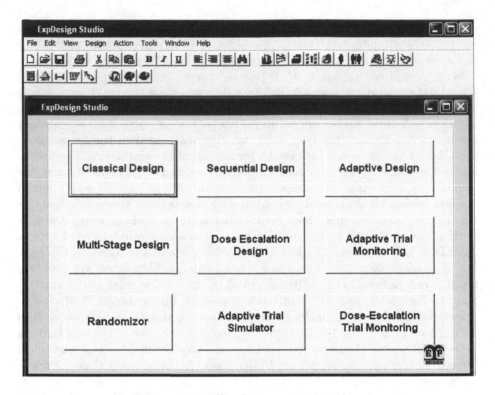

Figure 15.2.1: ExpDesign start window.

15.2.3 How to design a classical trial

Classical design with a fixed sample size can always be used for comparison when we design an adaptive trial. Let's use the following example to show how to use ExpDesign Studio to accomplish the task.

Example 15.2.1: Suppose that a pharmaceutical company is interested in conducting a clinical trial to compare the efficacy of two antimicrobial agents when administrated orally once daily in the treatment of patients with skin structure infections. We are considering three different scenarios (i) testing for superiority based on mean cure rate, (ii) testing noninferiority of the test drug as compared to the active control agent, and (iii) testing for therapeutical equivalence. We assume that the sample size is calculated to achieve a 90% power at the 5% level of significance, and the cure rates are 65% and 75% for the control and test groups, respectively. The noninferiority margin is assumed to be 1%. For equivalence design, we assume the cure rates of 65% are the same for both treatment groups and the equivalent margin is ±10%. To complete the sample size calculations in ExpDesign Studio, we simply follow the following steps.

- Step 1. Click *Classical Trial Design* on the toolbar (Figure 15.2.2).

- Step 2. Select the desired options for the Number of Groups, Analysis Basis, Trial Endpoint, and Sample Allocation from *Design Option Panel*.

- Step 3. Select a method from the list of methods available (e.g., "Pearson's Chi-square test" for the superiority design, "One-sided non-inferiority test for two proportions" for the noninferiority design, and "Equivalance for two proportions" for the equivalence design).

- Step 4. Enter appropriate values for the selected design (enter 0.025 for the significance level for the one-sided noninferiority test).

- Step 5. Click on *Compute* to calculate the required sample size.

- Step 6. Click on *Report* to view the report of the selected design.

- Step 7. Click on *Print* to print the desired output.

- Step 8. Click on *Copy-Graph* to copy the graph and use *Paste* or *Paste-Special* under *Edit* menu to paste it to other applications.

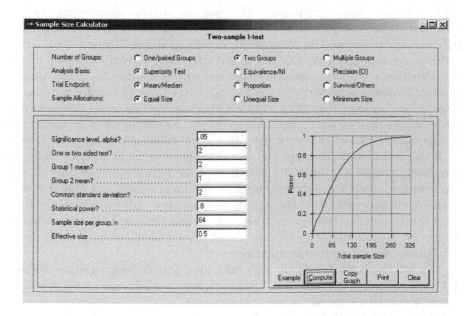

Figure 15.2.2: Example of classical design with ExpDesign Studio.

The sample calculations performed by the software provided the following results: 459 per group for the superiority design, 360 per group for the noninferiority design, and 492 for the equivalence design.

15.2.4   How to design a group sequential trial

A group sequential design involves multiple stages. At each stage an interim analysis is performed. An interim analysis is intended to compare treatment arms with respect to efficacy or safety at any time prior to formal completion of a trial. Because the number and methods of these comparisons will affect the interpretation of the trial, all interim analyses should be planned carefully in advance and described in the protocol, including the timing of the analyses and stopping rules. (Later we will see that these requirements may be eased in adaptive designs.) An interim analysis planned with the intention of deciding whether or not to terminate a trial is usually accomplished through the use of a group sequential design that employs statistical monitoring schemes or a data monitoring committee charter as guidelines. The goal of such an interim analysis is to stop the trial early if the superiority of the treatment under study is clearly established, if the demonstration of a relevant treatment difference has become unlikely, or if unacceptable adverse effects are apparent.

There are many factors that can be used to characterize a group sequential design, such as the expected sample size under the hypotheses and the maximum sample size in selecting a group sequential design. If you wish to reduce the expected cost, you might want to choose a design with a minimum expected sample size; if you wish to reduce the maximum possible cost, you might want to consider a design with a minimum total sample size. In any case, you should compare all the stopping probabilities between designs carefully before determining an appropriate design. O'Brien–Fleming boundaries, with the corresponding $\Delta = 0$, are very conservative in early rejection of the null hypothesis. Pocock's method, with the corresponding $\Delta = 0.5$, using a constant stopping boundary (on the z - scale) over time. Generally speaking, a large value of Δ (e.g., 0.8) will lead to a design that spends type I error more at earlier stages than at later stages. To increase the probability of accepting the null hypothesis at earlier stages, you can use the triangular inner boundaries.

If you don't want to accept the null hypothesis at all at interim analyses, you should choose a design with rejection of the null hypothesis only. If you don't want to reject the null hypothesis at interim analyses, you should choose a design with acceptance of the null hypothesis only. Adjusting the size fractions is also an effective way to achieve a desired design. Although balanced designs are commonly used, one can, if desired, use an unbalanced design with a difference size for each experimental group.

You will be shown below, through examples, how to design various sequential trials using ExpDesign Studio. However, before we discuss these, it will be helpful to explain some of the input parameters.

The potential early claim can be "the null hypothesis is true" (i.e., the futility design), "the alternative hypothesis is true" (i.e., the efficacy design), or "either of the hypotheses is true." The sample-size fractions at K analyses should be a sequence of numbers between 0 and 1, separated by commas. When you enter the number of stages, the fractions are filled into the textbox automatically based on an equal-sample-size design (an equal-information-interval design). You can change them anytime afterward. The stopping boundary shape parameter, delta, is the Δ in the Wang–Tsiatis boundary family, in which a low value will lead to a low probability of rejecting the alternative hypothesis. The allowable range for Δ is $(-0.5, 1)$. You can move the mouse over each input box and wait for a second to see the hint. You can always click the example button to see the input example.

Example 15.2.2: Consider a trial to test the effectiveness of a new drug, ABC, in treating patients with mild to moderate asthma. A parallel design with two treatment groups (placebo vs. ABC) is chosen for the design. The primary efficacy parameter is percentage change from baseline in FEV1. The mean difference in percentage change in FEV1 between placebo and ABC is estimated to be 6% (5% vs. 11%), with a standard deviation of 18%.

A single-stage design with a fixed sample of 282 will allow us to have 80% power to detect the difference at a one-sided significance level $\alpha = 0.025$. The sponsors believe that there is a good chance that the test drug will be superior to the placebo and want to stop the trial early if the superiority becomes evident.

To design a group sequential trial, we simply follow these steps.

- Step 1. Click on *Group Sequential Design* on the toolbar.

- Step 2. Select the desired option from the *Design Option Panel*.

- Step 3. Select a method from the list of methods available.

- Step 4. Enter appropriate values for the selected design.

- Step 5. Click on *Compute* to generate the design.

- Step 6. Click on *Report* to view the design report.

- Step 7. Click on *Print* to print the desired output.

- Step 8. Click on *Copy-Graph* to copy the graph and use *Paste* or *Paste-Special* under *Edit* menu to paste it to other application.

- Step 9. Click *Save* to save the design specification or report.

For the example, we specify the options in ExpDesign as follows: two groups, hypothesis test, mean/median, and alternative hypothesis. Enter "2" for the number of analyses, "1" for a one-sided analysis, "0.025" for α, "0.05" for the group 1 mean, "0.11" for the group 2 mean, "0.18" for the common standard deviation, "1" for the sample size ratio, "0.5,1" for the sample size fractions, "0.5" for the stopping boundary shape parameter Δ, and "0.8" for the power (Figure 15.2.3). Click to run the simulation. When it is finished, click on the toolbar; the outputs reported below will be generated.

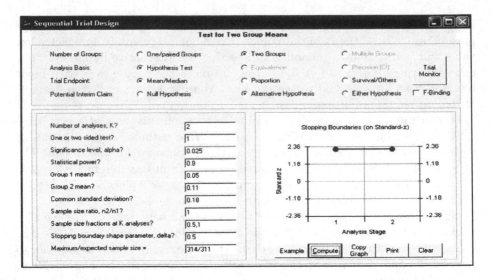

Figure 15.2.3: Two-stage group sequential design for two means.

Design Outputs - Sample size for the single-stage design = 282; maximum sample size (combined total) = 314; sample size expected under the null hypothesis H_0 is 311; sample size expected under the alternative hypothesis H_a is 241.

Report - This experimental design has one interim analysis and a final analysis. The sample sizes for the two analyses are 157 and 314, respectively. The sample size ratio between the two groups is 1. The maximum sample size for the design is 314, and the expected sample size is 311 under the null hypothesis and 241 under the alternative hypothesis. The calculation is based on a level of significance $\alpha = 0.025$, power = 0.8, mean difference = 0.06, and standard deviation = 0.18.

The decision rules are specified as follows:

At stage 1:

• Accept null hypothesis if p-value > 0.5.

• Reject null hypothesis if p-value < or = 0.0147.

• Otherwise, continue.

At stage 2:

• Accept null hypothesis if p-value > 0.0147.

• Reject null hypothesis if p-value < or = 0.0147.

It is important to know that the sponsors are more interested in the expected sample size (241) under the alternative hypothesis than the sample size (309) under the null hypothesis. The maximum sample size is 314, whereas it is 284 for the classical single-stage design. The sponsors believe that there is a good chance to stop the trial early, which means that only 157 patients are required. This will lead not only to a reduction in the number of patients but also a savings in time.

15.2.5 How to design an adaptive trial with SSR

To design an adaptive trial, we simply follow the following steps.

- Step 1. Click on *Adaptive Design* on the toolbar.The Adaptive Design – Step 1 window will appear (see Figure 15.2.4).

- Step 2. Select the Sample Size Re-estimation (SSR) option.

- Step 3. Specify parameters in each of the steps.

- Step 4. Select the option in the Endpoint.

- Step 5. Enter appropriate values for the Response Under Ha, the noninferiority margin for the noninferiority trial, One-Sided Alpha, and Power.

- Step 6. Click the Next button; the Adaptive Design – Step 2 window will appear (see Figure 15.2.5).

- Step 7. Enter values for the initial number of stages and Information Time for Analyses .

- Step 8. Choose stopping boundaries using the arrow button.

- Step 9. Enter values for N Simulations and N/group .

- Step 10. Select a statistical method in the panel.

- Step 11. Enter values for Maximum N/group Allowed for SSR and Targeted Conditional Power for SSR.

- Step 12. Click to start the simulation.

- Step 13. Click on *Save* to save the design specification or report.

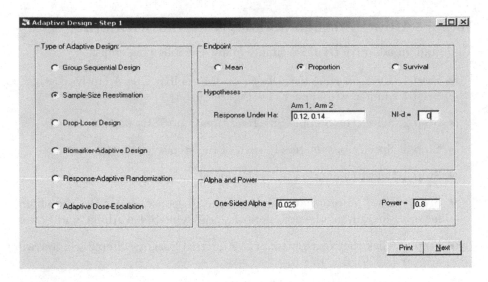

Figure 15.2.4: The adaptive design window - step 1.

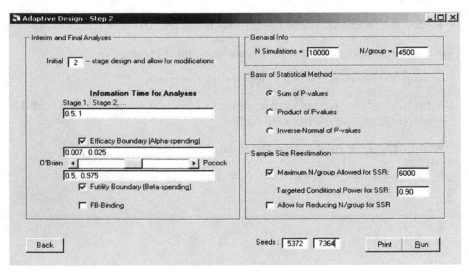

Figure 15.2.5: The adaptive design window - step 2.

How to Design a Adaptive Dose-Escalation Trial

To design a dose-escalation trial, we simply follow these steps (see Figure 15.2.6).

- Step 1. Click *Dose-Escalation Design* on the toolbar.

- Step 2. Select the CRM option.

- Step 3. Enter appropriate values for your design on the *Basic Spec Panel*.

- Step 4. Select *Dose-response Model, Escalation Scheme,* and *Dose Interval Spec* or open a existing design by clicking *Open.*

- Step 5. Click on *Compute* to generate the simulation results.

- Step 6. Click on *Report* to view the design report.

- Step 7. Click on *Print* to print the desired output.

- Step 8. Click on *Save* to save the design specification or report.

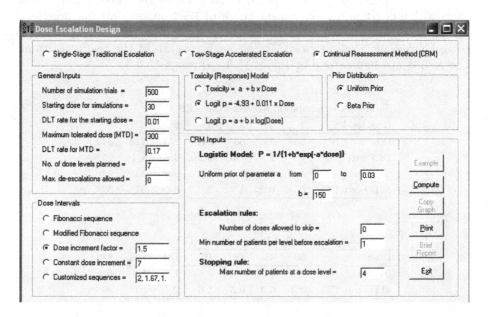

Figure 15.2.6: Dose-escalation design window.

15.3 Early Phases Development

To illustrate the application of clinical trial simulation in early phases of clinical development, we consider the example of dose-escalation trial as described in the previous section. Suppose the study objective is to determine the maximum tolerable dose (MTD) of newly developed test treatment. In what follows, the application of clinical trial simulation for dose escalation with different traditional escalation rules (TER) and continued reassessment method (CRM) are discussed.

Example 15.3.1: Simulation example using TER and TSER   For a planned dose-escalation trial, suppose we are interested in choosing an appropriate dose-escalation algorithm from the traditional escalation rule (TER) and the two-stage escalation rule (TSER) described earlier. Suppose that based on results from pre-clinical studies, it was estimated that the toxicity (DLT rate) is 1% for the starting dose of 30 mg/m^2 (1/10 of the lethal dose). The DLT rate at the MTD was defined as 17% and the MTD was estimated to be 300 mg/m^2. The true dose-toxicity was assumed to follow a logistic model, i.e.,

$$Logit(p) = -4.93 + 0.011Dose,$$

where p is the probability of DLT or DLT rate. There were seven planned dose levels with a constant dose increment factor of 1.5. Suppose only one dose level de-escalation was allowed. Twenty thousand simulation runs were conducted using ExpDesign Studio (www.CTriSoft.net) for each of the two algorithms. The results are summarized in Tables 15.3.1 through 15.3.3.

Table 15.3.1: Simulation Results from TER

Dose level	1	2	3	4	5	6	7
Dose	30	45	68	101	151	228	342
DLT rate (%)	1	1.2	1.5	2.2	3.8	8.4	25
mean n	3.1	3.1	3.1	3.2	3.5	5.0	5.0
MTD rate (%)	0	0	1	2	6	57	33

Table 15.3.2: Simulation Results from STER

Dose	30	45	68	101	151	228	342
mean n	1.1	1.1	1.2	1.3	1.5	5.9	5.2
MTD rate (%)	0.3	0.3	0.5	1.6	2	69	29

Table 15.3.3: Comparison of TER and STER

Method	MTD	$\overline{MTD}$	σ_{MTD}	N	DLTs	n
3+3 TER	300	257	67	24.3	1.84	5.0
Two-stage	300	276	58	10.8	1.26	4.1

$\overline{MTD}$ = Simulated MTD, σ_{MTD} = dispersion of MTDs, N = expected sample size, n = patients treated above MTD.

The true MTD is somewhere between dose level 6 and 7. As it can be seen from Tables 15.1 and 15.2, the two-stage design requires fewer patients at the dose levels lower than MTD. Table 15.3 indicates that there is a large gain in the expected sample size with TSER, i.e., 10.8 compared 24.6 in TSER. On average, the single-stage TSER has 1.84 DLTs and the two-stage design has 1.26 DLTs. The two-stage has fewer patients treated above MTD than the single-stage TSER. Two-stage increases precision compared to TER (58 vs. 67 in dispersion of simulated MTDs). In the given scenario, both TER and TSER underestimate the true MTD (about 13%). This bias can be reduced using continual re-assessment method (CRM), which will be discussed below.

Example 15.3.2: Simulation example using CRM   We repeat the above clinical trial simulation using the Bayesian continual re-assessment method (CRM). The logistic model considered to model the dose-toxicity relationship is given by

$$\Pr(x = 1) = (1 + 150e^{-ax})^{-1},$$

where parameter a follows an uniform prior distribution over the range of $[0, 0.3]$. The next patient is assigned to the dose level that has the predicted response rate closest to the target DLT rate of 0.17 as defined earlier for the MTD. No response-delay is considered. Due to safety concerns, no dose-jump is allowed, i.e., at least one patient has to be treated before escalating to the next higher dose level. The trial will be stopped when four patients are treated at any dose level. The simulations were conducted using *ExpDesign Studio*® *version 5*. The results are summarized in Table 15.3.4.

Table 15.3.4: Simulation Results with CRM

Dose level	1	2	3	4	5	6	7
Dose	30	45	68	101	151	228	342
$P_{DLT}(\%)$	1	1.2	1.5	2.2	3.7	8.4	25
$\hat{P}_{DLT}(\%)$	1	1.2	1.5	2.2	6.7	18.2	39
Percent MDTs	0	0	0	0	24.8	46.2	29
Expected N	1	1	1	1	1.9	2.9	1.9

$P_{DLT} = DLT$ rate, $\hat{P}_{DLT}$ and σ_{DLT} are the predicted rate and its standard deviation. N = number of patients.

In this example, the CRM produces excellent predictions for the DLT rates. We can see that one of the advantages with CRM is that it produces the posterior parameter distribution and predicted probability of DLT for each dose level (any dose) and allows us to select an unplanned dose level as the MTD. In the current case, the true MTD is 300 mg/m^2 with a DLT rate P_{DLT} = 0.17, which is an unplanned dose level. As long as the dose-response model is appropriately selected, bias can be avoided. This is an advantage compared to TER or TSER discussed in the previous example. The simulations also indicate that the number of DLTs per trial is 0.83. The number of patients treated with dose higher than MTD is 10.8 per trial, smaller than those from TSER and the two-stage designs.

15.4 Late Phases Development

To investigate the effect of the adaptations, we will compare the classic, group sequential and adaptive designs with regards to their operating characteristics using computer simulations.

Example 15.4.1: Adaptive Design for an Oncology Trial In a two-arm comparative oncology trial with time to progression (TTP) as the primary efficacy endpoint, the median TTP is estimated to be 8 months (hazard rate = 0.08664) for the control group and 10.5 months (hazard rate = 0.06601) for the test group. Assume a uniform enrollment with an accrual period of 9 months and a total study duration of 24 months. An exponential survival distribution is assumed for the purpose of sample-size calculation. The classical design requires a sample size of 321 subjects per group for 85% power. We design the trial with one interim analysis when 40% of patients have been enrolled. The interim analysis for efficacy is planned based on TTP, but it does not allow for futility stopping. Following are the steps for the trial design using ExpDesign Studio.

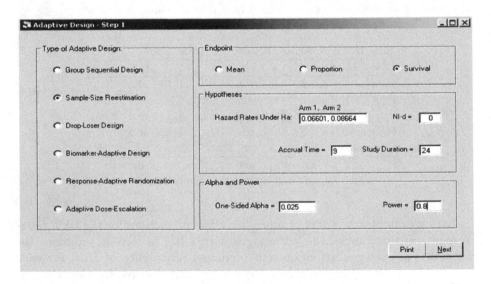

Figure 15.4.1: Adaptive design for the oncology trial.

Click the Adaptive Design button to bring up the Adaptive Design – Step 1 window (see Figure 15.4.1). In the Adaptive Design – Step 1 window, do the following:

- Select the Sample-Size Re-estimation option in the Type of Adaptive Design panel.

- Select the Survival option in the Endpoint window.

- Enter "0.06601, 0.08664" for Hazard Rates Under Ha in the Hypotheses panel.

- Enter "0" for NI-d , the noninferiority margin, because it is a superiority trial.

- Enter "9" for Accrual Time and "24" for Study Duration.

- Enter "0.025" for One-Sided Alpha and "0.8" for Power.

- Click the Next button to bring up the Adaptive Design – Step 2 window (see Figure 15.8).

In the Adaptive Design–Step 2 window, do the following:

- Enter "2" for the initial number of stages.

- Enter "0.4, 1" for Information Time for Analyses.

- Choose stopping boundaries using the arrow near O'Brien or Pocock.

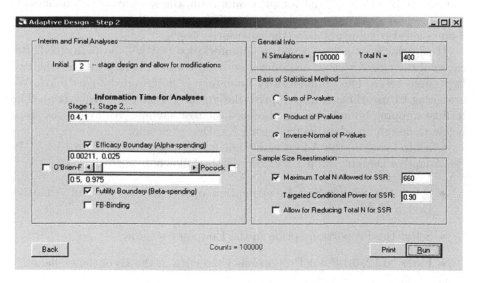

Figure 15.4.2: Input parameters for the adaptive oncology trial.

If you want to have futility boundaries, you can check the Futility Boundary (Beta-spending) checkbox.

- Enter " 100000" for N Simulations.

- Enter "400" for Total N (events).

- Select the Inverse-Normal of P-values option in the Basis of Statistical Method panel.

- Enter "660" for M aximum Total N Allowed for SSR (this is the number of events for a survival endpoint) and check the box.

- Enter "0.90" for the Targeted Conditional Power for SSR.

- Click the Run button to start the simulation.

After the simulation is completed, you can click the Report icon to view the design report. We can see that the sample size expected is 616 under the alternative hypothesis and the power is 87.4%. The classical design has 83.5% power with the same sample size. When the median TTP is 10 months instead of 10.5, this adaptive design will still have 73% power, whereas the classical design has only 70% power.

Example 15.4.2: Noninferiority Design with a Binary Endpoint   A phase III trial is to be designed for patients with acute ischemic stroke of recent onset. The primary endpoint is defined as the composite endpoint (death or MI) with an estimated event rate 14% for the control group and 12% for the test group. Based on a large-sample assumption, the sample size for a classical design is 4437 per group, which provides 80% power to detect the difference at a one - sided α value of 0.025 (the superiority test).

If superiority is not achieved, a noninferiority test will be performed. Because of the closed testing procedure, no α adjustment is required for the two hypothesis tests. The noninferiority boundary is determined to be 0.5%. We are going to use three-stage adaptive design for the noninferiority trial. The futility stopping boundaries are also used for cost savings. We follow the steps below to design an adaptive trial using ExpDesign Studio:

Click to bring up the Adaptive Design – Step 1 window (Figure 15.4.3). In the Adaptive Design – Step 1 window, do the following:

- Select the Sample-Size Re-estimation option in the Type of Adaptive Design panel.

- Select the Proportion option in the Endpoint window.

- Enter "0.12, 0.14" for Proportions Under Ha in the Hypotheses panel.

- Enter "0.005" for NI-d , the noninferiority margin, for the noninferiority trial.

- Enter "0.025" for One-Sided Alpha and "0.8" for Power.

- Click to bring up the Adaptive Design–Step 2 window.

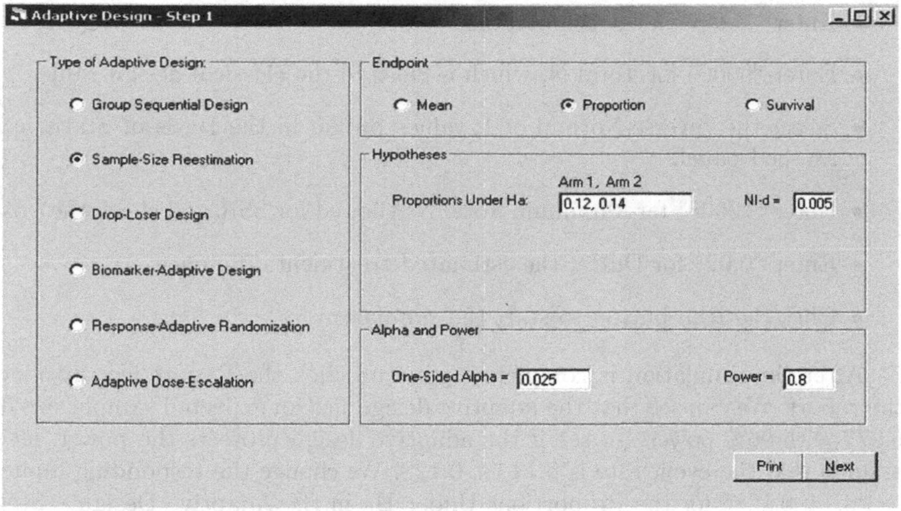

Figure 15.4.3: Adaptive design for the noninferiority trial - Step 1.

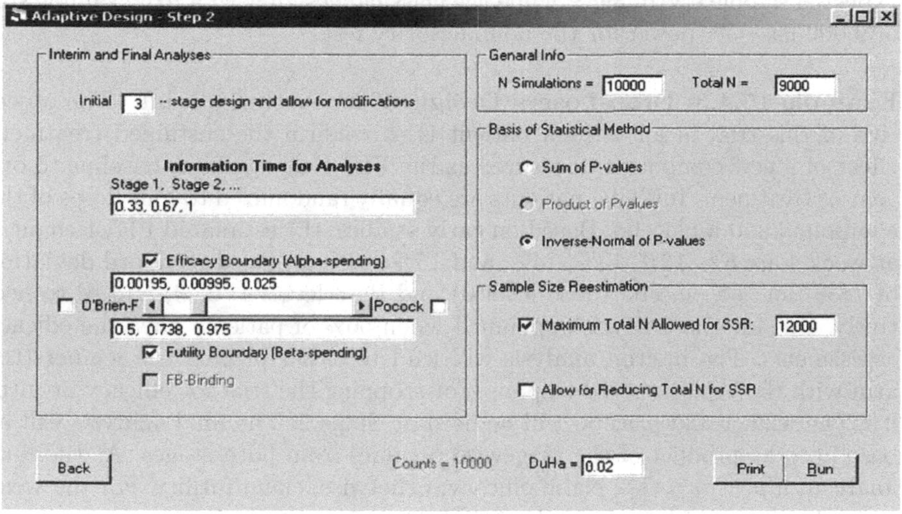

Figure 15.4.4: Adaptive design for the noninferiority trial - Step 2.

In the Adaptive Design – Step 2 window (Figure 15.4.4), do the following:

- Enter "3" for the initial number of stages.

- Enter "0.33, 0.67, 1" for Information Time for Analyses.

- Choose stopping boundaries by the arrow near O'Brien or Pocock .

- If you want to have futility boundaries, you can check the Futility Boundary (Beta-spending) checkbox.

- Enter "10000" for N Simulations.

- Enter "9000" for Total N, which is close to the classical design value.

- Select the Inverse-Normal of P-values option in the Basis of Statistical Method panel.

- Enter "12000" for Maximum Total N Allowed for SSR and check the box.

- Enter "0.02" for DuHa, the estimated treatment difference.

- Click the Run button to start the simulation.

After the simulation is completed, you can click the Report icon to view the report. We can see that the adaptive design has an expected sample size of 6,977 with 96% power. To see if the adaptive design protects the power, let's assume that the event rate is 0.14 vs. 0.128. We change the responding inputs to "0.14, 0.128" for the Proportions Under Ha in the Adaptive Design – Step 1 window. Keep everything else the same (DuHa = 0.02, not DuHa = 0.012). The simulation results show that the adaptive design has 72% power with an expected sample size of 8988, while the classical design with a fixed sample size of 9,000 has 65% power for the noninferiority test.

Example 15.4.3: Drop-Losers Design of an Asthma Trial The objective of this trial in an asthma patient is to confirm the sustained treatment effect of a new compound, measured as the FEV1 change from baseline to one year of treatment. Initially, patients are equally randomized to four doses of the compound and a placebo. Based on early studies, the estimated FEV1 changes at week 4 are 6%, 12%, 13%, 14%, and 15% (with a pooled standard deviation of 18%) for the placebo (dose level 0) and dose levels 1, 2, 3, and 4, respectively. One interim analysis is planned when 50% of patients have the efficacy assessments. The interim analysis will lead to either picking the winner (the arm with the best observed response) or stopping the trial for efficacy or futility. The winner and placebo will be used at Stage 2. The final analysis will be based on the product of the stagewise p-values from both stages. At the final analysis, if p_1 , $p_2 \leq \alpha_2$, claim efficacy; otherwise, claim futility. For the weak control, $p_1 = \hat{p}_1$, where $\hat{p}_1$ is the naive stagewise p-value from a contrast test based on a subsample from Stage 1. For the strong control, p_1 is the adjusted p-value (i.e., $p_1 = 4p_{min}$), where p_{min} is the smallest p-value among the four comparisons.

To do an adaptive design with ExpDesign, follow the steps below.

- Click the Adaptive Design button to bring up the Adaptive Design – Step 1 window (see Figure 15.4.5). In the Adaptive Design – Step 1 window, do the following:

- Select the Drop-Loser Design option in the Type of Adaptive Design panel.

- Select the Mean option in the Endpoint window.

- Enter "0.05, 0.12, 0.13, 0.14, 0.15" for Mean Under Ha and 0.18 for sigma in the Hypotheses panel.

- Enter "0" for NI-d, the noninferiority margin, for the noninferiority trial.

- Enter "0.025" for One-Sided Alpha and "0.90" for Power .

- Click the Next button to bring up the Adaptive Design – Step 2 window (Figure 15.4.6).

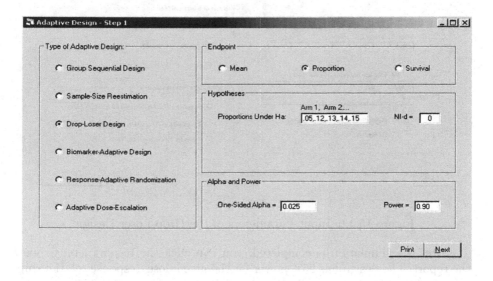

Figure 15.4.5: Drop-Loser Design.

In the Adaptive Design – Step 2 window, do the following:

- Enter "2" for the initial number of stages.

- Enter "0.5, 1" for Information Time for Analyses .

- Choose stopping boundaries by the arrow near O'Brien or Pocock.

- If you want to have futility boundaries, you can check the Futility Boundary (Beta-spending) checkbox.

- Enter "10000" for N Simulations.

- Enter "180" for Total N, which is close to the classical design.

- Select the Product of P-values option in the Basis of Statistical Method panel.

- Enter "400" for Maximum Total N Allowed for SSR and check the box.

- Enter "0.90" for Targeted Conditional Power for SSR, the estimated treatment difference.

- Click the Run button to start the simulation.

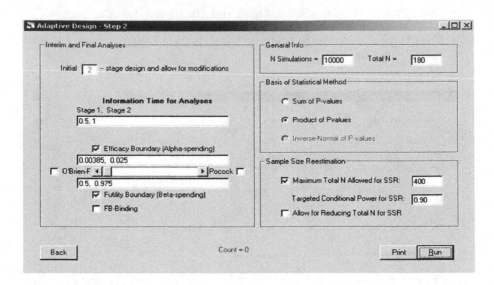

Figure 15.4.6: Input Parameters of the Drop-Loser Design.

After the simulation is completed, you can click the Report icon to view the report. The design has 95% power for the given dose–response relationship. Because the adaptive also allows for sample-size re-estimation, when the responses in arms 2 through 5 decrease to 0.12, the design still has 80% power with the expected sample size of 287—a very robust design.

Example 15.4.4: Response-adaptive design with multiple treatment groups   As discussed earlier, The randomized play-the-winner (RPW) model is a simple probabilistic model used to randomize subjects sequentially in a clinical trial. The RPW model can be used for randomized clinical trials with a binary endpoint. In the RPW model it is assumed that the previous subject's outcome will be available before the next patient is randomized. At the start of the clinical trial, an urn contains $a0$ balls representing treatment A and $b0$ balls representing treatment B, where $a0$ and $b0$ are positive integers. We denote these balls by either type A or type B balls. When a subject is recruited, a ball is drawn and replaced. If it is a type A ball, the subject receives treatment A; if it is a type B ball, the subject receives treatment B. When a subject's outcome is available, the urn is updated as follows: Success on treatment A (B) or a failure on treatment B (A) will generate additional $a1$ ($b1$) type A (B) balls in the urn. In this way the urn builds up more balls, representing the more successful treatment (see Figure 15.4.8).

Suppose that we are designing an oncology clinical study with tumor response as the primary endpoint. The response rate is estimated to be 0.3 in the control group and 0.5 in the test group. The response rate is 0.4 in both groups under the null condition. We want to design the trial with about 80% power at a one-sided α value of 0.025. We first check the type I error of a classical two-group design with n = 200 (100 per group), which is the sample size required for 83% power using a classical design. We now use the RPW design as specified in the following steps.

Click the Adaptive Design button to bring up the Adaptive Design – Step 1 window (see Figure 15.4.7). In the Adaptive Design – Step 1 window, do the following:

- Select the Response-Adaptive Randomization option in the Type of Adaptive Design panel.

- Select the Proportion option in the Endpoint window.

- Enter "0.4, 0.4" for Proportions Under Ha in the Hypotheses panel.

- Enter "0" for NI-d , the noninferiority margin, because it is a superiority trial.

- Enter "0.025" for One-Sided Alpha and any decimal value for Power (no effect in this version).

- Click the Next button to bring up the Response-Adaptive Randomization window (Figure 15.4.8).

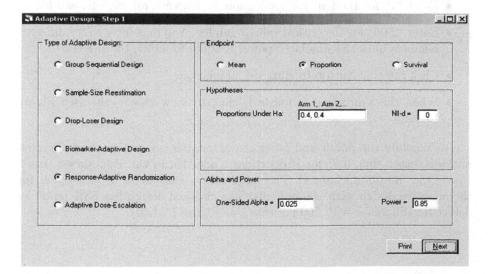

Figure 15.4.7: Response-adaptive randomization design.

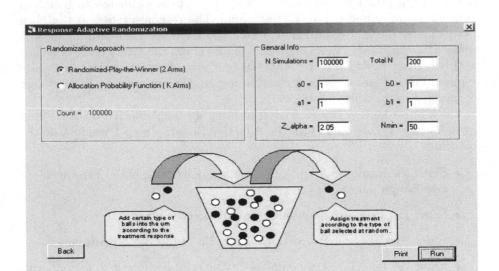

Figure 15.4.8: Input parameters for the binary RAR design.

- Enter "100000" for N Simulations in the General Info panel.

- Enter "200" for T otal N , which is based on a classical design for 83% power.

- Enter "1" for the four randomization parameters: $a0$, $b0$, $a1$, and $b1$.

- Enter "2.06" for the critical value Z _alpha . You may have to try different numbers until the simulated power is equal to 0.025, the α level.

- Click the Run button to start the simulation.

- When the simulation is finished, click to view the results (see Figure 15.4.9).

To simulate the power and other characteristics under the alternative hypothesis, enter "0.3, 0.5" for Proportions Under Ha in the Hypotheses panel. Keep other inputs unchanged. The results show that there is 74% power for the adaptive design with 200 patients. The classical design has 83% power to detect the difference with 200 patients (see Figure 15.4.10).

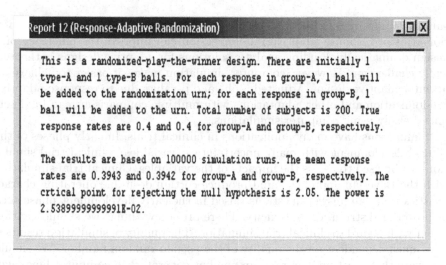

Figure 15.4.9: Determination of rejection region based type I error.

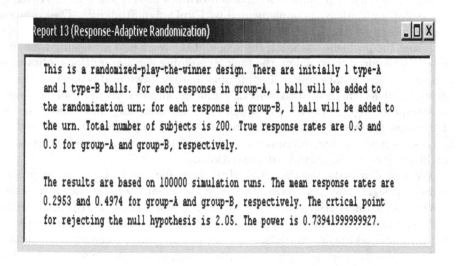

Figure 15.4.10: Simulation of power for the RAR design.

15.5 Concluding Remarks

From classic design to group sequential design to adaptive design, each step forward increases in complexity and at the same time, improves the efficiency of clinical trials as a whole. Adaptive designs can increase the number of responses in a trial and provide more benefits to the patient in comparison to the classic design. With sample size re-estimation, an adaptive design can preserve the power even when the initial estimations of treatment effect and its variability are inaccurate. In the case of a multiple-arm trial, dropping inferior arms or response-adaptive randomization can improve the efficiency of a design dramatically. Finding analytic solutions for adaptive designs is theoretically challenging. However, computer simulation makes it easier to achieve an optimal adaptive design. Adjusted alpha and p-values due to response-adaptive randomization and other adaptations with multiple comparisons can be determined easily using computer simulations.

Simulations have many applications in clinical trials. In early phases of the clinical development with many uncertainties (variables), clinical trial simulation can be used to assess the impacts of the variables. Clinical trial simulation with the Bayesian approach could produce certain desirable operating characteristics that can answer questions raised in the early development phase such as posterior distribution of toxicity. There are a few things we should caution about with regard to clinical trial simulation. The quality of simulation results is very much dependent on the quality of the pseudo-random number. We should be aware that most built-in random number generators in computer languages and software tools are poor in quality; therefore they should not be used directly if we are not sure about the algorithm. Implementing a high-quality of random number generator is as simple as a dozen of lines of computer code (Press et al., 2002; Gentle, 1998) as implemented by ExpDesign Studio$^{(R)}$. The common steps for conducting a clinical trial simulation include defining the objectives, analyzing the problem, assessing the scope of the work and proposing time and resources required to complete the task, examining the assumptions, obtaining and validating the data source if applicable, nailing down evaluation criteria for various trial designs/scenarios, selecting an appropriate software tool, outlining the computer algorithms for the simulation, implementing and validating the algorithms, proposing scenarios to simulate, conducting simulations, interpreting results and making recommendations, and last, but not least, addressing the limitations of the performed simulations.

We have demonstrated that clinical trial simulation can be used for various complex designs. By comparing the operating characteristics of each design provided by clinical trial simulation, we are able to choose an optimal design or development strategy. Computer simulation is commonly seen in statistics literature related to clinical trials, most of them for power calculations and data analyses. We will see more pharmaceutical companies using clinical trial simulation for their clinical development planning to streamline the drug process, increase the probability of success, and reduce the cost and time-to-market. Ultimately, clinical trial simulation will bring the best treatment to the patients. When conducting clinical trial simulation for an adaptive design, the following is recommended in order to protect the integrity of the trial: Specify in the trial protocol (i) the type of adaptive design, (ii) details of the adaptations to be used, (iii) the estimator for treatment effect, and (iv) the hypotheses and the test statistics. Run the simulation under the null hypothesis and construct the distribution of the test statistic. To estimate the sample size for the adaptive design, run the simulation under the alternative hypothesis and construct the distribution of the test statistic. Sensitivity analyses are suggested to simulate potential major protocol deviations that would impact the validity of the trial simulations. To achieve an optimal design, a Bayesian or frequentist-Bayesian hybrid adaptive approach should be used. There are several simulation tools available on the web. For adaptive designs discussed in this section, the ExpDesign Studio® can be used.

Chapter 16

Regulatory Perspectives - A Review of FDA Draft Guidance

16.1 Introduction

Immediately after the FDA released the draft guidance on adaptive clinical trial design in February 2010 (FDA, 2010b) the Journal of Biopharmaceutical Statistics (JBS) published a special theme issue for adaptive clinical trial design (Vol 20, No. 6, 2010). This special theme issue consists of three special articles. The first special article provides a summary of the morning session of a spring conference (sponsored by the Basel Biometric Section of the Austro-Swiss Region of the International Biometric Society) on *Perspectives on the Use of Adaptive Designs in Clinical Trials* held at the Basel University, Basel, Switzerland on March 12, 2010 (Wang, 2010; Benda et al., 2010). The second special article is a collection of papers containing a leading article by the United States Pharmaceutical Research and Manufacturers of America (PhRMA) Working Group on adaptive designs followed by a number of discussion papers on the FDA draft guidance (Gallo et al., 2010). The third special article attempts to provide a better understanding of the FDA draft guidance from a practitioner's point of view (Liu and Chi, 2010). This chapter will summarize some of the key points from the draft guidance and the experts. However, it should be noted that, as indicated in the draft guidance, the draft is not ready for implementation but for discussions and suggestions. Nevertheless, it reflects the FDA's current thinking. Thus, this guidance should be viewed as regulatory recommendations rather than regulatory requirements.

In the next section, a brief description of the FDA draft guidance is given. Further interpretations of the two categories of adaptive designs (i.e., well understood and less-well understood adaptive designs) are discussed in Sections

16.3 and 16.4, respectively. Some principles for implementation of an adaptive design are given in Section 16.5.

16.2   The FDA Draft Guidance

As indicated in the draft guidance, an adaptive design clinical study is defined as a study that includes a prospectively planned opportunity for modification of one or more specified aspects of the study design and hypotheses based on analysis of data (usually interim data) from subjects in the study. Analyses of the accumulating study data are performed at prospectively planned timepoints within the study, can be performed in a fully blinded manner or in an unblinded manner, and can occur with or without formal statistical hypothesis testing. The term prospective here means that the adaptation was planned (and details specified) before data were examined in an unblinded manner by any personnel involved in planning the revision. There is a critical distinction between adaptations based on an interim analysis of unblinded results of the controlled trial (generally involving comparative analyses of study endpoints or outcomes potentially correlated with these endpoints) and adaptations based on interim noncomparative analysis of blinded data (including study endpoint data but also including data such as discontinuation rates and baseline characteristics). Revisions not previously planned and made or proposed after an unblinded interim analysis raise major concerns about study integrity (i.e., potential introduction of bias). Protocol revisions intended to occur after any unblinded analysis should be prospectively defined and carefully implemented to avoid risking irresolvable uncertainty in the interpretation of study results. In contrast, revisions based on blinded interim evaluations of data (e.g., aggregate event rates, variance, discontinuation rates, baseline characteristics) do not introduce statistical bias to the study or into subsequent study revisions made by the same personnel. Certain blinded-analysis-based changes, such as sample size revisions based on aggregate event rates or variance of the endpoint, are advisable procedures that can be considered and planned at the protocol design stage, but can also be applied when not planned from the study outset, if the study has remained unequivocally blinded. Thus, the major focus of this guidance is adequate and well-controlled effectiveness (A&WC) studies intended to provide substantial evidence of effectiveness required by law to support a conclusion that a drug is effective.

As pointed out by the FDA, this draft guidance is to give advice on topics such as (i) what aspects of adaptive design trials (i.e., clinical, statistical, regulatory) call for special consideration, (ii) when to interact with FDA while planning and conducting adaptive design studies, (iii) what information to include in the adaptive design for FDA review, and (iv) issues to consider in the evaluation of a completed adaptive design study. This guidance is intended to assist sponsors in planning and conducting adaptive design clinical studies and to facilitate an efficient FDA review. The FDA raises two principal issues concerning adaptive design methods in clinical trials which are:

• whether or not the adaptation process has led to design, analysis, or conduct flaws that have introduced bias that increases the chance of a false conclusion that the treatment is effective (a type I error)

• whether or not the adaptation process has led to positive study results that are difficult to interpret irrespective of having control of type I error

Based on the level of familarties, the guidance divides adaptive trials into two large categories, *well-understood* and *less well-understood* designs. The FDA's draft guidance discusses clinical, statistical, and regulatory aspects of a wide range of adaptive design clinical studies that can be proposed as part of a drug development program, including both familiar and less familiar approaches. The familiar design methods are included because they represent, in many cases, well-established and relatively low-risk means of enhancing study efficiency and informativeness that may deserve wider use. The less familiar design methods incorporate methodological features with which there is little experience in drug development at this time.

To avoid the potentially false positive rate increase and minimize the induced bias, it is suggested that well-understood adaptive design can be used for pivotal studies, whereas those not well-understood adaptive features are encouraged to be adopted in early exploratory phases first before applying them to the pivotal trials. In what follows, further discussions regarding the two categories of adaptive designs are provided.

16.3 Well-Understood Designs

The guidance elaborates generally well-understood adaptive designs that have valid approaches to implement. The FDA believes that for such designs, a considerable experience in modern drug development provides confidence that these design features and procedures will enhance efficiency while limiting risk of introducing bias or impairing interpretability. In what follows, some characteristics that are commonly seen in generally well-understood adative designs are outlined.

16.3.1 Adaptive entry criteria based on baseline data

The inclusion and exclusion criteria defined a target population for a study drug. However, such criteria may be found inappropriate or impractical. For instance, as stated in the draft guidance, examination of baseline characteristics of the accumulating study population might show that the expected population is not being enrolled and that by modifying eligibility criteria, subsequent subject enrollment may be shifted towards a population with greater numbers of patients with the desired characteristics. Similarly, if the study enrollment rate is substantially slower than expected, the screening log can be examined for noncritical entry criteria that might be modified to allow greater numbers of screened patients to qualify. The guidance further states that such examination of baseline information and modification of study eligibility criteria can contribute to timely completion of informative studies. Knowing the baseline characteristics of the overall study population at any time during the study does not generate concerns of introducing statistical bias as long as the treatment assignment remains blinded.

However, a substantial modification of inclusion and exclusion criteria can impair the interpretation of the study result, especially when the study population changes mid-way and an important relationship of treatment effect to the changed patient characteristic exists (i.e., a treatment-patient factor interaction). Exploratory analyses of the data obtained before and after the eligibility change can help to identify such problems. The draft guidance states firmly that because post-baseline patient data are not involved in the analyses, the study sponsor or investigator steering committee can review the baseline-data summaries and make design changes to the eligibility criteria without risk to the integrity of the study.

16.3.2 Sample size adjustment without unblinding

The guidance asserts that in the interest of maintaining the desired power of statistical test, reviewing interim data in a blinded fashion for sample size adjustment does not introduce statistical bias, and hence no statistical adjustment is required. For studies with continuous endpoints, the guidance indicates that sample size may be adjusted based on pooled variance. For studies using a time-to-event analysis, the interim and final sample size, which are usually based on the total number of events observed or time of last evaluation, may be the preferred design feature for adaptation. For studies with progressive diseases, an interim analysis of the aggregate rate of progression can be used to assess whether the duration of the study should be adjusted to allow for sufficient time to distinguish responses between treatment groups (given an assumed treatment-effect size). A combination of sample size and duration modification can also be applied in this case for maintaining the desired study power.

It should be noted that blinded interim analyses can also be used to adjust sample size for a subpopulation within the stratified baseline (e.g., by a genetic or disease-phenotype characteristic). The draft guidance indicates that the blinded interim analysis of the event rate (or, e.g., variance) can be done by subset, and study eligibility criteria modified to focus the remainder of the study on the subset(s) with the advantageous tendency (e.g., greater event rate, lower variance). A sample size readjustment could be considered at the same time. However, in practice, the intention of blinded interim analyses is to make decision or justification for a sample size increase, not for sample size reduction.

The draft guidance emphasizes that blinded interim analyses should not contain any information potentially revealing the between-group differences. A typical example is that a data display showing the distribution of aggregate interim results might reveal the presence and suggest a size of a treatment effect (e.g., a histogram showing a bimodal distribution of the endpoint data), and might influence the personnel making these adaptations.

16.3.3 Adaptations based on outcomes unrelated to efficacy

When the interim analysis is not based on any unblinded effectiveness-related data, the Type I error rate is then maintained/controlled, which does not require statistical adjustment. As an example, as indicated in the draft guidance, in a multiple group dose-response study, some doses might cause an unacceptable rate of a serious adverse effect or a less serious adverse effect sufficient to make the treatment unattractive. It is therefore important to look for these events at an interim stage of the study, and discontinue a dose group with unacceptable observed toxicity. If the adverse effect is completely independent of the treatment's benefit, then an unblinded analysis of the rate of the adverse effect provides no knowledge of the efficacy results, and the Type I error rate remains controlled without an adjustment. Similarly, if an unexpected serious toxicity is observed in safety monitoring, dropping the dose groups with excessive toxicity is usually appropriate. To ensure full awareness of the process and avoid missteps that could compromise the study integrity, the design and analysis plan should specify the number of groups to be terminated, how they will be selected, and the appropriate analysis procedures for testing the final data. Study planning should ensure that the personnel who make the modification decision (e.g., a steering committee) have not previously seen any unblinded efficacy analyses.The concern is that because the interim results are related to efficacy, the DMC might be biased in making any subsequent decisions about study modification.

16.3.4 Group sequential futility design

As pointed out earlier, a typical group sequential trial design is considered a well-understood adaptive design. Thus, a group sequential trial design with futility and/or efficacy stopping boundaries is considered a valid adaptive design and is widely accepted by the regulatory agencies worldwide and it is well described in the ICH E9 guideline since 1990s. A group sequential futility design usually includes an error-spending approach and it is not limited to one or two groups. For group sequential designs with more than two groups, multiplicity adjustment for multiple comparison should be taken into consideration.

The draft guidance points out that for the group sequential methods to be valid, it is important to adhere to the prospective analytic plan, terminating the group if a futility criterion is met and not terminating the study for efficacy unless the prospective efficacy criterion is achieved. Failure to follow the prospective plan in either manner risks confounding interpretation of the study results. Also, it is important to bear in mind that early termination for efficacy should generally be reserved for circumstances where there is the combination of compelling ethical concern and robust statistical evidence. A study terminated early will have a smaller size than the initially planned study size. It will therefore provide fewer safety data than planned. A potential also exists for more difficulty with the efficacy analysis and interpretation related to issues that become apparent only during the later detailed analysis (e.g., related to loss to follow-up or debatable endpoint assessments) and decreased power to assess patient subsets of interest.

In practice, clinical trials utilizing group sequential designs often establish an independent data monintoring committee (IDMC) to ensure the validity and integrity of the trials. IDMC usually performs its role/responsibility and function/activity according to an IDMC charter, which is an integral part of the study protocol. The draft guidance emphasizes that an independent, nonsponsor-controlled data monitoring committee (DMC) is an inherent part of the group sequential method's protection of study integrity. However, it is not clear which parties should prepare the analyses for the DMC for maintaining independence of the DMC. The draft guidance does not reach firm conclusion on this issue, but it is critical that the analyses be carried out either externally (and independently) to the study sponsor or by a group within the sponsor that is unequivocally separated (independently) from all other parties related to the study team.

16.3.5   Adaptations independent of treatment differences

In practice, a statistical analytic plan (SAP) for the clinical trial is often developed prior to database lock and/or unblinding. The SAP is often developed under certain assumptions regarding the distribution of the outcome data. As indicated in the draft guidance, generally, a prospective SAP should be written carefully and completely, and implemented without further changes once the study has started. However, if blinding has been unequivocally maintained, *limited* changes to the SAP late in the study can be considered. The ICH E9 guideline suggests that after a blinded inspection of the data, the SAP can be updated regarding the appropriate data transformations, adding covariates identified from other research sources or reconsideration of parametric vs. nonparametric analysis methods.

In some cases, with unequivocal assurance that unblinding has not occurred, changes in the primary endpoint, composition of the defined endpoint-event, or endpoint analytic sequence ordering may be considered. For example, a change in the primary endpoint may be useful when the predefined primary endpoint proves difficult to obtain and a substantial amount of missing data may occur for this assessment. In certain situations, the optimal statistical analysis plan may be difficult to specify fully before completing the study and examining the relevant characteristics of the final outcome data. If these characteristics are examined for the entire study population in a blinded manner, analytic plan modifications based on these characteristics do not introduce bias. The prospective analysis plan should clearly specify the characteristics and the procedure for selecting the analysis methodology based on these data characteristics.

Regarding the SAP, the draft guidance also indicates that an analytic plan might direct that if the amount of missing data in the preferred outcome assessment exceeds some prospectively stated criterion, a specified alternative outcome would be used as the primary efficacy endpoint. Similarly, when a composite event endpoint is used but there is uncertainty regarding the event rates to expect for the possible components, an analytic plan accommodating inclusion of one or two specific additional types of events might be appropriate if an insufficient number of events within the initial composite were observed in the overall study. In a similar manner, selection or sequential order of secondary endpoints might also be adapted.

16.4 Less Well-Understood Designs

16.4.1 Less well-understood adaptive designs

The draft guidance defines a less well-understood adaptive study design as a trial design with the characteristics that (i) there is relatively little *regulatory* experience, and (ii) its properties are not fully understood at this time. In practice, a less well-understood design is often proposed under the circumstances where the primary study objective(s) cannot be achieved by other (standard or well-understood) study designs. Thus, statistical methods for less well-understood designs are usually not yet developed due to the fact that its statistical/clinical properties are not fully understood at this time. As indicated in the draft guidance, the less well-understood adaptive design methods should be all based on unblinded interim analyses that estimate the treatment effect(s). In what follows, some less well-understoond designs utilizing various adaptations that mentioned in the draft guidance are discussed.

Adaptive dose-finding design - A typical example for less well-understood adaptive designs would be adaptive dose-finding studies, which allow dropping, modifying, and/or adding dose arms or regimens. Such highly flexible modifications should generally be limited to an exploratory study, but some of these approaches, when used with rigorous protection of the Type I error rate, might have a role in A&WC studies as pointed out by the draft guidance. Using this approach in an A&WC study will call for careful statistical adjustment to control the Type I error rate and should be limited to modest pruning of the number of dose groups.

Adaptive randomization design - For response-adaptive randomization, the draft guidance recommends that sponsors maintain randomization to the placebo group to ensure that sufficient patients are enrolled into the placebo group along the entire duration of the study. Examining an exploratory analysis of response over time within the placebo group, and examining exploratory comparisons of response in the placebo group to drug-treated groups by dividing the study into periods of enrollment, may help evaluate this concern for a completed study. Maintaining the placebo group will also best maintain the power of the study to show a treatment effect. It is also prudent to consider the treatment-effect estimate obtained from an adaptive randomization exploratory study cautiously, and this estimate should probably be used more conservatively in setting the sample size of a subsequent A&WC study to offset the potential over-estimate of effect size.

Flexible sample size re-estimation design - For sample size re-estimation based on unblinded data, the draft guidance suggests that estimates of treatment effect observed early in the study, when there are relatively fewer patient data, are generally variable and can be misleadingly large or small. Thus, those responsible for monitoring the study should act conservatively when deciding upon study changes using the early estimates. This is similar in spirit to the approach used in group sequential design alpha spending functions, where more conservative alpha spending is used early in the study.

Population adaptive design - For a population adaptive design based on unblind data, adaptive methods that have been proposed include (1) changing only the eligibility criteria, with no change in the study overall sample size and with the final analysis including the entire study population, or (2) modifying the plan for the final analysis to include only patients with the preferred characteristic. Other methods can increase the sample size for the population subset with the desired characteristic. For such trials, the draft guidance pointed out that these designs are less well understood, pose challenges in avoiding introduction of bias, and generally call for statistical adjustment to avoid increasing the type I error rate. Caution should be exercised in planning studies where an interim analysis and eligibility modification are performed multiple times, because when multiple revisions to the study population are made it may be challenging to obtain adequate estimates of the treatment effect in the populations of interest, or to interpret to what patient population the results apply.

Adaptive endpoint selection - For adaptive endpoint selections based on unblinded data, the draft guidance states that the primary endpoint revision usually takes one of two forms, replacement of the designated primary endpoint with an entirely new endpoint, or modification of the primary endpoint by adding or removing data elements to the endpoint (e.g., the discrete event types included in a composite event endpoint). In addition to prospectively stating all possible endpoint modifications, study designers should ensure that all possible choices are appropriate for the objective of the study (e.g., all possible primary endpoints in an A&WC study are clinical efficacy endpoints). It should be noted that this adaptive design approach is an alternative to a fixed design with two (or more) primary endpoints. The guidance suggested that "sponsors conducting an endpoint-adaptive study should be particularly alert to ensuring that the data on each endpoint are collected in a uniform manner with good quality, both before and after the interim analysis and design modification.

Adaptive noninferiority design - For adaptive noninferiorty design, the draft guidance mentioned that many design features of a noninferiority study may not be suitable for adaptation. The selection of the noninferiority margin is the key issue for noninferiority trials. Besides, the patient population enrolled in the study may also be difficult to change. The noninferiority margin is based on historical studies that had enrolled patients meeting specified criteria, and may apply only to a study population that is similar in important characteristics. Changing the enrolled patient population (e.g., to increase the rate of enrollment) to a population substantially different from that enrolled in the historical studies may compromise the validity of the noninferiority comparison. Similarly, adequate historical data on which to base a noninferiority margin are often available for only one endpoint, so that endpoint selection cannot be adaptively modified in the study.

Other less well-understood designs - Note that combinations of adaptations of various types in a single trial are included in the less well-understood category in the draft guidance. These adaptive designs include, but are not limited to, biomarker-adaptive design, adaptive-hypothesis design, adaptive drop-the-loser (or adaptive pick-the-winner) design, seamless adaptive design, two-stage adaptive design with different study objectives/endpoints, and multiple adaptive design as described in the previous chapters. For less well-understood adaptive designs, if accepted by the regulatory agency, statistical inference is often difficult, if not impossible, to obtain.

16.4.2 Statistical considerations

Control of type I error rate - As indicated earlier, the issue regarding the control of the overall type I error rate in a clinical trial utilizing an adaptive design regardless of whether it is well-understood or less well-understood is a great concern to both the investigator and the regulatory agency. The control of the overall type I error rate is a good clinical practice for patient protection. Thus, in the draft guidance, the FDA emphasizes that controlling the type I error rate for all involved hypotheses is best accomplished by prospectively specifying and including in the SAP all possible adaptations that may be considered during the course of the trial. The flexibility to apply such late changes should be reserved for situations where the change is limited in scope and is particularly important and should not to be proposed repeatedly during a study.

Statistical bias in estimates of treatment effect - For a clinical trial utilizing an adaptive design method, the possible introduction of operational biases after the adaptations is also a great concern to both the investigator and the regulatory agency. Major or significant operational bias would decrease the validity, reliability, and integrity of the study, and consequently the conclusion drawn could be misleading. Thus, the draft guidance states that inconsistent treatment effect estimates among the stages (before and after adaptations) of the study can make the overall treatment effect estimate difficult to interpret. The estimate of treatment effect(s) for an adaptive design A&WC study should be critically assessed at the completion of the study. It should be noted that in classical design, we almost never split data into several stages and examine the consistency across stages.

Clinical trial simulation - As pointed out by the FDA, many of the less well-understood and complex adaptive designs involve several adaptation decision points and many potential adaptations. For study designs that have multiple factors to be simultaneously considered in the adaptive process, it is difficult to assess design performance characteristics and guide sample size planning or optimal design choices because these characteristics might depend upon the adaptations that actually occur. In these cases, trial simulations performed before conducting the study can help evaluate the multiple-trial design options and the clinical scenarios that might occur when the study is actually conducted, and can be an important planning tool in assessing the statistical properties of a trial design and the inferential statistics used in the data analysis. Section IX of the draft guidance provides guidance for the format and content for the reporting of clinical trial simulation studies to be included in the adaptive design protocol and the SAP.

In general, clinical trial simulations rely on a statistical model of recognized important design features and other factors, including the posited rate of occurrence of clinical events or endpoint distribution, the variability of these factors among patient subsets, postulated relationships between outcomes and prognostic factors, correlation among endpoints, the time course of endpoint occurrence or disease progression, and the postulated patient withdrawal or dropout patterns, among others. More complex disease models or drug models might attempt to account for changing doses, changing exposure duration, or variability in bioavailability. The multiple ways to adapt, and the multiple ways to declare a study as positive can be simulated as part of study planning.

Some modeling and simulation strategies lend themselves to a Bayesian approach that might be useful. The Bayesian framework provides a way to posit models (i.e., priors) for the study design and the adaptive choices as they might probabilistically occur, and may aid in evaluating the impact of different assumed distributions for the parameters of the model and modeled sources of uncertainty. The Bayesian approach can be a useful planning tool at the study design stage to accommodate a range of plausible scenarios. Using Bayesian predictive probability, which depends upon probabilities of outcomes conditional on what has been observed up to an interim point in the adaptive study, may aid in deciding which adaptation should be selected, while the study design is still able to maintain statistical control of the Type I error rate in the frequentist design.

The draft guidance indicates that trial simulations can be helpful in comparing the performance characteristics among several competing designs under different scenarios (e.g., assumptions about drug effect such as the shape and location of the dose-response relationship, the magnitude of the response, differing responses in subgroups, the distribution of the subgroups in the enrolled population, the clinical course of the comparison group (usually the placebo group), and study dropout rate and pattern). The simulations will allow between-design comparisons of the probability of success of the trial for the objective (e.g., to lead to correct dose selection, to identify a response above a specific threshold, to identify the correct subgroup), and comparisons of the potential size of bias in the treatment-effect estimates. For drug development programs where there is little prior experience with the product, drug class, patient population, or other critical characteristics, clinical trial simulations can be performed with a range of potential values for relevant parameters encompassing the uncertainty in current knowledge.

In general, every adaptation may create a new hypothesis whose type I error rate should be controlled. There have been suggestions that because of the complexity resulting from multiple adaptations and the difficulty in forming an analytical evaluation, modeling and simulation provide a solution for demonstrating control of the type I error rate for these multiple hypotheses. Using simulations to demonstrate control of the type I error rate, however, is controversial and not fully understood.

For safety concern, the draft guidance recommends that sponsors should explore the features of different study designs with regard to the balance of efficiency (study size) and subject safety. Study simulations with multiple combinations of escalation criteria, dose-step size, and hypothetical-assumed relationships of exposure to severity and frequency of adverse events may be useful in evaluating different designs. These simulations can assist in assessing the risks and selecting a design that offers improved efficiency without increasing risk excessively. Depending on the rapidity of dose escalation in the design, it may be important to submit these simulations and analyses to FDA when the selected design is submitted.

For earlier design, with major extension sample size, the draft guidance suggests that development programs using adaptive design methods are sometimes intended to condense the development program into fewer fully independent studies, with more rapid advancement from small early studies into the large A&WC studies. This approach may lead to having only a limited amount of safety data available at the time that a large adaptive study is being planned that will entail a great increase in the number of patients exposed to the drug. This circumstance is in contrast to a typical non-adaptive development program where a large A&WC study would be preceded by shorter, moderate-sized exploratory studies and the safety data analyzed and considered to inform design of the larger study. There are advantages to the usual sequential approach that should be considered in selecting a study design. If there is a significant adverse effect that is inadequately understood or unrecognized because of the limited safety data of the very early studies, evaluating the data from a moderate-sized study might indicate that effect and lead to design changes to the large A&WC study to improve safety for patients within the A&WC study.

16.5   Adaptive Design Implementation

16.5.1   Content of an adaptive design protocol

When the FDA is asked to evaluate an adaptive design study (see also Section X of the draft guidance), the process is more challenging because of the complex decision criteria and processes inherent in some of these designs. The protocol and supporting documentation should contain all the information critical to allow a thorough FDA evaluation of the planned study. This documentation should include the rationale for the design, justification of design features, evaluation of the performance characteristics of the selected design (particularly less well-understood features), and plans to ensure study integrity when unblinded analyses are involved. Documentation of the rules of operation of the DMC (or other involved groups) should usually be more extensive than for conventional studies and should include a description of the responsibilities of each entity involved in the process.

16.5.2   Adequate documentation in adaptive trials

As indicated by the FDA, a complex adaptive design protocol cannot be carried out without an adequately detailed protocol, SAP, and supportive information. Protocols for adaptive design studies intended to be A&WC should include a detailed description of all of the important design and decision features of the proposed trial, such as the study's planned endpoints, design, criteria for success, hypotheses to be tested, conduct procedures, data management, and quality control. The SAP is an important part of that documentation because it states in detail the prospective hypotheses and statistical methods of analysis. The draft guidance recommends that the documentation for an adaptive design A&WC study should include the following:

• A summary of the relevant information about the drug product, including what is known at the present stage of development about the drug from other studies, and why an adaptive study design, in contrast to a non-adaptive design, has been chosen in this situation. The role of the chosen adaptive study design in the overall development strategy should also be discussed.

• A complete description of all the objectives and design features of the adaptive design, including each of the possible adaptations envisioned, the assumptions made in the study design with regard to these adaptations, the statistical analytical approaches to be used and/or evaluated, the clinical outcomes and quantitative decision models for assessing the outcomes, the relevant calculations that describe treatment effects, and the quantitative justifications for the conclusions reached in planning the trial.

• A summary of each adaptation and its impact upon critical statistical issues such as hypotheses tested, type I errors, power for each of the hypotheses, parameter estimates and confidence intervals, and sample size. In general, the study design should be planned in a frequentist framework to control the overall study type I error rate. A Bayesian framework that incorporates uncertainty into planning parameters in a quantitative manner (i.e., prior distributions on parameters) can also be useful for planning purposes to evaluate model assumptions and decision criteria. If models are used to characterize the event rates, disease progression, multiplicity of outcomes, or patient withdrawal rates, these models should be summarized clearly to allow evaluation of their underlying assumptions. Summary tables and figures should be included that incorporate all the important quantitative characteristics and metrics that inform the adaptive design.

- Computer simulations intended to characterize and quantify the level of statistical uncertainty in each adaptation and its impact on the type I error, study power (conditional, unconditional) or bias (in hypothesis testing and estimates of the treatment effect). The simulations should consider the impact of changes in a single design feature (e.g., the number of dose groups to be dropped), as well as the combination of all proposed adaptive features. The computer programs used in the simulations should be included in the documentation, as should graphical flowcharts depicting the different adaptive pathways that might occur, the probabilities of their occurrence, and the various choices for combining information from the choices.

- Full detail of the analytic derivations, if appropriate. For some adaptations, statistical calculations of the type I error and/or statistical bias in treatment-effect estimates can be performed analytically without using simulations. If the analytic approaches are based on published literature, the portions of the analytic approaches specifically relevant to the adaptive design employed should be provided in detail.

- The composition, written charter, and operating procedures for the personnel assigned responsibility for carrying out the interim analyses, adaptation selection, and any other forms of study monitoring. This information should include all the written agreements that the sponsor has in place and written assurances from the involved parties for the protection of information that should not be shared outside of the limited team with access to the unblinded data. A description of whether a sponsor-involved statistician will perform the unblinded analysis and/or whether sponsor-involved personnel (e.g., sponsor employees or contract research organization (CRO) staff) will make recommendations for the adaptation should be included. A well-trusted firewall established for trial conduct beyond those established for conventional group sequential clinical trials can help provide assurance that statistical and operational biases have not been introduced.

16.5.3 Interactions with FDA

As indicated in the draft guidance, FDA's review of an exploratory study protocol is usually focused upon the safety of the study participants and does not typically scrutinize the protocol as closely for design elements related to assessment of pharmacologic activity, efficacy, and strength of inferences. As resources allow, however, FDA might review exploratory protocols to consider the relevance of the information being gathered to guide the design of later studies (e.g., do the doses being examined seem reasonable for early efficacy evaluations; are the endpoints or biomarkers being examined reasonable for the stage of drug development).

For late stages of drug development, the FDA has a more extensive role in assessing the design of studies that contribute to substantial evidence of effectiveness. FDA's review focus in later stages of drug development continues to include safety of study subjects, but also includes ensuring that studies performed at this stage contain plans for assessment of safety and efficacy that will result in data of sufficient quality and quantity to inform a regulatory decision. Regulatory mechanisms for obtaining formal, substantive, feedback from FDA on design of the later stage trials and their place in the drug development program are well established, e.g., the End-of-Phase 2 (EOP2) meeting and Special Protocol Assessments (SPA).

Due to the complexity of adaptive design, the FDA suggested sponsors to work with the FDA in the protocol design as early as possible. The draft guidance reminds the sponsors that it is important to recognize that the use of less well-understood adaptive methods may limit the FDA's ability to offer such an assessment. FDA may be unable to assess in advance whether the adaptively selected aspects of drug use (e.g., dose, regimen, population) will be sufficiently justified by the study results. As usual, FDA will review and comment to the extent possible on aspects of the drug's use that the sponsor considers well defined, as well as non-adaptive aspects of the study.

16.5.4   Special protocol assessments

As indicated in the draft guidance, special protocol assessments (SPA) entail timelines (45-day responses) and commitments that may not be best suited for adaptive design studies. The full review and assessment of a study using less well-understood adaptive design methods can be complex, will involve a multidisciplinary evaluation team, and might involve extended discussions among individuals within different FDA offices before reaching a conclusion. If there has been little or no prior discussion between FDA and the study sponsor regarding the proposed study and its adaptive design features, other information requests following initial FDA evaluation are likely and full completion of study assessment within the SPA 45-day time frame is unlikely. Sponsors are therefore encouraged to have thorough discussions with FDA regarding the study design and the study's place within the development program before considering submitting an SPA request.

FDA also indicates that even when adequate advance discussion has occurred, the nature of a full protocol assessment of an adaptive design study may not be the same as for an SPA request for a conventional study, as one or more critical final decisions regarding study design are made after the study has started. FDA cannot realistically commit to accepting aspects of study design yet to be determined. Thus, although an adaptive design SPA request that had been preceded by adequate advance discussion, enabling a complete protocol review, the FDA response may have certain limitations that an SPA regarding a non-adaptive study would not require.

16.5.5   Execution and documentation

As indicated in the draft guidance, SOPs for clinical trials utilizing adaptive trial designs are necessarily developed. It is well recognized that SOPs for an adaptive design study with an unblinded interim analysis are likely to be more complex than SOPs for nonadaptive studies to ensure that there is no possibility of bias introduction. This written documentation should include (1) identification of the personnel who will perform the interim analyses, and who will have access to the interim results, (2) how that access will be controlled and verified, and how the interim analyses will be performed, including how any potential irregularities in the data (e.g., withdrawals, missing values) will be managed, and (3) how adaptation decisions will be made. Other issues that should be addressed in these SOPs are (1) whether or not there are any foreseeable impediments to complying with the SOPs, (2) how compliance with the SOPs will be documented and monitored, and (3) what information, under what circumstances, is permitted to be passed from the DMC to the sponsor or investigators. It is likely that the measures defined by the SOPs will be related to the type of adaptation and the potential for impairing study integrity.

The FDA suggests that the sponsor summarize comprehensive information regarding the whole adaptive trial. Complete information describing the study conduct should include the following:

• information on compliance with the planned adaptive process and procedures for maintaining study integrity,

• description of the processes and procedures actually carried out when there were any deviations from those planned,

• records of the deliberations and participants in the internal discussions by any committees (e.g., DMC meeting minutes, steering or executive committee meeting minutes) involved in the adaptive process,

• results of the interim analysis used for the adaptation decisions (including estimates of treatment effects, uncertainty of the estimates, and hypothesis tests at that time),

• assessment of adequacy of any firewalls established to limit dissemination of information in prospectively designed adaptive trials and postpectively designed adaptive trials.

16.6 Concluding Remarks

The intention of the FDA draft guidance on adaptive clinical trial designs is to assist the sponsors for maintaning the quality, validity, and integrity of the clinical trials utilizing adaptive trial design. Due to its flixibility, the use of adaptive design methods in clinical trials has become very popular in clinical research. However, adaptive design methods are often misused or abused in clinical trials especially for those less well-understood and complicated designs. Misuse and/or abuse of the adaptive design methods in clinical trials could have negative impact on the intended clinical research. It could not only lead to the failure of the intended clinical research, but also cause a disaster to the medical community and public health. Thus, it is strongly suggested that the FDA draft guidance be followed by closely monitoring the quality, validity, and integrity of the clinical trials utilizing adaptive trial designs.

Based on recent experience regarding some regulatory submissions of clinical trials utilizing adaptive design, the following questions are commonly asked by the FDA for maintaining the quality, validity, and integrity of the clinical trials. First, the FDA requires possible operational biases be identified and clinical strategies for preventing/reducing and/or controlling these operational biases be provided. In addition, the FDA requires that detailed information regarding how the overall type I error rate is controlled be provided, especially when a less well-understood adaptive trial designs is used. Moreover, the FDA also requires that detailed information regarding valid statistical methods for assessment of the treatment effect under investigation be provided. This is critical, especially when those less well-understood adaptive trial designs are used.

Chapter 17

Case Studies

As indicated earlier, the adaptation or modification made to a clinical trial includes prospective adaptation (by design), concurrent or on-going adaptation (ad hoc), and retrospective adaptation (at the end of the trial and prior to database lock or unblinding). Different adaptations or modifications could lead to different adaptive designs with different levels of complexity. In practice, it is suggested that by design prospective adaptation be considered at the planning stage of a clinical trial (Gallo et al. 2006) although it may not reflect real practice in the conduct of clinical trials. Li (2006) pointed out that the use of adaptive design methods (either by design adaptation or ad hoc adaptation) provides a second chance to re-design the trial after seeing data internally or externally at interim. However, it may introduce so-called operational biases such as selection bias, method of evaluations, early withdrawal, and modification of treatments. Consequently, the adaptation employed may inflate type I error rate. Uchida (2006) also indicated that these biases could be translated to information (assessment) biases, which may include (i) patient enrollment, (ii) differential dropouts in favor of one treatment, (iii) crossover to the other treatment, (iv) protocol deviation due to additional medications/treatments, and (v) differential assessment of the treatments. As a result, it is difficult to interpret the clinically meaningful effect size for the treatments under study (see also, Quinlan, Gallo, and Krams, 2006).

In the next section, basic considerations when implementing adaptive design methods in clinical trials are given. Successful experience for the implementation of adaptive group sequential design (see, e.g., Cui, Hung, and Wang, 1999), adaptive dose-escalation design (see, e.g., Chang and Chow, 2005), and seamless adaptive phase II/III trial design (see, e.g., Maca, et al., 2006) are discussed in Section 17.2, Section 17.3, and Section 17.4, respectively.

313

17.1   Basic Considerations

As discussed in the early chapters of this book, the motivation behind the use of adaptive design methods in clinical trials includes (i) the flexibility in modifying trial and statistical procedures for detecting any signals or trends (preferably identifying best clinical benefits) of a test treatment under investigation, and (ii) the efficiency in shorten the development time of the test treatment. In addition, adaptive designs provide the investigator a second chance to re-design the trial with more relevant data observed (internally) or clinical information available (externally) at interim. The flexibility and efficiency are very attractive to investigators and/or sponsors. However, major adaptation may alter trial conduct and consequently result in a biased assessment of the treatment effect. Li (2006) suggested a couple of principles when implementing adaptive designs in clinical trials: (i) adaptation should not alter trial conduct and (ii) type I error should be preserved. Following these principles and FDA's draft guidance, some studies with complicated adaptation may be more successful than others. In what follows, some basic considerations when implementing adaptive design methods in clinical trials are discussed.

Dose and Dose Regimen

Dose selection is an integral part of clinical development. An inadequate selection of dose for a large confirmatory trial could lead to a failure of the development of the compound under study. Traditional dose-escalation and/or dose de-escalation studies are not efficient. The objective of dose or dose regimen selection is not only to select the best dose group but also to drop the least efficacious or unsafe dose group with a limited number of patients available. Under this consideration, adaptive designs with appropriate adaptation in selection criteria and decision rules are useful.

Study Endpoints

Maca et al. (2006) suggested that well-established and well-understood study endpoints or surrogate markers be considered when implementing adaptive design methods in clinical trials, especially when the trial is to learn about the primary endpoints to be carried forward into later phase clinical trials. An adaptive design would not be feasible for clinical trials with not well-established or not well-understood study endpoints due to (i) uncertainty of the treatment effect, and (ii) a clinically meaningful difference cannot be determined.

Treatment Duration

For a given study endpoint, treatment duration is critical in order to reach the optimal therapeutic effect. If the treatment duration is short relative to the time needed to enroll all patients planned for the study, then an adaptive design such as response-adaptive randomization design is feasible. On the other hand, if the treatment duration is too long, too many patients would be randomized during the period which could result in unacceptable inefficiencies. In this case, it is suggested that an adaptive biomarker design be considered.

Logistical Considerations

Logistical considerations relative to the feasibility of adaptive designs in clinical trials include, but are not limited to (i) drug management, (ii) site management, and (iii) procedural consideration. For costly and/or complicated dose regimen, drug packaging and drug supply could be a challenge to the use of adaptive design methods in clinical trials, especially when the adaptive design allows dropping the inferior dose groups. Site management is referred to the selection of qualified study sites and patient recruitment for the trial. For some adaptive designs, recruitment rate is crucial to the success of the trial, especially when the intention of the trial is to shorten the time of development. Procedural consideration is referred to decision processes and dissemination of information in order to maintain the validity and integrity of the trial.

Independent Data Monitoring Committee

When implementing an adaptive design in a clinical trial, an independent data monitoring committee (IDMC) is necessarily considered for maintaining the validity and integrity of the clinical trial. A typical example is the implementation of an adaptive group sequential design which cannot only allow stopping a trial early due to safety and/or futility/efficacy, but also address sample size re-estimation based on the review of unblinded data. In addition, IDMC conveys some limited information to investigators or sponsors about treatment effects, procedural conventions, and statistical methods with recommendations so that the adaptive design methods can be implemented with less difficulty.

17.2   Adaptive Group Sequential Design

Group Sequential Design

Group sequential design is probably one of the most commonly used clinical trial designs in clinical research and development. As indicated in Chapter 6, the primary reasons for conducting interim analyses of accrued data are probably due to (i) ethical consideration, (ii) administrative reasons, and (iii) economic constraints. Group sequential design is very attractive because it allows stopping a trial early due to (i) safety, (ii) futility, and/or (iii) efficacy. Moreover, it also allows adaptive sample size adjustment at interim either blinding or unblinding through an independent data monitoring committee (DMC).

Adaptation

Basic adaptation strategy for an adaptive group sequential design is that one or more interim analyses may be planned. In practice, it is desirable to stop a trial early if the test compound is found to be ineffective or not safe. However, it is not desirable to terminate a trial early if the test compound is promising. To achieve these goals, data safety monitoring and interim analyses for efficacy are necessarily performed. Note that how to control the overall type I error rate and how to determine treatment effect that the trial should be powered at the time of interim analyses would be the critical issues for this adaptation.

At each interim analysis, an adaptive sample size adjustment based on un-blinded interim results and/or external clinical information available at interim may be performed. In practice, at the planning stage of a clinical trial, a pre-study power analysis is usually conducted based on some initial estimates of the within or between patient variation and the clinically meaningful differ-ence to be detected. This crucial information is usually not available or it is available (e.g., data from small pilot studies) with a high degree of uncertainty (Chuang-Stein et al., 2006). Lee, Wang, and Chow (2006) showed that sample size obtained based on estimates from small pilot studies is highly instable. Thus, there is a need to adjust sample size adaptively at interim. Mehta and Patel (2006) and Offen et al. (2006) also discussed other situations where sam-ple size re-estimation at interim are necessary. The use of an independent data monitoring committee (DMC) would be the critical issue for this adaptation.

Other adaptation such as adaptive hypotheses from a superiority trial to a non-inferiority trial may be considered. In practice, interim results may indicate that the trial will never achieve statistical significance at the end of the trial. In this case, the sponsors may consider changing the hypotheses or study endpoints to increase the probability of success of the trial. A typical example is to switch from superiority hypotheses to noninferiority hypotheses. At the end of the trial, final analysis will be performed for testing noninferiority rather than superiority. Note that superiority can still be tested after the noninferiority has been established without paying any statistical penalty due to the closed testing procedure. Note that the determination of the noninferiority margin would be the challenge for this adaptation.

Statistical Methods

For the adaptation of interim analyses, statistical methods as described in Chapter 6 for controlling the overall type I error rate are useful. For the adap-tation of sample size re-estimation, the methods proposed by Cui, Hung, and

Wang (1999), Fisher's combination of p-values, error function method, inverse normal method, or linear combination of p-values can be used. For the adaptation of switching hypotheses, statistical methods discussed in Chapter 4 are useful. As indicated by Chuang-Stein et al. (2006), since the weighting of the normal statistics will not, in general, be proportional to the sample size for that stage, the method does not use the sufficient statistics (the unweighted mean difference and estimated standard deviation from combined stages) for testing, and is therefore less efficient (Tsiatis and Mehta, 2003). Additional discussion on efficiency can be found in Burman and Sonesson (2006) and Jennison and Turnbull (2006a).

Case Study - An Example

For illustration purposes, consider the example given in Cui, Hung, and Wang (1999). This example considers a phase III two-arm trial for evaluating the effect of a new drug for prevention of myocardial infection (MI) in patients undergoing coronary artery bypass graft surgery. It was estimated that a sample size of 300 patients per group would give a 95% power for detecting a 50% reduction in incidence rate from 22% to 11% at the one-sided significance level of $\alpha = 0.025$. Although the sponsor was confident about the incidence rate of 11% in the control group, they were not sure about the 11% incidence rate in the test group. Thus, an interim analysis was planned to allow for sample size re-estimation based on observed treatment difference. The interim analysis was scheduled when 50% of the patients were enrolled and had their efficacy assessment. The adaptive group sequential using the method of Fisher's combination of stage-wise p-values was considered. The decision rules were: at Stage 1, stop for futility if the stage-wise p-value $p_1 > \alpha_0$ and stop for efficacy if $p_1 \leq \alpha_1$; at the final stage, if $p_1 p_2 \leq C_\alpha$, claim efficacy; otherwise claim futility. The stopping boundary was chosen from Table 8.5.1. The futility boundary $\alpha_0 = 0.5$, the efficacy stopping boundary $\alpha_1 = 0.0102$ at Stage 1 and $C_\alpha = 0.0038$ at the final stage. The upper limit of the sample size is $N_{max} = 800$ per group. The futility boundary was used to stop the trial in the case of a very small effect size because in such a case, to continue the trial would result in a unrealistic large sample size or N_{max} with insufficient power. The adaptive group sequential design would have a 99.6% power when the incidence rates were 22% and 11%, and an 80% power when the incidence rates were 22% and 16.5%.

At interim analysis based on data from 300 patients, it was observed that the test group had an incidence rate of 16.5% and 11% in the control group. If these incidence rates were the true incidence rates, the power for the classical design would be about 40%. Under the adaptive group sequential design, the sample size was re-estimated to be 533 per group. If the 16.5% and 11% are the true incidence rates, the conditional power is given by 88.6%.

Remarks Note that the trial was originally designed not allowing for sample size re-estimation. The sponsor requested sample size re-estimation and was rejected by the FDA. The trial eventually failed to demonstrate statistical significance. In practice, it is recommended that the adaptation for sample size re-estimation be considered in the study protocol and an independent data monitoring committee (IDMC) be established to perform sample size re-estimation based on the review of unblinded date at interim for maintaining the validity and integrity of the trial.

17.3   Adaptive Dose-Escalation Design

Traditional Dose-Escalation Design

As discussed in Chapter 5, the traditional "3+3" escalation rule is commonly considered in phase I dose-escalation trials for oncology The "3+3" rule is to enter three patients at a new dose level and then enter another three patients when dose limiting toxicity is observed. The assessment of the six patients is then performed to determine whether the trial should be stopped at the level or to increase the dose. The goal is to find the maximum tolerated dose (MTD). The traditional "3+3" rule (TER) is not efficient with respect to the number of dose-limiting toxicities and the estimation of MTD. There is a practical need to have a better design method that will reduce the number of patients and number of DLTs, and at the same time, have a more precise estimation of MTD. We will use the Bayesian continual reassessment method (CRM) to achieve our goals.

Adaptation

The basic adaptation strategy for an adaptive dose-escalation trial design is change in the traditional escalation rule (TER). As discussed in Chapter 5, the traditional "3+3" dose-escalation rule is not efficient. As a result, a m+n dose-escalation rule may be considered with some pre-specified selection criteria based on the dose limiting toxicity (DLT). Other adaptations that are commonly considered include the application of adaptation to the design characteristics such as the selection of starting dose, the determination of dose levels, prior information on the maximum tolerable dose (MTD), dose toxicity model, stopping rules, and statistical methods.

Statistical Methods

As indicated earlier, many methods such as the assessment of dose response using multiple-stage designs (Crowley, 2001) and the continued re-assessment method (CRM) are available in the literature for assessment of dose-escalation trials. For the method of CRM, the dose-response relationship is continually re-assessed based on accumulative data collected from the trial. The next patient who enters the trial is then assigned to the potential MTD level. This approach is more efficient than that of the usual TER with respect to the allocation of the MTD. However, the efficiency of CRM may be at risk due to delayed response and/or a constraint on dose-jump in practice (Babb and Rogatko, 2004). Chang and Chow (2005) proposed an adaptive method that combines CRM and utility-adaptive randomization (UAR) for multiple-endpoint trials. The proposed UAR is an extension of the response-adaptive randomization (RAR). Note that the CRM could be a Bayesian, a frequentist, or a hybrid frequentist-Bayesian based approach. As pointed out by Chang and Chow (2005), this method has the advantage for achieving the optimal design by means of the adaptation to the accrued data of the on-going trial. In addition, CRM could provide a better prediction of dose-response relationship by selecting an appropriate model as compared to the method simply based on the observed response.

Case Study - An Example

A trial is designed to establish the dose-toxicity relationship and to identify maximum tolerable dose (MTD) for a compound in treatment of patients with metastatic androgen independent prostate cancer. Based on pre-clinical data, the estimated MTD is about 400 mg/m^2. The modified Fibonacci series is chosen for the dose levels (in Table 17.3.1). Eight dose levels are considered in this trial with the option of adding more dose levels if necessary. The initial dose level is chosen to be 30 mg/m^2, at which about 10% of deaths (MELD10) occur in mice after the verification that no lethal and no life-threatening effects were seen in another species. The toxicity rate (i.e., the DLT rate) at MTD defined for this indication/population is 17%.

We compare the operating characteristics between the traditional escalation rule (TER) design and the CRM design. In CRM, the following logistic model is used

$$p = \frac{1}{1 + 150 \exp(-ax)},$$

where the prior distribution for parameter a is flat over (0,0.12).

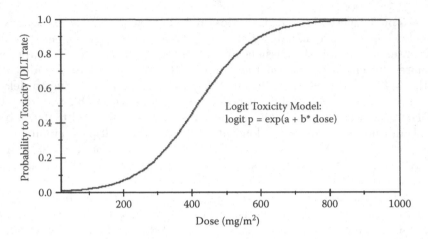

Figure 17.3.1: Example of dose-toxicity model.

Using ExpDesign Studio®, the simulation results are presented as follows. The TER predicts the MTD at dose level 7 (lowest dose level to the true MTD) with a probability of 75%. The CRM predicted the MTD at dose level 7 with a probability of 100% (5,000 out of 5,000 simulations). The TER requires an average of 18.2 patients and 2.4 DLTs per trial. CRM requires only 12 patients with 4 DLTs per trial.

Table 17.3.1: Dose Levels and DLT Rates

Dose level	1	2	3	4	5	6	7	8
dose	30	60	99	150	211	280	373	496
DLT rate	0.010	0.012	0.017	0.026	0.042	0.071	0.141	0.309

Remarks A dose-escalation trial is an early phase trial with flexible adaptation for dose selection using CRM. It is suggested that the protocol should be submitted to the Regulatory Agencies for review and approval prior to the initiation of the trial. The design characteristics such as starting dose, dose levels, prior information on the MTD, dose toxicity model, escalation rule, and stopping rule should be clearly stated in the study protocol. In practice, there may be a situation that the next patient has enrolled before the response from the previous patient is obtained. In this case, the efficiency of the TER and CRM may be reduced. There may also be limitation for dose escape which may also reduce the efficiency of the CRM. To investigate this, a simulation was conducted using ExpDesign Studio with cluster randomization of size 3 patients (i.e., 2 patients have enrolled before the response is obtained). In the simulation, we allow for one level of dose escape. Under this scenario, the CRM requires only 12 patients with 1.8 DLTs. It can be seen that with the limitation of dose escalation, the average DLTs per trial is reduced from 4 to 2 without sacrificing the precision. This is because with 12 patients there is enough precision to eliminate the precision loss due to the delayed response. Note that when we use CRM, we need to do the modeling or simulation at real time such that the next dose level can be determined quickly.

17.4 Two-Stage Phase II/III Adaptive Design

Seamless Phase II/III Design

A seamless phase II/III trial design is a design that combines a traditional phase IIb trial and a traditional phase III trial into a single trial. As a result, the study objectives of a seamless design are the combination of the objectives which have been traditionally addressed in separate trials. This type of design closes the gap of the time that would have occurred between the two trials which are traditional trials conducted separately. Maca et al. (2006) defines an seamless adaptive phase II/III design as a seamless phase II/III design that would use data from patients enrolled before and after the adaptation in the final analysis. Thus, the feasibility and/or efficiency of an seamless adaptive phase II/III trial design depend upon the adaptation employed. In practice, it is possible to combine studies into a seamless design within or across phases of clinical development. Seamless designs are useful in early clinical development since there are opportunities in the seamless transition between phase IIb (learning phase) and phase III (confirming phase).

Adaptation

The basic adaptation strategy for a seamless phase II/III trial design is to drop the inferior arms (or drop the losers) based on some pre-specified criteria at the learning phase. The best arms and the control arm will be retained and advanced to the confirming phase. Other commonly employed adaptations include (i) enrichment process at the learning phase of the trial and (ii) change in treatment allocation at the confirming phase. The enrichment process is commonly employed to identify sub-populations, which are most likely to response to the treatment or to suffer from adverse events based on some pre-specified criteria on genomic biomarkers. Change in treatment allocation at the confirming phase is to not only to have more patients assigned to superior arms but also to increase the probability of success of the trial. In practice, it is not uncommon to apply an adaptation on the primary study endpoint. For example, at the learning phase, the treatment effect may be assessed based on a short-term primary efficacy endpoint (or a surrogate endpoint or some biomarkers), while a long-term primary study endpoint is considered at the confirming phase. It should be noted that the impact on statistical inference should be carefully evaluated when implementing an adaptation to a seamless trial design.

Methods

For a seamless adaptive phase II/III trial design, if the trial is not stopped for lack of efficacy after the first stage, we proceed into the second stage. At the end of the second stage, we may calculate the second stage p-value based upon the disjoint sample of the second stage only. The final analysis is conducted by combining the two p-values into a single test statistic using a predefined combination function. The method proposed by Sampson and Sill (2005) for dropping the losers in normal case, and the contrast test with p-value combination method suggested by Chang, Chow and Pong (2006) are useful. Note that a data-dependent combination rule should not be used after the first stage. It is suggested that a prior be considered at the planning phase.

Thall, Simon, and Ellenberg (1989) proposed a two-stage design for trials with binary outcomes. In their proposed two-stage design, the first stage is used to select the best treatment, and the second stage includes just the selected treatment together with the control. As indicated by Thall, Simon and Ellenberg (1989), the inclusion of the control in the first stage is crucial because it allows results from that stage to be pooled with the data observed in the second stage. On the other hand, Schaid, Wieand, and Therneau (1990) considered a time-to-event endpoint. Their design not only allows stopping the trial early for efficacy after the first stage, but also allows more than one treatment to continue into the second stage. Stallard and Todd (2003) generalized these designs to allow for the possibility of more than two stages by using error spending functions. The design is applicable for general endpoint such as normal, binary, ordinal, or survival time. These methods are useful for seamless adaptive phase II/III trial designs.

Remarks   Note that the methods considered above are based on the same primary endpoint. As an alternative, Todd and Stallard (2005) considered an adaptive group sequential design that incorporates treatment selection based upon a short-term endpoint, followed by a confirmation stage comparing the selected treatment with control in terms of a long-term primary endpoint.

Case Study - Some Examples

In what follows, several examples are provided to illustrate the implementation of seamless adaptive phase II/III trial designs in clinical trials. The first three examples are adopted from Maca et al. (2006).

Example 17.4.1: Adaptive Treatment Selection Similar to the study design described in Bauer and Kieser (1999), a seamless adaptive phase II/III two-stage design is considered to evaluate the efficacy and safety of a compound when given in combination with methotrexate to patients with active rheumatoid arthritis (RA) who have had two or more inadequate responses to anti-TNF therapy (Maca et al., 2006). The objectives of this trial include treatment selection and efficacy confirmation. The primary clinical endpoint is ACR-20 (American College of Rheumatology 20 score) at 6 months. The first stage will be used for dose selection, while the second stage is for efficacy confirmation. At the end of the second stage, data obtained from the second stage and the relevant data from the first stage will be combined for final analysis using Fisher's combination test at the significance level of 0.025. In this adaptive seamless phase II/III two-stage design, early stopping is allowed for futility, but not for efficacy.

Qualified subjects will be randomly assigned to five treatment arms (four active and one placebo) in equal ratio. At the end of the first stage, a planned interim analysis will be conducted. The best active treatment arm and the placebo arm will be retained and advanced to the second stage for efficacy confirmation. The best treatment arm will be selected based on a set of predefined efficacy, safety, and immunogenicity criteria. Based on interim results, the following decisions (i) the best treatment group (safe and efficacious) will be advanced to the second stage, (ii) the least efficacious and/or unsafe treatment groups will be dropped, and (iii) the futility requirement will be evaluated. All these decisions will be made based upon the clinical endpoint in conjunction with information obtained from early endpoint. To ensure the validity and integrity of the trial design, two committees will be established: one is an external independent Data Monitoring Committee (DMC) and the other one is an internal Executive Decision Committee (EDC).

Example 17.4.2: Confirming Treatment Effect A seamless phase II/III trial design is employed to confirm substantial treatment effect in patients with neuropathic pain (Maca, et al., 2006). The primary endpoint considered in this trial is the PI-NRS score change from baseline to the 8th week of treatment. Qualified patients will be randomly assigned to four treatment groups (three active doses and one placebo) at equal ratio. An adaptation for having two interim analyses is planned prior to the end of the enrollment period. Another adaptation to select best dose and change treatment allocation at first interim is also made. Note that patients are initially equally randomized to three doses of the new compound and placebo. Two interim analyses are planned before the end of enrollment period. At the second interim, one dose will be selected to continue for confirmation of treatment effect. Final analysis will use a p-value combination test to confirm the superiority of the selected dose over placebo.

As compared to the traditional approach of a phase IIb trial with three doses and placebo based on a short-term endpoint (e.g., 2 weeks change from baseline) followed by a confirmatory phase III trial with a long-term (e.g., 8-week) endpoint, this adaptive design combines the two trials in one study with a single protocol and uses information on the long-term endpoint from patients in the first (learning) and the second (confirmatory) phases of the study. Note that a longitudinal model for the primary endpoint in time (i.e., at 2 weeks, 4 weeks, 6 weeks, and 8 weeks) can be used to improve the estimate of the sustained treatment effect.

Example 17.4.3: Confirming Efficacy in Subpopulation Maca et al. (2006) presented an example concerning a clinical trial using a two stage adaptive design trial for patients with metastatic breast cancer. This trial has two objectives. First, it is to select patient population at the first stage. Second, it is to confirm the efficacy based on the hazard ratio between treatment and control at the second stage. In addition, a genomic biomarker (expression level) was used. Patients were initially randomized into three treatment arms (two actives and one control) in equal ratio. One interim analysis was planned for this study when the trial reached approximately 60% of the targeted events. During the interim analysis, two subpopulations were defined based on whether the biomarker expression level of each subject of that population exceeds a pre-defined cutoff value. Data were analyzed for efficacy evaluation and safety assessment for both populations. A decision was made based on patients advanced to the second stage. Moreover, a futility was also assessed at this interim analysis. The final analysis was performed using the inverse normal p-value combination test for the selected population to confirm the superiority of the selected dose over control. In contrast to a conventional design with one phase IIb for population selection followed by a confirmatory Phase III study, this trial design was able to achieve the same objectives

Example 17.4.4 The objective of this trial in patients with asthma is to confirm sustained treatment effect, measured as FEV1 change from baseline to the one-year of treatment. Initially, patients are equally randomized to four doses of the new compound and placebo. Based on early studies, the estimated FEV1 change at four-weeks are 6%, 13%, 15%, 16%, and 17% (with pooled standard deviation 18%) for the placebo (dose level 0), dose level 2, 3, and 4, respectively. One interim analysis is planned when 50% patients have their short term efficacy assessment (4-week change from baseline). The interim analysis will lead to either picking the winner (arm with best observed response) or early stopping for futility with a very conservative stopping boundary. The selected dose and placebo will be used at Stage 2. The final analysis will use a sum of the stage-wise p-values from both stages. (Note that the Fisher's combination of p-values was not used because it does not provide a design with futility stopping only. In other work, Fisher's combination is not efficient for adaptive design with no early efficacy stopping). The stopping boundaries are shortened from Table 17.4.2: $\alpha_1 = 0$, $\beta_1 = 0.25$, $\alpha_2 = 0.2236$. The decision rule will be: if $p_1 > \beta_1$, stop the trial; if $p_1 \leq \beta_1$, proceed to the second stage. At the final analysis, if $p_1 + p_2 \leq 0.2236$, claim efficacy, otherwise claim futility. The p_1 is the p-value from a contrast test based on sub-sample from stage 1.

Table 17.4.1: Seamless Design

Arms	0	1	2	3	4
4-week FEV1 change	0.06	0.12	0.13	0.14	0.15
Contrasts		-0.54	0.12	0.13	0.14	0.15

With the maximum sample size of 120 per group, the power is 91.2% at overall one-sided α−level of 0.025. The expected total sample size is 240 and 353 under the null hypothesis and the alternative hypothesis, respectively. As mentioned early the method controled the type I error under a global null hypothesis.

Issues and Recommendations

Seamless adaptive trial designs are very attractive to the sponsors in pharmaceutical development. It helps in identifying best treatment in a more efficient way with certain accuracy and reliability within a relatively short timeframe. In practice, the following issues are commonly encountered when implementing a seamless trial design.

Clinical development time As indicated earlier, the primary rationale behind the use of an adaptive seamless trial design is to shorten the time of development. Thus, it is important to consider whether a seamless development program would accomplish the goal for reducing the development time. In practice, it is clear if the seamless trial is the only pivotal trial required for regulatory submission. However, if the seamless trial is one of the two pivotal trials required for registration, the second pivotal trial should be completed in a timely fashion, which can shorten the overall development time. During the planning stage, the additional time required for the second seamless trial must be included in the evaluation of the overall clinical development time.

Statistical Inference   As indicated by Maca et al. (2006), data analysis for seamless trials may be problematic due to bias induced by the adaptation employed. This bias of the maximum likelihood estimate of the effect of the selected treatment over the control could lead to an inaccurate coverage for the associated confidence interval. As a result, it is suggested that the test comparing the selected treatment with the control must be adjusted to give a correct type I error rate. Estimates of treatment effect must also be adjusted to avoid statistical bias and produce confidence intervals with correct coverage probability. Brannath, Koening, and Bauer (2003) derived a set of repeated confidence intervals by exploiting the duality of hypothesis tests and confidence intervals. This approach, however, is strictly conservative if the trial stops at the interim analysis. Alternatively, Posch et al. (2005) proposed a more general approach is to use for each null hypothesis a different combination test. Stallard and Todd (2005) evaluated the bias of the maximum likelihood estimate and proposed a bias adjusted estimate. Using a stage-wise ordering of the sample space, they also construct a confidence region for the selected treatment effect.

Decision Process   Seamless Phase II/III trials usually involve critical decision making at the end of the learning phase. A typical approach is to establish an independent data monitoring committee (IDMC) to monitor ongoing trials. For an adaptive seamless phase II/III trial design, the decision process may require additional expertise not usually represented on IDMCs, which may require sponsor's input or at least sponsor's ratification on IDMC's recommendation. Maca et al. (2006) pointed out several critical aspects that are relevant to the decision process in seamless phase II/III designs. These critical aspects include (i) composition of the decision board, (ii) process for producing analysis results, (iii) sponsor representation, (iv) information inferable from the selection decision, and (v) regulatory perspectives.

For the composition of the decision board, it is not clear whether all of the study objectives or adaptation of a seamless trial at the learning phase should be addressed by the same board or by separate boards. There seems to be no universal agreement on which approach is a correct approach. Maca et al. (2006) suggested that if it is decided that a single board would suffice, then at a minimum, it should be strongly considered whether the composition of the board should be broadened to include individuals not normally represented on a DMC who have proper perspective and experience in making the selection decision; for example, individuals with safety monitoring expertise may not have relevant experience in dose selection. On the other hand, if separate boards are used, then the members of the board making the selection decision should in general only review unblinded data at the selection point and should only see results relevant to the decision they are charged to make. For the process of producing analysis results, results should be produced by an independent statistician and/or programmer who should provide the results directly to the appropriate IDMC for review. For sponsor representation, as indicated in a recent FDA guidance, the following principles should be followed (FDA, 2005c):

- Sponsor representatives who will participate in the recommendation, or be allowed to ratify the recommendation, are adequately distanced from trial activities, i.e., they do not have other trial responsibilities, and should have limited direct contact with people who are involved in the day-to-day management of the trial.

- Sponsor representation is minimal to meet the needs, i.e., the smallest number of sponsor representatives which can provide the necessary perspective is involved, these individuals see the minimum amount of unblinded information needed to participate in the decision process, and only at the decision point.

- Appropriate protections and firewalls are in place to ensure that knowledge is appropriately limited, e.g., procedures and responsibilities are clearly documented and understood by all parties involved, confidentiality agreements reflecting these are produced, secure data access and transfer processes are in place, etc.

For information inferable from the selection decision, as a general principle, knowledge regarding which treatment groups continuing into the confirming phase should be perceived to provide only minimal information without potentially biasing the conduct of the trial. Care should be taken to limit the information to personnel who may infer from a particular selection decision. For regulatory perspectives, it is strongly recommended that a regulatory reviewer be consulted when implementing seamless adaptive trial designs in appropriate clinical development programs in order to maintain the validity and integrity of the trial.

Bibliography

[1] Arbuck, S. G. (1996). Workshop on phase I study design. *Annals of Oncology*, 7, 567-573.

[2] ASCO Special Article. (1997). Critical role of phase I clinical trials in cancer treatment. *Journal of Clinical Oncology*, I5, 853–859.

[3] Atkinson, A.C. (1982). Optimum biased coin designs for sequential clinical trials with prognostic factors. *Biometrika*, 69, 61-67.

[4] Atkinson, A.C., and Donev, A.N. (1992). *Optimum Experimental Designs*. Oxford University Press, New York, New York.

[5] Babb, J. S., and Rogatko, A. (2001). Patient specific dosing in a cancer phase I clinical trial. *Statistics in Medicine*, 20, 2079-2090.

[6] Babb, J.S., and Rogatko, A. (2004). Bayesian methods for cancer phase I clinical trials, *Advances in Clinical Trial Biostatistics*, Nancy L. Geller (ed.), Marcel Dekker, New York, New York.

[7] Babb, J., Rogatko, A., and Zacks. S. (1998). Cancer phase I clinical trials. Efficient dose escalation with overdose control. *Statistics in Medicine*, 17, 1103-1120.

[8] Bandyopadhyay, U., and Biswas A. (1997). Some sequential tests in clinical trials based on randomized play-the-winner rule. *Calcutta. Stat. Assoc. Bull.*, 47, 67-89.

[9] Banerjee, A., and Tsiatis, A.A. (2006). Adaptive two-stage designs in phase II clinical trials. *Statistics in Medicine*, In press.

[10] Basford K.E., Greenway D.R., McLachlan G.J., and Peel D. (1997). Standard Errors of Fitted Component Means of Normal Mixtures. *Computational Statistics*, 12, 1-17.

[11] Bauer, P. (1999). Multistage testing with adaptive designs (with discussion). *Biometrie und Informatik in Medizin und Biologie*, 20, 130-148.

[12] Bauer, P., and Kieser, M. (1999). Combining different phases in development of medical treatments within a single trial. *Statistics in Medicine*, 18, 1833-1848.

[13] Bauer, P., and Köhne, K (1994). Evaluation of experiments with adaptive interim analysis. *Biometrics*, 50, 1029-1041.

[14] Bauer, P., and Köhne, K. (1996). Evaluation of experiments with adaptive interim analyses. *Biometrics*, 52, 380 (Correction).

[15] Bauer, P., and König, F. (2006). The reassessment of trial perspectives from interim data – a critical view. *Statistics in Medicine*, 25, 23-36.

[16] Bauer, P., and Röhmel, J. (1995). An adaptive method for establishing a dose-response relationship. *Statistics in Medicine*, 14, 1595-1607.

[17] Bechhofer, R.E., Kiefer, J., and Sobel, M. (1968). *Sequential Identification and Ranking Problems*. University of Chicago Press, Chicago, Illinois.

[18] Benda, N., Brannath, W., Bretz, F., Burger, H.-U., Friede, T., Maurer, W., and Wang, S.J. (2010). Perspectives on the use of adaptive designs in clinical trials. Part II. Panel Discussion. *Journal of Biopharmaceutical Statistics*, 20, 1098-1112.

[19] Berry, D.A. (2005). Introduction to Bayesian methods III: use and interpretation of Bayesian tools in design and analysis. *Clinical Trials*, 2, 295-300.

[20] Berry, D.A., and Eick, S.G. (1995). Adaptive assignment versus balanced randomization in clinical trials: a decision analysis. *Statistics in Medicine*, 14, 231-246.

[21] Berry, D.A., and Fristedt, B. (1985). *Bandit Problems: Sequential Allocation of Experiments*. Chapman Hall, London.

[22] Berry, D.A., Müller, P., Grieve, A.P., Smith, M., Parke, T., Blazek, R., Mitchard, N., and Krams, M. (2002). Adaptive Bayesian designs for dose-ranging drug trials. In *Case Studies in Bayesian Statistics V*. Lecture Notes in Statistics. Springer, New York. 162 –181.

[23] Berry, D.A., and Stangl, D.K. (1996). *Bayesian Biostatistics*. Marcel Dekker, Inc. New York, New York.

[24] Berry, S.M., Carlin, B.P., Lee, J.J., and Muller, P. (2011). *Bayesian Adaptive Methods for Clinical Trials*. Chapman and Hall/CRC Press, Taylor & Francis, New York.

[25] Birkett, N.J. (1985). Adaptive allocation in randomized controlled trials. *Controlled Clinical Trials*, 6, 146-155.

[26] Bischoff, W., and Miller, F. (2005). Adaptive two-stage test procedures to find the best treatment in clinical trials. *Biometrika*, 92, 197-212.

[27] Blackwell, D., and Hodges, J.L., Jr. (1957). Design for the control of selection bias. *Annal of Mathematical Statistics*, 28, 449-460.

[28] Brannath, W., Koening, F., and Bauer, P. (2003). Improved repeated confidence bounds in trials with a maximal goal. *Biometrical Journal*, 45, 311–324.

[29] Brannath, W., Posch, M., and Bauer, P. (2002). Recursive combination tests. *Journal of American Statistical Association*, 97, 236–244.

[30] Branson M., and Whitehead W. (2002). Estimating a treatment effect in survival studies in which patients switch treatment. *Statistics in Medicine*, 21, 2449-2463.

[31] Bretz, F., and Hothorn, L.A. (2002). Detecting dose-response using contrasts: asymptotic power and sample size determination for binary data. *Statistics in Medicine*, 21, 3325-3335.

[32] Bronshtein, I.N., Semendyayev, K.A., Musiol, G., and Muehlig, H. (2004). *Handbook of Mathematics*. Springer-Verlag Berlin Heidelberg.

[33] Brophy, J.M., and Joseph, L. (1995). Placing trials in context using Bayesian analysis. GUSTO revisited by reverend Bayes [see comments]. *Journal of American Medical Association*, 273, 871-875.

[34] Burman, C.F., and Sonesson, C. (2006). Are flexible designs sound? *Biometrics*, In press.

[35] Casciano, D.A., and Woodcock, J. (2006). Empowering microarrays in the regulatory setting. *Nature Biotechnology*, 24, 1103.

[36] Chaloner, K., and Larntz, K. (1989). Optimal Bayesian design applied to logistic regression experiments. *Journal of Planning and Inference*, 21, 191-208.

[37] Chang, M. (2005a). Bayesian adaptive design with biomarkers. Presented at IBC's Second Annual Conference on *Implementing Adaptive Designs for Drug Development*, November 7-8, 2005, Nassau Inn, Princeton, New Jersey.

[38] Chang, M. (2005b). A simple n-stage adaptive design, submitted.

[39] Chang, M. (2007). Adaptive design method based on sum of p-values, *Statistics in Medicine*, 26, 2772–2784.

[40] Chang, M. (2010). *Monte Carlo Simulation for the Pharmaceutical Industry: Concepts, Algorithms, and Case Studies*. Chapman and Hall/CRC press, Taylor & Frances, New York.

[41] Chang, M., and Chow, S.C. (2005). A hybrid Bayesian adaptive design for dose response trials. *Journal of Biopharmaceutical Statistics*, 15, 667-691.

[42] Chang, M., and Chow, S.C. (2006a). Power and sample size for dose response studies. In *Dose Finding in Drug Development*. Ed. Ting, N. Springer, New York, New York.

[43] Chang, M., and Chow, S.C. (2006b). An innovative approach in clinical development - utilization of adaptive design methods in clinical trials. Unpublished manuscript.

[44] Chang, M., and Chow, S.C. (2007). Analysis strategies for multiple-endpoint adaptive design. *Journal of Biopharmaceutical Statistics*, 17, 1189-1200.

[45] Chang, M., Chow, S.C., and Pong, A. (2006). Adaptive design – issues, opportunities, and recommendations. *Journal of Biopharmaceutical Statistics*, 16, 299-309.

[46] Chang, M.N. (1989). Confidence intervals for a normal mean following group sequential test. *Biometrics*, 45, 249-254.

[47] Chang, M.N., and O'Brien, P.C. (1986). Confidence intervals following group sequential test. *Controlled Clinical Trials*, 7, 18-26.

[48] Chang, M.N., Wieand, H.S., and Chang, V.T. (1989). The bias of the sample proportion following a group sequential phase II trial. *Statistics in Medicine*, 8, 563-570.

[49] Chang, M., and Chow, S.C. (2007). Analysis strategies for multiple-endpoint adaptive designs. Journal of Biopharmaceutical Statistics, 17, 1189-1200.

[50] Channon, E.J. (2000). Equivalence testing in dose-reponse study, *Drug Information Journal*, 34, 551–562.

[51] Chen, J.J., Tsong, Y., and Kang S. (2000). Tests for equivalence or non-inferiority between two proportions, *Drug Information Journal*, 34, 569-578.

[52] Chen, T.T. (1997). Optimal three-stage designs for phase II cancer clinical trials. *Statistics in Medicine*, 16, 2701-2711.

[53] Chen, T.T., and Ng, T.H. (1998). Optimal flexible designs in phase II cancer clinical trials. *Statistics in Medicine*, 17, 2301-2312.

[54] Cheng, B., and Chow, S.C. (2010). On flexibility of adaptive designs and criteria for choosing a good one – a discussion of FDA draft guidance. *Journal of Biopharmaceutical Statistics*, 20, 1171-1177.

[55] Cheng, B., and Chow, S.C. (2011). Multi-stage transitional seamless trial designs with different objectives and endpoints. Submitted.

[56] Chevret, S. (1993). The continual reassessment method in cancer phase I clinical trials: A simulation study. *Statistics in Medicine*, 12, 1093-1108.

[57] Chow, S.C. (2005). Randomized trials stopped early for benefit. Presented at Journal Club, Infectious Diseases Division, Duke University School of medicine, Durham, North Carolina.

[58] Chow, S.C. (2006). Adaptive design methods in clinical trials. *International Chinese Statistical Association* bulletin January, 2006, 37-41.

[59] Chow, S.C. (2010). Changing with the times. *European Biopharmaceutical Review*, October Issue, 48-52.

[60] Chow, S.C. (2011). *Controversial Statistical Issues in Clinical Trials*. Chapman and Hall/CRC Press, Taylor & Francis, New York.

[61] Chow, S.C., and Chang, M. (2006). *Adaptive Design Methods in Clinical Trials*. Chapman and Hall/CRC Press, Taylor & Francis, New York.

[62] Chow, S.C., and Chang, M. (2008). Adaptive design methods in clinical trials – a review. *The Orphanet Journal of Rare Diseases*, 3, 11-18.

[63] Chow, S.C., Chang, M., and Pong, A. (2005). Statistical consideration of adaptive methods in clinical development. *Journal of Biopharmaceutical Statistics*, 15, 575-591.

[64] Chow, S.C., and Liu, J.P. (2004). *Design and Analysis of Clinical Trials*. 2nd edition, John Wiley & Sons, New York, New York.

[65] Chow, S.C., and Shao, J. (2002). *Statistics in Drug Research*. Marcel Dekker, Inc., New York, New York.

[66] Chow, S.C., and Shao, J. (2005). Inference for clinical trials with some protocol amendments. *Journal of Biopharmaceutical Statistics*, 15, 659-666.

[67] Chow, S.C., and Shao, J. (2006). On margin and statistical test for non-inferiority in active control trials. *Statistics in Medicine*, 25, 1101-1113.

[68] Chow, S.C., Shao, J., and Hu, Y.P. (2002). Assessing sensitivity and similarity in bridging studies. *Journal of Biopharmaceutical Statistics*, 12, 385-400.

[69] Chow, S.C., Shao, J., and Wang, H. (2003). *Sample Size Calculation in Clinical Research*. Marcel Dekker, Inc., New York, New York.

[70] Chow, S.C., Shao, J., and Wang, H. (2008). *Sample Size Calculation in Clinical Research.* 2nd Edition, Chapman Hall/CRC Press, Taylor & Francis, New York, New York.

[71] Chow, S.C., and Tu, Y.H. (2008). On two-stage seamless adaptive design in clinical trials. *Journal of Formosan Medical Association*, 107, No. 12, S51-S59.

[72] Chow, S.C., Lu, Q., and Tse, S.K. (2007). Statistical analysis for two-stage adaptive design with different study endpoints. *Journal of Biopharmaceutical Statistics*, 17, 1163-1176.

[73] Chuang-Stein, C. and Agresti A. (1997). A review of tests for detecting a monotone dose-response relationship with ordinal response data. *Statistics in Medicine*, 16, 2599-2618.

[74] Chuang-Stein, C. Anderson, K., Gallo, P., and Collins, S. (2006). Sample size re-estimation. Submitted.

[75] Coad, D.S., and Rosenberger, W.F. (1999). A comparison of the randomized play-the-winner and the trianglar test for clinical trials with binary responses. *Statistics in Medicine*, 18, 761-769.

[76] Coburger, S., and Wassmer, G. (2003). Sample size reassessment in adaptive clinical trials using a bias corrected estimate. *Biometrical Journal*, 45, 812–825.

[77] Cohen, A., and Sackrowitz, H.B. (1989). Exact tests that recover interblock information in balanced incomplete block design. *Journal of American Statistical Association*, 84, 556-559.

[78] Conawav, M. R., and Petroni, G. R. (1996). Designs for phase I I trials allowing for a trade-off between response and toxicity. *Biometrics*, 52, 1375-1386.

[79] Conley, B.A., and Taube, S.E. (2004). Prognostic and predictive markers in cancer. *Dis Markers*, 20, 35-43.

[80] Cox, D.R. (1952). A note of the sequential estimation of means. *Proc. Camb. Phil. Soc.*, 48, 447-450.

[81] Cox, D.R., and Oakes, D. (1984). *Analysis of Survival Data.* Monographs on Statistics and Applied Probability. Chapman & Hall, London.

[82] Cox, D.R., and Snell, E.J. (1968). A general definition of residuals (with discussion). *Journal of the Royal Statistical Society*, 8, 30, 248-275.

[83] Crowley, J. (2001). *Handbook of Statistics in Clinical Oncology*, Marcel Dekker, Inc., New York, New York.

[84] CTriSoft Intl. (2002). Clinical Trial Design with ExpDesign Studio, www.ctrisoft.net.

[85] Cui. L., Hung, H.M.J., and Wang, S.J. (1999). Modification of sample size in group sequential trials. *Biometrics*, 55, 853-857.

[86] Decoster, G., Stein, G., and Ioldener. E. E. (1990). Responses and toxic deaths in phase I clinical trials. *Annals of Oncology*, 1, 175-181.

[87] DeMets, D.L., and Ware, J.H. (1980). Group sequential methods for clinical trials with a one-sided hypothesis. *Biometrika*, 67, 651-660.

[88] DeMets, D.L., and Ware, J.H. (1982). Asymmetric group sequential boundaries for monitoring clinical trials. *Biometrika*, 69, 661-663.

[89] Demidenko , E. (2007). Sample site determination for logistic regression revisited. *Statistics in Medicine*, 26, 3385-3397.

[90] Dempster A.P., Laird N.M., and Rubin D.B. (1977). Maximum likelihood estimation from incomplete data via the EM algorithm (with discussion). *J. Roy. Statist. Soc.* B, 39, 1–38.

[91] Dent. S. F. and Fisenhauer, F. A. (1996). Phase I trial design: Are new methodologies being put into practice? *Annals of Oncology*, 6, 561-566.

[92] Dunnett, C.W. (1955). A multiple comparison procedure for comparing several treatments with a control. *Journal of American Statistical Association*, 50, 1076-1121.

[93] East (2010). Cytel, Inc., EastSurvAdapt, Cambridge, MA, (2010).

[94] Efron, B. (1971). Forcing a sequential experiment to be balanced. *Biometrika*, 58, 403-417.

[95] Efron, B. (1980). Discussion of Minimum chi-square, not maximumlikelihood. *Annal of Statistics*, 8, 469-471.

[96] Efron B., and Tibshirani R.J. (1993). *An Introduction to the Bootstrap.* Chapman and Hall, New York, New York.

[97] Eichhorn, B. H., and Lacks. S. (1981). Bayes sequential search of an optimal dosage: Linear regression with both parameters unknown. *Communications in Statistics - Theory and Methods*, 10, 931-953.

[98] Ellenberg, S.S., Fleming, T.R., and DeMts, D.L. (2002). *Data Monitoring Committees in Clinical Trials – A Practical Perspective*, John Wiley and Sons, New York, New York.

[99] EMEA. (2002). Point to Consider on *Methodological Issues in Confirmatory Clinical Trials with Flexible Design and Analysis Plan.* The European Agency for the Evaluation of Medicinal Products Evaluation of Medicines for Human Use. CPMP/EWP/2459/02, London, UK.

[100] EMEA. (2004). Point to Consider on the *Choice of Non-inferiority Margin*. The European Agency for the Evaluation of Medicinal Products Evaluation of Medicines for Human Use. London, UK.

[101] EMEA. (2006). Reflection paper on *Methodological Issues in Confirmatory Clinical Trials with Flexible Design and Analysis Plan*. The European Agency for the Evaluation of Medicinal Products Evaluation of Medicines for Human Use. CPMP/EWP/2459/02, London, UK.

[102] Ensign, L.G., Gehan, E.A., Kamen, D.S., and Thall, P.F. (1994). An optimal three-stage design for phase II clinical trials. *Statistics in Medicine*, 13, 1727-1736.

[103] Faries, D. (1994). Practical modifications of the continual reassessment method for phase I cancer cliitical trials. *Journal of Biopharmaceutical Statistics*, 4, 147-164.

[104] FDA. (1988). Guideline for *Format and Content of the Clinical and Statistical Sections of New Drug Applications*. The United States Food and Drug Administration, Rockville, Maryland.

[105] FDA. (2000). Guidance for *Clinical Trial Sponsors On the Establishment and Operation of Clinical Trial Data Monitoring Committees*. The United States Food and Drug Administration, Rockville, Maryland.

[106] FDA. (2005a) Draft Guidance on *Multiplex Tests for Heritable DNA Markers, Mutations, and Expression Patterns*, The United States Food and Drug Administration, Rockville, Maryland, USA.

[107] FDA. (2005b). The draft concept paper on Drug-Diagnostic Co-Development, The United States Food and Drug Administration, Rockville, Maryland, USA.

[108] FDA. (2005c). Draft Guidance for *Clinical Trial Sponsors. Establishment and Operation of Clinical Trial Data Monitoring Committees*. The United States Food and Drug Administration, Rockville Maryland. http://www.fda.gov/cber/qdlns/clintrialdmc.htm.

[109] FDA. (2007) Draft Guidance on *In Vitro Diagnostic Multivariate Index Assays*, The United States Food and Drug Administration, Rockville, Maryland, USA.

[110] FDA. (2010a). Draft Guidance for Industry – *Adaptive Design Clinical Trials for Drugs and Biologics*, The United States Food and Drug Administration, Rockville Maryland, Feb, 2010.

[111] FDA. (2010b). Guidance for Industry – *Noninferiority Clinical Trials*. The United States Food and Drug Administration, Rockville, Maryland.

[112] Feng, H., Shao, J., and Chow, S.C. (2007). Adaptive group sequential test for clinical trials with changing patient population. *Journal of Biopharmaceutical Statistics*, 17, 1227-1238.

[113] Fleiss J.L., Levin B., and Paik M.C. (2003). *Statistical Methods for Rates and Proportions.* John Wiley and Sons, New York.

[114] Follman, D.A., Proschan M.A., and Geller, N.L. (1994). Monitoring pairwise comparisons in multi-armed clinical trials. *Biometrics*, 50, 325–336.

[115] Friedman, B. (1949). A simple urn model. *Comm. Pure Appl. Math.*, 2, 59-70.

[116] Gallo, P., Anderson, K., Chuang-Stein, C., Dragalin, V., Gaydos, B., Krams, M., and Pinheiro, J. (2010). Viewpoint on the FDA draft adaptive designs guidance from the PhRMA working group (with discussions). *Journal of Biopharmaceutical Statistics*, 20, 1115-1177.

[117] Gallo, P., Chuang-Stein, C., Dragalin, V., Gaydos, B., Krams, M., and Pinheiro, J. (2006). Adaptive design in clinical drug drug development - an executive summary of the PhRMA Working Group (with discussions). *Journal of Biopharmaceutical Statistics*, 16, No. 3, 275-283.

[118] Gasprini, M., and Eisele, J. (2000). A curve-free method for phase I clinical trials. *Biometrics*, 56, 609-615.

[119] Gatsonis. C., and Ireenlmuse, B. (1992). Bayesian methods For phase I clinical trials. *Statistics in Medicine*, 11, 1377-1389.

[120] Gelman, A., Carlin, J.B., and Rubin, D.B. (2003). *Bayesain Data Analysis.* 2nd Ed. Chapman & Hall/CRC. New York, New York.

[121] Gillis,P.R., and Ratkowsky, D.A. (1978). The behaviour of estmators of the parameters of various yield-density relationships. *Biometrics*, 34, 191-198.

[122] Goodman, S.N. (1999). Towards evidence-based medical statistics I: the p-value fallacy. *Annals of Internal Medicine*, 130, 995-1004.

[123] Goodman, S.N.(2005). Introduction to Bayesian methods I: measuring the strength of evidence. *Clinical Trials*, 2, 282-290.

[124] Goodman, S. N., Lahurak, M.L., and Piantadosi, S. (1995). Some practical improvements in the continual reassessment method for phase I studies. *Statistics in Medicine*, 5, 1149-1161.

[125] Gould, A.L. (1992). Interim analyses for monitoring clinical trials that do not maternally affect the type I error rate. *Statistics in Medicine,* 11, 55-66.

[126] Gould, A.L. (1995). Planning and revising the sample size for a trial. *Statistics in Medicine*, 14, 1039-1051.

[127] Gould, A.L. (2001). Sample size re-estimation: recent developments and practical considerations. *Statistics in Medicine*, 20, 2625-2643.

[128] Gould, A.L., and Shih, W.J. (1992). Sample size re-estimation without unblinding for normally distributed outcomes with unknown variance. *Communications in Statistics - Theory and Methodology*, 21, 2833-2853.

[129] Hallstron, A., and Davis, K. (1988). Imbalance in treatment assignments in stratified blocked randomization. *Controlled Clinical Trials*, 9, 375-382.

[130] Hamasaki, T., Isomura, T., Baba, M., and Goto, M. (2000). Statistical approaches to detecting dose–response relationships. *Drug Information Journal*, 34, 579–590.

[131] Hardwick, J.P., and Stout, Q. F. (1991). Bandit strategies for ethical sequential allocation. *Computing Science and Stat.*, 23, 421-424.

[132] Hardwick, J.P., and Stout, Q. F. (1993). Optimal allocation for estimating the product of two means. *Computing Science and Stat.*, 24, 592-596.

[133] Hardwick, J.P., and Stout, Q.F. (2002). Optimal few-stage designs. *Journal of Statistical Planning and Inference*, 104, 121-145.

[134] Hawkins, M. J. (1993). Early cancer clinical trials: safety, numbers, and consent. *Journal of the National Cancer Institute*, 85, 1618-1619.

[135] Hedges. L.V., and Olkin, I. (1985). *Statistical Methods for Meta-analysis*. Academic Press, New York, New York.

[136] Hellmich, M. (2001). Monitoring clinical trials with multiple arms. *Biometrics*, 57, 892-898.

[137] Hochberg, Y. (1988). A sharper Bonferroni's procedure for multiple tests of significance. *Biometrika*, 75, 800-803.

[138] Holmgren, E.B. (1999). Establishing equivalence by showing that a specified percentage of the effect of the active control over placebo is maintained. *Journal of Biopharmaceutical Statistics*, 9, 651-659.

[139] Hommel, G. (2001). Adaptive modifications of hypotheses after an interim analysis. *Biometrical Journal*, 43, 581-589.

[140] Hommel, G., and Kropf, S. (2001). Clinical trials with an adaptive choice of hypotheses. *Drug Information Journal*, 33, 1205-1218.

[141] Hommel, G., Lindig, V., and Faldum, A. (2005). Two stage adaptive designs with correlated test statistics. *Journal of Biopharmaceutical Statistics*, 15, 613-623.

[142] Horwitz, R.I. and Horwitz, S.M. (1993). Adherence to treatment and health outcomes. *Annals of Internal Medicine*, 153, 1863–1868.

[143] Hothorn, L. A. (2000). Evaluation of animal carcinogenicity studies: Cochran-Armitage trend test vs. multiple contrast tests. *Biometrical Journal*, 42, 553-567.

[144] Hu, F.F., and Rosenberger , W.F. (2007). *The Theory of Response-Adaptive Randomization in Clinical Trials.* John Wiley. Hoboken, NJ.

[145] Hughes, M.D. (1993). Stopping guidelines for clinical trials with multiple treatments. *Statistics in Medicine*, 12, 901-913.

[146] Hughes, M.D., and Pocock, S.J. (1988). Stopping rules and estimation problems in clinical trials. *Statistics in Medicine*, 7, 1231-1242.

[147] Hung, H.M.J., Wang, S.J., and O'Neill, R. (2007). Statistical considerations for testing multiple endpoints in group sequential or adaptive clinical trials. *Journal of Biopharmaceutical Statistics*, 17, 1201-1210.

[148] Hung, H.M.J., Wang, S.J., Tsong, Y., Lawrence, J., and O'Neil, R.T. (2003). Some fundmental issues with noninferiority testing in active controlled trials. *Statistics in Medicine*, 22, 213-225.

[149] Hung, H.M.J., Cui, L, Wang, S.J., and Lawrence, J. (2005). Adaptive statistical analysis following sample size modification based on interim review of effect size. *Journal of Biopharmaceutical Statistics*, 15, 693-706.

[150] ICH (1996). International Conference on Harmonization tripartite Guideline for Good Clinical Practice.

[151] ICH E9 Expert Working Group (1999). Statistical principles for clinical trials (ICH Harmonized Tripartite Guideline E9). *Statistics in Medicine*, 18, 1905-1942.

[152] Inoue, L.Y.T., Thall, P.F. and Berry, D.A. (2002). Seamlessly expanding a randomized phase II trial to phase III. *Biometrics*, 58, 823–831.

[153] Ivanova, A. (2006). Escalation, up-and-down and A+B designs for dose-finding trials, *Statistics in Medicine*, 25, 3668-3678.

[154] Ivanova, A., and Flournoy, N. (2001). A birth and death urn for ternary outcomes: stochastic processes applied to urn models. In *Probability and Statistical Models with Applications*. Ed. Charalambides, C. A., Koutras, M. V., and Balakrishnan, N. Chapman and Hall/CRC Press, Boca Raton, 583-600.

[155] Ivanova, A., Liu, K., Snyder, E., and Snavely, D. (2009). An adaptive design for identifying the dose with best efficacy/tolerability profile with application to crossover dose-finding study. *Statistics in Medicine*, 28, 2941-2951.

[156] Jennison, C., and Turnbull, B.W. (1990). Statistical approaches to interim monitoring of medical trials: a review and commentary. *Statistics in Medicine*, 5, 299-317.

[157] Jennison, C., and Turnbull, B.W. (2000). *Group Sequential Method with Applications to Clinical Trials*, Chapman & Hall/CRC, New York, New York.

[158] Jennison, C., and Turnbull, B.W. (2003). Mid-course sample size modification in clinical trials based on the observed treatment effect. *Statistics in Medicine*, 22, 971-993.

[159] Jennison, C., and Turnbull, B.W. (2005). Meta-analysis and adaptive group sequential design in the clinical development process. *Journal of Biopharmaceutical Statistics*, 15, 537-558.

[160] Jennison, C., and Turnbull, B.W. (2006a). Adaptive and non-adaptive group sequential tests. *Biometrika*, 93, 1-21.

[161] Jennison, C., and Turnbull, B.W. (2006b). Efficient group sequential designs when there are several effect sizes under consideration. *Statistics in Medicine*, 25, 917-932.

[162] Johnson, N.L., and Kotz, S. (1972). *Distribution in Statistics*. Houghton Mifflin Company, Boston, MA.

[163] Johnson, N. L., Kotz, S., and Balakrishnan, N. (1994). *Continuous Univariate Distributions*, Vol. 1, John Wiley & Sons, New York, New York.

[164] Kalbfleisch, J.D., and Prentice, R.T. (1980). *The Statistical Analysis of Failure Time Data*. Wiley, New York, New York.

[165] Kelly, P.J., Sooriyarachchi, M.R., Stallard, N., and Todd, S. (2005). A practical comparison of group-sequential and adaptive designs. *Journal of Biopharmaceutical Statistics*, 15, 719-738.

[166] Kelly, P.J., Stallard, N., and Todd, S. (2005). An adaptive group sequential design for phase II/III clinical trials that select a single treatment from several. *Journal of Biopharmaceutical Statistics*, 15, 641-658.

[167] Khatri, C.G., and Shah, K.R. (1974). Estimation of location of parameters from two linear models under normality. *Communications in Statistics*, 3, 647-663.

[168] Kieser, M., Bauer, P., and Lehmacher, W. (1999). Inference on multiple endpoints in clinical trials with adaptive interim analyses. *Biometrical Journal*, 41, 261-277.

[169] Kieser, M., and Friede, T. (2000). Re-calculating the sample size in internal pilot study designs with control of the type I error rate. *Statistics in Medicine*, 19, 901-911.

[170] Kieser, M., and Friede, T. (2003). Simple procedures for blinded sample size adjustment that do not affect the type I error rate. *Statistics in Medicine*, 22, 3571-3581.

[171] Kim, K. (1989). Point estimation following group sequential tests. *Biometrics*, 45, 613-617.

[172] Kimko, H.C., and Duffull, S.B. (2003). *Simulation for Designing Clinical Trials*, Marcel Dekker, Inc., New York, New York.

[173] Kramar, A., Lehecq, A., and Candalli, E. (1999). Continual reassessment methods in phase I trials of the combination of two drugs in oncology. *Statistics in Medicine*, 18, 1849-1864.

[174] Krams, M., Burman, C.F., Dragalin, V., Gaydos, B., Grieve, A.P., Pinheiro, J., and Maurer, W. (2007). Adaptive designs in clinical drug development: opportunities, challenges, and scope reflections following PhRMA's November 2006 Workshop. *Journal of Biopharmaceutical Statistics*, 17, 957-964.

[175] Lachin, J.M. (1988). Statistical properties of randomization in clinical trials. *Controlled Clinical Trials*, 9, 289-311.

[176] Lan, G.K.K. (2002). Problems and issues in adaptive clinical trial design. Presented at New Jersey Chapter of the American Statistical Association, Piscataway, New Jersey, June 4, 2002.

[177] Lan, K.K.G., and DeMets, D.L. (1983). Discrete sequential boundaries for clinical trials. *Biometrika*, 70, 659-663.

[178] Lan, K.K.G., and DeMets, D.L. (1987). Group sequential procedures: calendar versus information time. *Statistics in Medicine*, 8, 1191-1198.

[179] Lee, Y., Wang, H., and Chow. S.C. (2006). A bootstrap-median approach for stable sample size determination based on information from a small pilot study. Unpublished manuscript.

[180] Lehmacher, W., Kieser, M., and Hothorn, L. (2000). Sequential and multiple testing for dose-response analysis. *Drug Information Journal*, 34, 591-597.

[181] Lehmacher, W., and Wassmer, G. (1999). Adaptive sample size calculations in group sequential trials. *Biometrics*, 55, 1286-1290.

[182] Lehmann, E.L. (1975). *Nonparametric: Statistical Methods Based on Ranks*. Holden-Day, San Francisco, California.

[183] Lehmann, E.L. (1983). *The Theory of Point Estimation*. Wiley, New York, New York.

[184] Li, H.I., and Lai, P.Y. (2003). Clinical trial simulation. In *Encyclopedia of Biopharmaceutical Statistics*, Ed. Chow, S.C., Marcel Dekker, Inc., New York, New York, 200-201.

[185] Li, N. (2006). Adaptive trial design - FDA statistical reviewer's view. Presented at the CRT 2006 Workshop with the FDA, Arlington, Virginia, April 4, 2006.

[186] Li, W.J., Shih, W.J., and Wang, Y. (2005), Two-stage adaptive design for clinical trials with survival data. *Journal of Biopharmaceutical Statistics*, 15, 707-718.

[187] Lilford, R.J., and Braunholtz, D. (1996). For debate: The statistical basis of public policy: a paradigm shift is overdue. *British Medical Journal*, 313, 603-607.

[188] Lin, Y., and Shih, W. J. (2001). Statistical properties of the traditional algorithm-based designs for phase I cancer clinical trials. *Biostatistics*, 2, 203-215.

[189] Liu, Q., (1998). An order-directed score test for trend in ordered 2xK Tables. *Biometrics*, 54, 1147-1154.

[190] Liu, Q., and Chi, G.Y.H. (2001). On sample size and inference for two-stage adaptive designs. *Biometrics*, 57, 172-177.

[191] Liu, Q., and Chi, G.Y.H. (2010). Understanding the FDA guidance on adaptive designs: historical, legal, and statistical perspectives. *Journal of Biopharmaceutical Statistics*, 20, 1178-1219.

[192] Liu, Q., and Pledger, G.W. (2005). Phase 2 and 3 combination designs to accelerate drug development. *Journal of American Statistical Association*, 100, 493-502.

[193] Liu, J.P., and Chow, S.C. (2008). Statistical issues on the diagnostics multivariate index assay for target clinical trials. *Journal of Biopharmaceutical Statistics*, 18, 167-182.

[194] Liu, J.P., Lin, J.R., and Chow, S.C. (2009). Inference on treatment effects for target clinical trials under enrichment design. *Pharmaceutical Statistics*, 8, 356-370.

[195] Liu, Q., Proschan, M.A., and Pledger, G.W. (2002). A unified theory of two-stage adaptive designs. *Journal of American Statistical Association*, 97, 1034-1041.

[196] Lu, Q., Tse, S.K., Chow, S.C., Chi, Y., and Yang, L.Y. (2009). Sample size estimation based on event data for a two-stage survival adaptive trial with different durations. *Journal of Biopharmaceutical Statistics*, 19, 311-323.

[197] Lu, Q., Tse, S.K., and Chow, S.C. (2010). Analysis of Time-to-Event Data Under a Two-stage Survival Adaptive Design in Clinical Trials. *Journal of Biopharmaceutical Statistics*, 20, 705-719.

[198] Lu, Q., Tse, S.K., and Chow, S.C. (2011). Analysis of time-to-event data with non-uniform patient entry and loss to follow-up under a two-stage seamless adaptive design with weibull distribution. Submitted.

[199] Lu, Y., Chow, S.C., and Zhang, Z. (2010). Statistical inference for clinical trials with random shift in scale parameter of target patient population. Submitted.

[200] Lokhnygina, Y. (2004). Topics in design and analysis of clinical trials. Ph.D. Thesis, Department of Statistics, North Carolina State Univeristy. Raleigh, North Carolina.

[201] Louis, T.A. (2005). Introduction to Bayesian methods II: fundamental concepts. *Clinical Trials*, 2, 291-294.

[202] Maca, J., Bhattacharya, S., Dragalin, V., Gallo, P., and Krams, M. (2006). Adaptive seamless phase II/III designs - background, operational aspects, and examples. *Drug Information Journal*, 40, 463-474.

[203] Maitournam A., and Simon R. (2005). On the efficiency of target clinical trials. *Statistics in Medicine*, 24, 329-339.

[204] Marubini, E., and Valsecchi, M.G. (1995). *Analysis Survival Data from Clinical Trials and Observational Studies*, John Wiley & Sons, New York, New York.

[205] Maxwell, C., Domenet, J.G., and Joyce, C.R.R. (1971). Instant experience in clinical trials: a novel aid to teaching by simulation. *J. Clin. Pharmacol.*, 11, 323-331.

[206] McCullagh, P. (1980). Regression models for ordinal data (with discussion). *J. Royal Stat Soc.*, B., 42, 109-142.

[207] Watson A. B., and Pelli D. G. (1983). QUEST: A Bayesian adaptive psychometric method. *Perception & Psychophysics*, 33(2), 113–120.

[208] McLachlan G.J., and Krishnan T. (1997). *The EM algorithm and Extensions*, Wiley, New York, New York.

[209] McLachlan G.J., and Peel D. (2000). *Finite Mixture Models*, Wiley, New York, New York.

[210] Melfi, V., and Page, C. (1998). Variability in adaptive designs for estimation of success probabilities. In New Developments and Applications in Experimental Design, *IMS Lecture Notes Monograph Series*, 34, 106-114.

[211] Mendelhall, W., and Hader, R.J. (1985). Estimation of parameters of mixed exponentially distributed failure time distributions from censored life test data. *Biometrika*, 45, 504-520.

[212] Mehta, C.R., and Tsiatis, A.A. (2001). Flexible sample size considerations using information-based interim monitor. *Drug Information Journal*, 35,1095-1112.

[213] Mehta, C.R., and Patel, N.R. (2006). Adaptive, group sequential and decision theoretic approaches to sample size determination. *Statistics in Medicine*, 25, 3250-3269.

[214] Meier, P. (1953). Variance a weighted mean. *Biometrics*, 9, 59-73.

[215] Montori, V.M., Devereaux, P.J., Adhikari, N.K.J., Burns, K.E.A., et al. (2005). Randomized trials stopped early for benefit - a systematic review. *Journal of American Medical Association*, 294, 2203-2209.

[216] Müller, H.H., and Schäfer, H. (2001). Adaptive group sequential designs for clinical trials: combining the advantages of adaptive and classical group sequential approaches. *Biometrics*, 57, 886-891.

[217] Neuhauser, M., and Hothorn, L. (1999). An exact Cochran-Armitage test for trend when dose-response shapes are a priori unknown. *Computational Statistics & Data Analysis*, 30, 403-412.

[218] Nityasuddhi D., and Böhning D. (2003). Asymptotic properties of the EM algorithm estimate for normal mixture models with component specific variances. *Computational Statistics & Data Analysis*, 41, 591-601.

[219] O'Brien, P.C., and Fleming, T.R. (1979). A multiple testing procedure for clinical trials. *Biometrics*, 35, 549-556.

[220] Offen, W.W. (2003). Data Monitoring Committees (DMC). In *Encyclopedia of Biopharmaceutical Statistics*. Ed. S.C. Chow, Marcel Dekker, Inc., New York, New York.

[221] Offen, W., Chuang-Stein, C., Dmitrienko, A., Littman, G., Maca, J., Meyerson, L., Muirhead, R., Stryszak, P., Boddy, A., Chen, K., Copley-Merriman, K., Dere, W., Givens, S., Hall, D., Henry, D., Jackson, J.D., Krishen, A., Liu, T., Ryder, S., Sankoh, A.J., Wang, J., and Yeh, C.H. (2006). Multiple co-primary endpoints: Medical and statistical solutions. *Drug Information Journal*, In press.

[222] O'Quigley, J., Pepe, M., and Fisher, L. (1990). Continual reassessment method: A practical design for phase I clinical trial in cancer. *Biometrics*, 46, 33-48.

[223] O'Quigley, J., and Shen, L. (1996). Continual reassessment method: A likelihood approach. *Biometrics*, 52, 673-684.

[224] Parmigiani, G. (2002). *Modeling in Medical Decision Making.* John Wiley and Sons, West Sussex, England.

[225] Paulson, E. (1964). A selection procedure for selecting the population with the largest mean from k normal populations. *Annals of Mathematical Statistics*, 35, 174–180.

[226] Pizzo, P.A. (2006). The Dean's Newsletter. Stanford University School of Medicine, Stanford, California.

[227] Pocock, S.J. (2005). When (not) to stop a clinical trial for benefit. *Journal of American Medical Association*, 294, 2228-2230.

[228] Pocock, S.J., and Simon, R. (1975). Sequential treatment assignment with balancing for prognostic factors in the controlled clinical trials. *Biometrics*, 31, 103-115.

[229] Pong, A., and Chow, S.C. (2010). *Handbook of Adaptive Designs in Pharmaceutical and Clinical Development.* Chapman and Hall/CRC Press, Taylor & Francis, New York.

[230] Pong, A., and Luo, Z. (2005). Adaptive Design in Clinical Research. A special issue of the *Journal of Biopharmaceutical Statistics*, 15, No. 4.

[231] Posch, M., and Bauer, P. (1999). Adaptive two stage designs and the conditional error function. *Biometrical Journal*, 41, 689-696.

[232] Posch, M., and Bauer, P. (2000). Interim analysis and sample size reassessment. *Biometrics*, 56, 1170-1176.

[233] Posch, M., Bauer, P., and Brannath, W. (2003). Issues in designing flexible trials. *Statistics in Medicine*, 22, 953-969.

[234] Posch, M., König, F., Brannath, W., Dunger-Baldauf, C., and Bauer, P. (2005). Testing and estimation in flexible group sequential designs with adaptive treatment selection. *Statistics in Medicine*, 24, 3697-3714.

[235] Prentice, R.L. (1989). Surrogate endpoints in clinical trials: definitions and operational criteria. *Statistics in Medicine*, 8, 431-440.

[236] Proschan, M.A. and Hunsberger, S.A. (1995). Designed extension of studies based on conditional power. *Biometrics*, 51, 1315-1324.

[237] Proschan, M.A., Lan, K.K.G., and Wittes, J.T. (2006). *Statistical Monitoring of Clinical Trials: A Unified Approach.* Springer, New York. New York.

[238] Proschan, M.A. (2005). Two-stage sample size re-estimation based on a nuisance parameter: a review. *Journal of Biopharmaceutical Statistics*, 15, 539-574.

[239] Proschan, M.A., Leifer, E., and Liu, Q. (2005). Adaptive regression. *Journal of Biopharmaceutical Statistics*, 15, 593-603.

[240] Proschan, M.A., and Wittes, J. (2000). An improved double sampling procedure based on the variance. *Biometrics*, 56, 1183-1187.

[241] Proschan, M. A., Follmann, D. A., and Waclawiw, M. A. (1992). Effects of assumption violations on type I error rate in group sequential monitoring. *Biometrics*, 48, 1131-1143.

[242] Proschan, M.A., Follmann, D.A., and Geller, N.L. (1994). Monitoring multiarmed trials. *Statistics in Medicine*, 13, 1441-1452.

[243] Quinlan, J.A., Gallo, P., and Krams, M. (2006). Implementing adaptive designs: logistical and operational consideration. Submitted.

[244] Ravaris, C.L., Nies, A., Robinson, D.S., and Ives, J.O. (1976). Multiple dose controlled study of phenelzine in depression anxiety states. *Arch Gen Psychiatry*, 33, 347-350.

[245] Robins, J.M., and Tsiatis, A.A. (1991). Correcting for non-compliance in randomized trials using rank preserving structural failure time models. *Communications in Statistics – Theory and Methods*, 20, 2609–2631.

[246] Rom, D.M. (1990). A sequentially rejective test procedure based on a modified Bonferroni inequality. *Biometrika*, 77, 663-665.

[247] Rosenberger, W.F., and Lachin, J. (2002). *Randomization in Clinical Trials*, John Wiley and Sons, New York, New York. New York.

[248] Rosenberger, W.F., and Seshaiyer, P. (1997). Adaptive survival trials. *Journal of Biopharmaceutical Statistics*, 7, 617-624.

[249] Rosenberger, W. F., Stallard, N., Ivanova, A., Harper, C. N., and Ricks, M. L. (2001). Optimal adaptive designs for binary response trials. *Biometrics*, 57, 909-913.

[250] Sampson, A.R., and Sill, M.W. (2005). Drop-the-loser design: normal case (with discussions). *Biometrical Journal*, 47, 257-281.

[251] Sargent, D.J., and Goldberg, R.M. (2001). A flexible design for multiple armed screening trials. *Statistics in Medicine*, 20, 1051-1060.

[252] Schaid, D.J., Wieand, S., and Therneau, T.M. (1990). Optimal two stage screening designs for survival comparisons. *Biometrika*, 77, 659–663.

[253] Serfling, R.J. (1980). *Approximation Theorems of Mathematical Statistics*. John Wiley & Sons, New York, New York.

[254] Shao, J., Chang, M., and Chow, S.C. (2005). Statistical inference for cancer trials with treatment switching. *Statistics in Medicine*, 24, 1783-1790.

[255] Shao, J., and Chow, S.C. (2007). Variable screening in predicting Clinical outcome with high-dimensional microarrays. *Journal of Multivariate Analysis*, 98, 1529-1538.

[256] Shen, Y., and Fisher, L. (1999). Statistical inference for self-designing clinical trials with a one-sided hypothesis. *Biometrics*, 55, 190-197.

[257] Shih, W.J. (2001). Sample size re-estimation - a journey for a decade. *Statistics in Medicine*, 20, 515-518.

[258] Shirley, E. (1977). A non-parametric equivalent of Williams' test for contrasting increasing dose levels of treatment. *Biometrics*, 33, 386-389.

[259] Siegmund, D. (1985). *Sequential Analysis: Tests and Confidence Intervals*. Springer.

[260] Simon, R. (1979). Restricted randomization designs in clinical trials. *Biometrics*, 35, 503-512.

[261] Simon, R. (1989). Optimal two-stage designs for phase II clinical trials. *Controlled Clinical Trials*, 10, 1-10.

[262] Sommer, A., and Zeger, S.L. (1991). On estimating efficacy from clinical trials. *Statistics in Medicine*, 10, 45-52.

[263] Sonnesmann, E. (1991). Kombination unabhängiger Tests. In Biometrie in der chemisch-pharmazeutischen Industrie 4, Stand und Perspektiven, J. Vollmar (ed.). Stuttgart: Gustav-Fischer.

[264] Spiegelhalter, D.J., Abrams, K.R, and Myles, J.P. (2004). *Bayesian Approach to Clinical Trials and Health-care Evaluation*. John Wiley & Sons, Ltd., The Atrium, Southern Gate, Chrichester, West Sussex PO19 8SQ, England.

[265] Stallard, N., and Todd, S. (2003). Sequential designs for phase III clinical trials incorporating treatment selection. *Statistics in Medicine*, 22, 689-703.

[266] Stallard, N., and Todd, S. (2005). Point estimates and confidence regions for sequential trials involving selection. *Journal of Statististical Planning and Inference*, 135, 402-419.

[267] Stewart, W., and Ruberg, S. J. (2000). Detecting dose response with contrasts. *Statistics in Medicine*, 19, 913-921.

[268] Susarla, V., and Pathala, K.S. (1965). A probability distribution for time of first birth. *Journal of Scientific Research*, Banaras Hindu University, 16, 59-62.

[269] Taves, D.R. (1974). Minimization - a new method of assessing patients and control groups. *Clinical Pharmacol. Ther.*, 15, 443-453.

[270] Temple, R. (2005). How FDA currently makes decisions on clinical studies. *Clinical Trials*, 2, 276-281.

[271] Thall, P.F., Simon, R., and Ellenberg, S.S. (1989). A two-stage design for choosing among several experimental treatments and a control in clinical trials. *Biometrics*, 45, 537–547.

[272] Todd, S. (2003). An adaptive approach to implementing bivariate group sequential clinical trial designs. *Journal of Biopharmaceutical Statistics*, 13, 605-619.

[273] Todd, S., and Stallard, N. (2005). A new clinical trial design combining Phases 2 and 3: sequential designs with treatment selection and a change of endpoint. *Drug Information Journal*, 39, 109-118.

[274] Tsiatis, A.A., and Mehta, C. (2003). On the inefficiency of the adaptive design for monitoring clinical trials. *Biometrika* 90:367-378.

[275] Tsiatis, A.A., Rosner, G.L., and Mehta, C.R. (1984). Exact confidence interval following a group sequential test. *Biometrics*, 40, 797-803.

[276] Tukey, J.W., and Heyse, J.F. (1985). Testing the statistical certainty of a response to increasing doses of a drug. *Biometrics*, 41, 295-301.

[277] Uchida, T. (2006). Adaptive trial design - FDA view. Presented at the CRT 2006 Workshop with the FDA, Arlington, Virginia, April 4, 2006.

[278] Wald, A. (1947). *Sequential Analysis*. Dover Publications, New York.

[279] Wang, S.J. (2010). Perspectives on the use of adaptive designs in clinical trials, Part I. Statistical considerations and issues. *Journal of Biopharmaceutical Statistics*, 20, 1090-1097.

[280] Wang, S.J., and Hung, H.M.J. (2005). Adaptive covariate adjustment in clinical trials. *Journal of Biopharmaceutical Statistics*, 15, 605-611.

[281] Wang, S.J., Hung, H.M.J., and O'Neill, R.T. (2009). Adaptive patient enrichment designs in therapeutic trials. *Biometrical Journal*, 51, 358-374.

[282] Wang, S.K., and Tsiatis, A.A. (1987). Approximately optimal one-parameter boundaries for a sequential trials. *Biometrics*, 43, 193-200.

[283] Wassmer, G. (1998), A Comparison of two methods for adaptive interim analyses in clinical trials. *Biometrics*, 54, 696-705

[284] Wassmer, G., Eisebitt, R., and Coburger, S. (2001). Flexible interim analyses in clinical trials using multistage adaptive test designs. *Drug information Journal*, 35, 1131-1146.

[285] Wassmer, G., and Vandemeulebroecke, M. (2006). A brief review on software development for group sequential and adaptive designs. *Biometrical Journal*, 48, 732-737.

[286] Wei, L.J. (1977). A class of designs for sequential clinical trials. *Journal of American Statistical Association*, 72, 382-386.

[287] Wei, L.J. (1978). The adaptive biased-coin design for sequential experiments. *Annals of Statistics*, 9, 92-100.

[288] Wei, L.J., and Durham, S. (1978). The randomized play-the-winner rule in medical trials. *Journal of American Statistical Association*, 73, 840-843.

[289] Wei, L.J., Smythe, R.T., and Smith, R.L. (1986). K-treatment comparisons with restricted randomization rules in clinical trials. *Annals of Statistics*, 14, 265-274.

[290] Weinthrau, M., Jacox, R.F., Angevine, C.D., and Atwater, E.C. (1977). Piroxicam (CP 16171) in rheumatoid arthritis: A controlled clinical trial with novel assessment features. *J Rheum*, 4, 393-404.

[291] White, I. R. (2006). Estimating treatment effects in randomized trials with treatment switching. *Statistics in Medicine*, 25, 1619–1622.

[292] White, I.R., Babiker, A.G., Walker, S., and Darbyshire, J.H. (1999). Randomisation-based methods for correcting for treatment changes: examples from the Concorde trial. *Statistics in Medicine*, 18, 2617–2634.

[293] White, I.R., Walker, S., and Babiker, A.G. (2002). strbee: Randomisation-based efficacy estimator. *Stata Journal*, 2, 140–150.

[294] Whitehead, J. (1983). *The Design and Analysis of Sequential Clinical Trials*. Haisted Press. New York.

[295] Whitehead, J. (1993). Sample size calculation for ordered categorical data. *Statistics in Medicine*, 12, 2257-2271.

[296] Whitehead, J. (1994). Sequential methods based on the boundaries approach for the clinical comparison of survival times (with discussions). *Statistics in Medicine*, 13, 1357-1368.

[297] Whitehead, J. (1997). Bayesian decision procedures with application to dose-finding studies. *International Journal of Pharmaceutical Medicine*, 11, 201-208.

[298] Williams, D.A. (1971). A test for difference between treatment means when several dose levels are compared with a zero dose control. *Biometrics*, 27, 103-117.

[299] Williams, D.A. (1972). Comparison of several dose levels with a zero dose control. *Biometrics*, 28, 519-531.

[300] Williams, G., Pazdur, R., and Temple, R. (2004). Assessing tumor-related signs and symptoms to support cancer drug approval. *Journal of Biopharmaceutical Statistics*, 14, 5-21.

[301] Woodcock, J. (2005). DFA introduction comments: clinical studies design and evaluation issues. *Clinical Trials*, 2, 273-275.

[302] Yang, L.Y, Chi, Y., and Chow, S.C. (2011). Statistical inference for clinical trials with random shift in scale parameter for target patient population. *Journal of Biopharmaceutical Statistics*, 21, 437-452.

[303] Zelen, M. (1974). The randomization and stratification of patients to clinical trials. *Journal of Chronic Diseases*, 28, 365-375.

[304] Zucker, D.M., Wittes, J.T., Schabenberger, O., and Brittain, E. (1999). Internal pilot studies II: comparison of various procedures. *Statistics in Medicine*, 19, 901-911.

Index

Printed in the United States
by Baker & Taylor Publisher Services